Depression and Heart Failure

Guest Editors

PHILIP F. BINKLEY, MD, MPH
STEPHEN S. GOTTLIEB, MD

HEART FAILURE CLINICS

www.heartfailure.theclinics.com

Consulting Editors

RAGAVENDRA R. BALIGA, MD, MBA
JAMES B. YOUNG, MD

Founding Editor

JAGAT NARULA, MD, PhD

January 2011 • Volume 7 • Number 1

SAUNDERS an imprint of ELSEVIER, Inc.

W.B. SAUNDERS COMPANY
A Division of Elsevier Inc.

1600 John F. Kennedy Boulevard • Suite 1800 • Philadelphia, Pennsylvania 19103-2899

http://www.theclinics.com

HEART FAILURE CLINICS Volume 7, Number 1
January 2011 ISSN 1551-7136, ISBN-13: 978-1-4557-0457-6

Editor: Barbara Cohen-Kligerman

Heart Failure Clinics (ISSN 1551-7136) is published quarterly by Elsevier Inc., 360 Park Avenue South, New York, NY 10010-1710. Months of publication are January, April, July, and October. Business and editorial offices: 1600 John F. Kennedy Boulevard, Suite 1800, Philadelphia, PA 19103-2899. Periodicals postage paid at New York, NY, and additional mailing offices. Subscription prices are USD 207.00 per year for US individuals, USD 326.00 per year for US institutions, USD 70.00 per year for US students and residents, USD 248.00 per year for Canadian individuals, USD 374.00 per year for Canadian institutions, USD 264.00 per year for international individuals, USD 374.00 per year for international institutions, and USD 89.00 per year for Canadian and foreign students/residents. To receive student and resident rate, orders must be accompanied by name of affiliated institution, date of term, and the *signature* of program/residency coordinator on institution letterhead. Orders will be billed at individual rate until proof of status is received. Foreign air speed delivery is included in all *Clinics* subscription prices. All prices are subject to change without notice. **POSTMASTER:** Send address changes to *Heart Failure Clinics*, Elsevier Health Sciences Division, Subscription Customer Service, 3251 Riverport Lane, Maryland Heights, MO 63043. **Customer Service: 1-800-654-2452 (US and Canada). From outside of the US and Canada, call 314-447-8871. Fax: 314-447-8029. For print support, e-mail: JournalsCustomerService-usa@elsevier.com. For online support, e-mail: JournalsOnlineSupport-usa@elsevier.com.**

Reprints. For copies of 100 or more of articles in this publication, please contact the Commercial Reprints Department, Elsevier Inc., 360 Park Avenue South, New York, NY 10010-1710. Tel.: 212-633-3812; Fax: 212-462-1935; E-mail: reprints@elsevier.com.

Heart Failure Clinics is covered in *MEDLINE/PubMed (Index Medicus).*

Cover artwork courtesy of Umberto M. Jezek.

Printed and bound in the United Kingdom

Transferred to Digital Print 2011

Contributors

CONSULTING EDITORS

RAGAVENDRA R. BALIGA, MD, MBA
Professor of Internal Medicine, Vice Chief and Assistant Division Director, Professor of Medicine, Division of Cardiovascular Medicine, The Ohio State University Medical Center, Columbus, Ohio

JAMES B. YOUNG, MD
Professor of Medicine and Executive Dean, Cleveland Clinic Lerner College of Medicine; George and Linda Kaufman Chair, Chairman, Endocrinology and Metabolism Institute, Cleveland Clinic, Cleveland, Ohio

GUEST EDITORS

PHILIP F. BINKLEY, MD, MPH
Wilson Professor of Medicine and Vice Chair for Academic Affairs, The OSU Department of Internal Medicine; Associate Dean for Faculty Affairs, The Division of Cardiovascular Medicine, The OSU College of Medicine; Professor of Epidemiology, The OSU College of Public Health, Columbus, Ohio

STEPHEN S. GOTTLIEB, MD
Professor of Medicine; Director, Cardiomyopathy and Pulmonary Hypertension Program; Director, Clinical Research Program in Cardiology, University of Maryland Medical Center and University of Maryland School of Medicine, Baltimore, Maryland

AUTHORS

PHILIP F. BINKLEY, MD, MPH
Wilson Professor of Medicine and Vice Chair for Academic Affairs, The OSU Department of Internal Medicine; Associate Dean for Faculty Affairs, The Division of Cardiovascular Medicine, The OSU College of Medicine; Professor of Epidemiology, The OSU College of Public Health, Columbus, Ohio

MARY BLAZEK, MD
Instructor, Section of Geriatric Psychiatry, Department of Psychiatry, University of Michigan, Ann Arbor, Michigan

J. MICHAEL BOSTWICK, MD
Consultant, Department of Psychiatry and Psychology, Mayo Clinic; and Professor of Psychiatry, Mayo Clinic College of Medicine, Rochester, Minnesota

ROBERT M. CARNEY, PhD
Professor of Psychiatry, Department of Psychiatry, Behavioral Medicine Center, Washington University School of Medicine, St Louis, Missouri

RUDOLF A. DE BOER, MD, PhD
Cardiologist, Assistant Professor, Department of Cardiology, Thorax Center, University Medical Center Groningen, Groningen, The Netherlands

PETER DE JONGE, PhD
Professor, Interdisciplinary Center for Psychiatric Epidemiology, University Medical Centre Groningen, University of Groningen, Groningen; Professor, Faculty of Social and Behavioural Sciences, University of Tilburg, Tilburg, The Netherlands

REBECCA L. DEKKER, PhD, ARNP, ACNS-BC
Assistant Professor, University of Kentucky College of Nursing, Lexington, Kentucky

ALLARD E. DEMBE, ScD
Chair, Division of Health Services Management & Policy, College of Public Health, The Ohio State University, Columbus, Ohio

CHIRAG V. DESAI, MD
Assistant Professor, Medical Director, Consultation & Liaison Service, Department of Psychiatry, University of Florida, College of Medicine, Jacksonville, Florida

MELVIN R. ECHOLS, MD
Department of Internal Medicine, Duke Clinical Research Institute, Duke University Medical Center, Durham, North Carolina

LUCY A. EPSTEIN, MD
Assistant Professor of Clinical Psychiatry, Columbia University; Women's Mental Health Program and Consultation-Liaison Psychiatry Service, New York Presbyterian Hospital-Columbia University Medical Center, New York, New York

DAVID A. FEDORONKO, MD
Assistant Clinical Professor of Psychiatry, Department of Psychiatry, Columbia University; Psychiatric Consultant, Heart and Lung Transplant Programs, New York Presbyterian Hospital-Columbia University Medical Center, New York, New York

VICKI FREEDENBERG, RN, MSN
Electrophysiology Nurse Clinician, Department of Cardiology, Children's National Medical Center, Washington, District of Columbia

KENNETH E. FREEDLAND, PhD
Professor of Psychiatry, Department of Psychiatry, Behavioral Medicine Center, Washington University School of Medicine, St Louis, Missouri

ERIKA FRIEDMANN, PhD
Professor, University of Maryland School of Nursing, Baltimore, Maryland

DEANNA M. GOLDEN-KREUTZ, PhD
Administrative Director, Cardiovascular Clinical Research; Clinical Assistant Professor, Internal Medicine, The Ohio State University, Columbus, Ohio

STEPHEN S. GOTTLIEB, MD
Professor of Medicine; Director, Cardiomyopathy and Pulmonary Hypertension Program; Director, Clinical Research Program in Cardiology, University of Maryland Medical Center and University of Maryland School of Medicine, Baltimore, Maryland

GOWRISHANKAR GNANASEKARAN, MD, MPH
Clinical Assistant Professor, Division of General Internal Medicine and Geriatrics, Department of Internal Medicine, Ohio State University Medical Center, Columbus, Ohio

WEI JIANG, MD
Associate Professor, Departments of Psychiatry and Behavioral Sciences and Internal Medicine, Duke University Medical Center, Duke Clinical Research Institute, Durham, North Carolina

HELEN C. KALES, MD
Section of Geriatric Psychiatry, Department of Psychiatry, University of Michigan; Associate Professor, Department of Veterans Affairs, Ann Arbor Center of Excellence (COE); Research Investigator, Department of Veterans Affairs, Serious Mental Illness Treatment, Research, and Evaluation Center (SMITREC), Ann Arbor, Michigan

WILLEM J. KOP, PhD
Division of Cardiology, Department of Medicine, University of Maryland School of Medicine, Baltimore, Maryland; Department of Medical Psychology and Neuropsychology, Center of Research on Psychology in Somatic Diseases (CoRPS), Tilburg, the Netherlands

SUSAN M. MAIXNER, MD
Assistant Professor, Section of Geriatric Psychiatry, Department of Psychiatry, University of Michigan, Ann Arbor, Michigan

TARA MAYES, MD
Clinical Assistant Professor of Psychiatry, The Ohio State University; Psychiatrist, Twin Valley Behavioral Health, Columbus, Ohio

LAXMI S. MEHTA, MD, FACC
Director, Women's Cardiovascular Health Clinic; Assistant Professor, Department of Clinical Internal Medicine, The Ohio State University, Columbus, Ohio

ELSA G.E. MIRASOL, MD
Attending Psychiatrist, Primary Care Mental Health Service, Department of Psychiatry, Veterans Administration Medical Center, Northport, New York

MICHAEL W. RICH, MD
Professor of Medicine, Division of Cardiology, Washington University School of Medicine; Director, Cardiac Rapid Evaluation Unit, Barnes-Jewish Hospital, St Louis, Missouri

RADU V. SAVEANU, MD
Chairman, Department of Psychiatry, The Ohio State University Medical Center, Columbus, Ohio

PETER A. SHAPIRO, MD
Professor of Clinical Psychiatry, Department of Psychiatry, Columbia University; Director, Fellowship Training Program in Psychosomatic Medicine, and Associate Director, Consultation-Liaison Psychiatry Service, New York Presbyterian Hospital-Columbia University Medical Center, New York, New York

CHRISTOPHER L. SOLA, DO
Consultant, Department of Psychiatry and Psychology, Mayo Clinic; Assistant Professor of Psychiatry, Mayo Clinic College of Medicine, Rochester, Minnesota

LAURA STRUBLE, PhD, GNP, BC
Clinical Assistant Professor, School of Nursing; Section of Geriatric Psychiatry, Department of Psychiatry, University of Michigan, Ann Arbor, Michigan

STEPHEN J. SYNOWSKI, PhD
Division of Cardiology, Department of Medicine, University of Maryland School of Medicine, Baltimore, Maryland

SUE A. THOMAS, RN, PhD
Assistant Dean for the PhD Program, University of Maryland School of Nursing, Baltimore, Maryland

JOOST P. VAN MELLE, MD, PhD
Cardiologist, Department of Cardiology, Thorax Center, University Medical Center Groningen, Groningen, The Netherlands

JERRY VAN RIEZEN, MD
Student of Psychiatry, Interdisciplinary Center for Psychiatric Epidemiology, University Medical Center Groningen, University of Groningen, Groningen, The Netherlands

DANIËLLE E.P. VERBEEK, MD
Medical Resident, Internal Medicine, Department of Internal Medicine, Ziekenhuisgroep Twente, Almelo; Medical Resident, Internal Medicine, Department of Internal Medicine, University Medical Center Groningen, Groningen, The Netherlands

SUBHDEEP VIRK, MD
Assistant Professor-Clinical, Department of Psychiatry, The Ohio State University, Columbus, Ohio

KENNETH R. YEAGER, PhD
Clinical Associate Professor, Department of Psychiatry, The Ohio State University, Columbus, Ohio

Contents

Editorial: Depression in Heart Failure is Double Trouble: Warding off the Blues Requires Early Screening **xiii**

Ragavendra R. Baliga and James B. Young

Preface: Depression and Heart Failure **xix**

Philip F. Binkley and Stephen S. Gottlieb

Epidemiology of Depression in Heart Failure **1**

Gowrishankar Gnanasekaran

Depression in heart failure recently has become a topic of great interest because of the high prevalence of the diseases and their tendency to worsen medical prognosis. This article reviews the epidemiology of depression in heart failure and provides the necessary knowledge and insight for understanding the complex burden of the disease in terms of mortality, morbidity, health-care costs and impact on quality of life (QOL). Early detection and treatment of this comorbid association is important for patients to improve QOL and regain function. The article also highlights the wide heterogeneity in the prevalence of depression in heart failure across the various studies done and emphasizes the need for future research to address these gaps.

Effect of Depression on Prognosis in Heart Failure **11**

Kenneth E. Freedland, Robert M. Carney, and Michael W. Rich

Depression is a common comorbid condition in heart failure, and there is growing evidence that it increases the risks of mortality and other adverse outcomes, including rehospitalization and functional decline. The prognostic value of depression depends, in part, on how it is defined and measured. The few studies that have compared different subsets of patients with depression suggest that major (or severe) depression is a stronger predictor of mortality than is minor (or mild) depression. Whether depression is a causal risk factor for heart failure mortality, or simply a risk marker, has not yet been established, but mechanistic research has identified several plausible behavioral and biologic pathways. Further research is needed to clarify the relationships among depression, heart failure, and adverse outcomes, as well as to develop efficacious interventions for depressive disorders in patients with heart failure.

Depression in Heart Failure: Biobehavioral Mechanisms **23**

Willem J. Kop, Stephen J. Synowski, and Stephen S. Gottlieb

The etiology, predictive value, and biobehavioral aspects of depression in heart failure (HF) are described in this article. Clinically elevated levels of depressive symptoms are present in approximately 1 out of 5 patients with HF. Depression is associated with poor quality of life and a greater than 2-fold risk of clinical HF progression and mortality. The biobehavioral mechanisms accounting for these adverse outcomes include biological processes (elevated neurohormones, autonomic nervous system dysregulation, and inflammation) and adverse health behaviors (physical inactivity, medication nonadherence, poor dietary control, and smoking). Depression often remains undetected because of its partial overlap with HF-related

disease (CHD). These studies have demonstrated relatively consistent results and suggest an important connection between cardiovascular morbidity and mortality in patients with depressive symptoms or major depression. This article discusses the current best practices for the screening, identification, and treatment of depression in patients with CHD and coronary heart failure, as well as the financial aspects associated with care management.

Diagnosing Depression in Congestive Heart Failure 75

Radu V. Saveanu and Tara Mayes

Depression is an all too common occurrence in heart failure patients. Depressive symptoms, however, sometimes are confused with the physical repercussions of heart failure. This article highlights different screening assessments for major depression and recommends treatment for this population.

Clinical Trial Evidence for Treatment of Depression in Heart Failure 81

Melvin R. Echols and Wei Jiang

Depression is an important disease state that requires a significant amount of time and resources for proper management. The presence of depression in patients with cardiovascular disease has been strongly associated with detrimental effects in terms of morbidity and mortality. Little is known about the management of depression in heart failure patients, although several investigators continue to pursue optimal treatment strategies for depression in this population. While limited, the prospective clinical trial data evaluating interventions for depression management in patients with heart failure continue to produce promising findings for progressive and improved management of both depression and heart failure.

A Review on the Putative Association Between Beta-Blockers and Depression 89

Daniëlle E.P. Verbeek, Jerry van Riezen, Rudolf A. de Boer, Joost P. van Melle, and Peter de Jonge

Several kinds of systematic studies have been conducted verifying the putative association between β-blockers and depressive symptoms. However, many of these studies had important limitations in their design. In most of the studies, no effect of β-blockers on depressive symptoms was seen. Because individual susceptibility cannot be ruled out, clinicians must stay vigilant, especially with patients who have a positive personal or family history and who have been prescribed lipophilic β-blockers. However, fear for depression should not be the reason for reluctance in prescribing β-blockers to cardiovascular patients.

Special Articles

An Updated Review of Implantable Cardioverter/Defibrillators, Induced Anxiety, and Quality of Life 101

J. Michael Bostwick and Christopher L. Sola

Despite overall favorable acceptance of implantable cardioverter-defibrillators (ICDs), patients may experience discharges as frightening and painful. The authors reviewed ICD-induced psychopathology in 2005. During the past 2 years the number of studies examining psychopathology and quality of life after ICD implantation has increased dramatically, warranting this update of that review. Variables assessed have included recipient age, gender, social support network, perception of control and predictability of shocks, and personality style. Now the picture of what is known is, if anything, cloudier than it was 2 years ago, with little definitive and much contradictory data emerging in most of these categories.

Psychiatric Aspects of Heart and Lung Disease in Critical Care **109**

Peter A. Shapiro, David A. Fedoronko, Lucy A. Epstein, Elsa G.E. Mirasol, and Chirag V. Desai

Psychiatric issues are important in the management of patients with heart and lung disease in acute, intensive, and critical care. Adjustment disorders, anxiety disorders, depression, and delirium, sometimes in association with substance abuse and withdrawal problems, are the most common issues, and may affect risk and prognosis of the associated general medical conditions and management in the acute care setting. In children with lung and heart diseases requiring critical care, appreciation of cognitive and social-psychologic developmental milestones is necessary to provide adequate care.

Cognitive Therapy for Depression in Patients with Heart Failure: A Critical Review **127**

Rebecca L. Dekker

Depression is a significant problem in patients with heart failure (HF). This article examines the evidence for the use of cognitive therapy (CT) in treating depression and depressive symptoms in patients with HF and cardiovascular related illnesses. In 8 of the 14 studies reviewed, researchers found that CT reduced depressive symptoms; however, the limitations of the studies prevent wide generalization of the results. Evidence to support the use of CT for the treatment of depressive symptoms in patients with cardiovascular illness is insufficient at this time. Large randomized controlled trials that demonstrate the efficacy of CT are needed before clinicians routinely refer patients with HF to CT for the purpose of improving depression or depressive symptoms.

Index **143**

Heart Failure Clinics

FORTHCOMING ISSUES

April 2011

Sudden Cardiac Death and Heart Failure
Raul Weiss, MD, and Emile Daoud, MD,
Guest Editors

July 2011

Cardio-oncology Related to Heart Failure
Daniel Lenihan, MD, and
Douglas B. Sawyer, MD, PhD,
Guest Editors

October 2011

Conducting and Interpreting Clinical Trials in Heart Failure
Mona Fiuzat, PharmD, and Christopher O'Connor, MD, *Guest Editors*

RECENT ISSUES

October 2010

Heart Failure in Children
Jeffrey A. Towbin, MD, FACC, FAAP, FAHA,
Guest Editor

July 2010

Anemia and Heart Failure
Anil K. Agarwal, MD, FACP, FASN,
Stuart D. Katz, MD, and
Ajay K. Singh, MB, FRCP,
Guest Editors

April 2010

Genetics of Cardiomyopathy and Heart Failure
Calum A. MacRae, MD, PhD,
Guest Editor

ISSUES OF RELATED INTEREST

Cardiology Clinics November 2010 (Volume 28, Issue 4)
Hypertension and Hypertensive Heart Disease
George A. Mensah, MD, FACC, *Guest Editor*
Available at: http://www.cardiology.theclinics.com/

Cardiac Electrophysiology Clinics December 2010 (Volume 2, Issue 4)
Genetics of Cardiac Arrhythmias
Silvia G. Priori, MD, PhD, *Guest Editor*
Available at: http://www.cardiacep.theclinics.com/

Editorial: Depression in Heart Failure is Double Trouble: Warding off the Blues Requires Early Screening

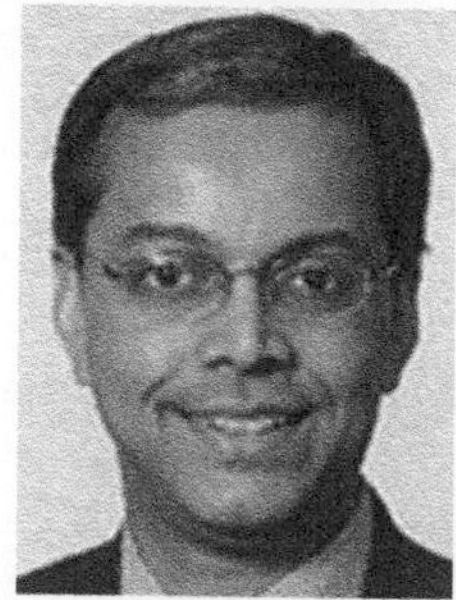

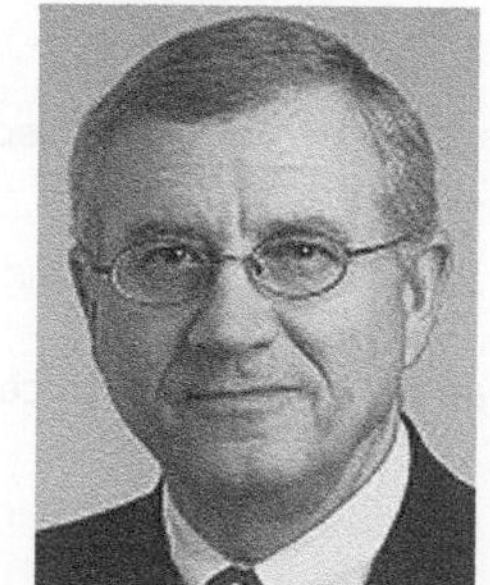

Ragavendra R. Baliga, MD, MBA James B. Young, MD
Consulting Editors

The prevalence of depression in heart failure (HF) is 21.5%[1] and it is one of many factors that contributes to adverse outcomes (**Fig. 1**), including mortality.[2,3] Depression affects both caregivers and family members, making management of depression challenging. Depression is also associated with increased costs; up to $5 billion of the total $20 billion in costs associated with HF during 1998 was ascribed to depression.[4] Increased costs were attributed to increased inpatient and outpatient use and not caused by increased use of mental health care.

Typical symptoms in heart failure include shortness of breath, tiredness, and fatigue; each can wear down even the most exuberant individual. These manifestations, however, overlap with features of depression, with the result that the diagnosis of depression is often overlooked. Moreover, the high prevalence of sleep apnea in heart failure, which also manifests with fatigue, makes depression difficult to diagnose. A diagnosis of major depression requires the presence of 5 or more of the following 9 symptoms for a 2-week period: sleep disturbance, psychomotor agitation or retardation, appetite disturbance, concentration impairment, low energy level, depressed mood, lost interest in activities, guilt or worthlessness, and suicidal ideation (**Box 1**). One of the symptoms must include depressed mood or loss of interest or pleasure, and the symptoms must reflect a change in functioning resulting in social, occupational, or other life impairment.

Depression and heart failure not only have similar symptoms but also have overlapping pathophysiological mechanisms, including increased

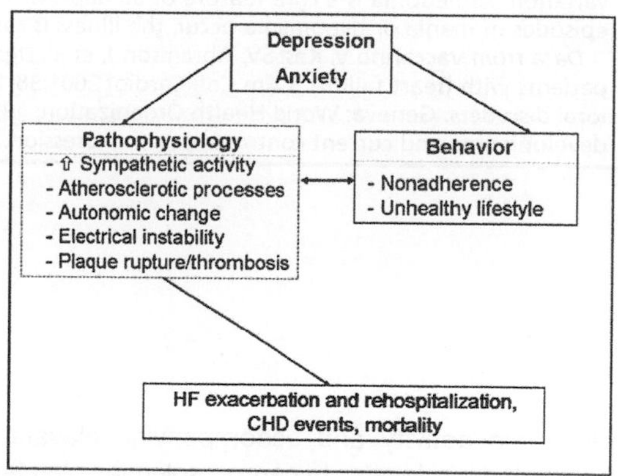

Fig. 1. Potential mechanisms linking depression and anxiety with adverse cardiac outcomes. CHD, coronary heart disease. (*From* Konstam V, Moser DK, De Jong MJ. Depression and anxiety in heart failure. J Card Fail 2005;11(6):455–63; with permission.)

Heart Failure Clin 7 (2011) xiii–xvii
doi:10.1016/j.hfc.2010.10.004
1551-7136/11/$ – see front matter

Box 1
Panel: *International Classification of Diseases, Tenth Revision* criteria for depression

Depressive episode

At least 2 weeks of depressed mood, loss of interest and enjoyment, reduced energy, increased fatigability, diminished activity, reduced concentration and attention, reduced self-esteem and self-confidence, ideas of guilt and unworthiness, bleak view of the future, ideas or acts of self-harm, disturbed sleep, diminished appetite

Mild depression

Two of depressed mood, loss of interest and enjoyment, reduced energy, and 2 others

Patient will not cease to function completely

Moderate depression

Two of depressed mood, loss of interest and enjoyment, reduced energy, and at least 3 others, some at marked intensity

Considerable difficulty functioning

Severe depression

Two of depressed mood, loss of interest and enjoyment, reduced energy, and at least 4 others (some of severe intensity), plus considerable distress and agitation or psychomotor retardation, sometimes with psychotic symptoms (eg, hallucinations or delusions)

Dysthymia

Depression of mood, which is never or only rarely severe enough to fulfill the criteria for recurrent depressive disorder, mild or moderate severity

Long standing

Usually begins in early adult life, lasts at least several years

Low mood varies little from day to day, is often unresponsive to circumstances, yet may show a characteristic diurnal variation. Anhedonia is a core feature of all depressive illnesses. Anxiety symptoms and weight loss are common. If episodes of mania or hypomania occur, the illness is called bipolar affective disorder.

Data from Vaccarino V, Kasl SV, Abramson J, et al. Depressive symptoms and risk of functional decline and death in patients with heart failure. J Am Coll Cardiol 2001;38(1):199–205; WHO. ICD-10 classification of mental and behavioral disorders. Geneva: World Health Organization; 1992; and quoted in Ebmeier KP, Donaghey C, Steele JD. Recent developments and current controversies in depression. Lancet 2006;367:153–67.

adrenergic activity and accompanying elevated catecholamine levels, hypercortisolemia, platelet activation,[5,6] increased inflammatory markers, and endothelial dysfunction (**Fig. 2** and **Box 2**).[7,8] The overlapping pathophysiological mechanisms have made it difficult to develop pharmacologic agents that will add incremental value to the current standard of care.[9]

In this issue, Phillip Binkley, MD, and Stephen Gottlieb, MD, have put together a multidisciplinary team of experts, including psychiatrists, psychologists, nurses, and cardiologists, to discuss the challenge of depression in heart failure. Recognition of depression at an early stage, before it progresses to major depression, is important so that the support of family, behavioral therapy, physical exercise, spirituality, and pharmacologic therapy can be used in a timely fashion. Recent guidelines[8,10] recommend the use of The Patient Health Questionnaire (PHQ-9) (**Fig. 3**) in cardiovascular disease. This questionnaire is self-administered and should be offered to all patients with heart failure to assist the physician in making an early diagnosis of depression. In addition, the US Preventive Services Task Force Recommendation Statement[11–13] opines that simply asking 2 questions is both sensitive and specific for depression

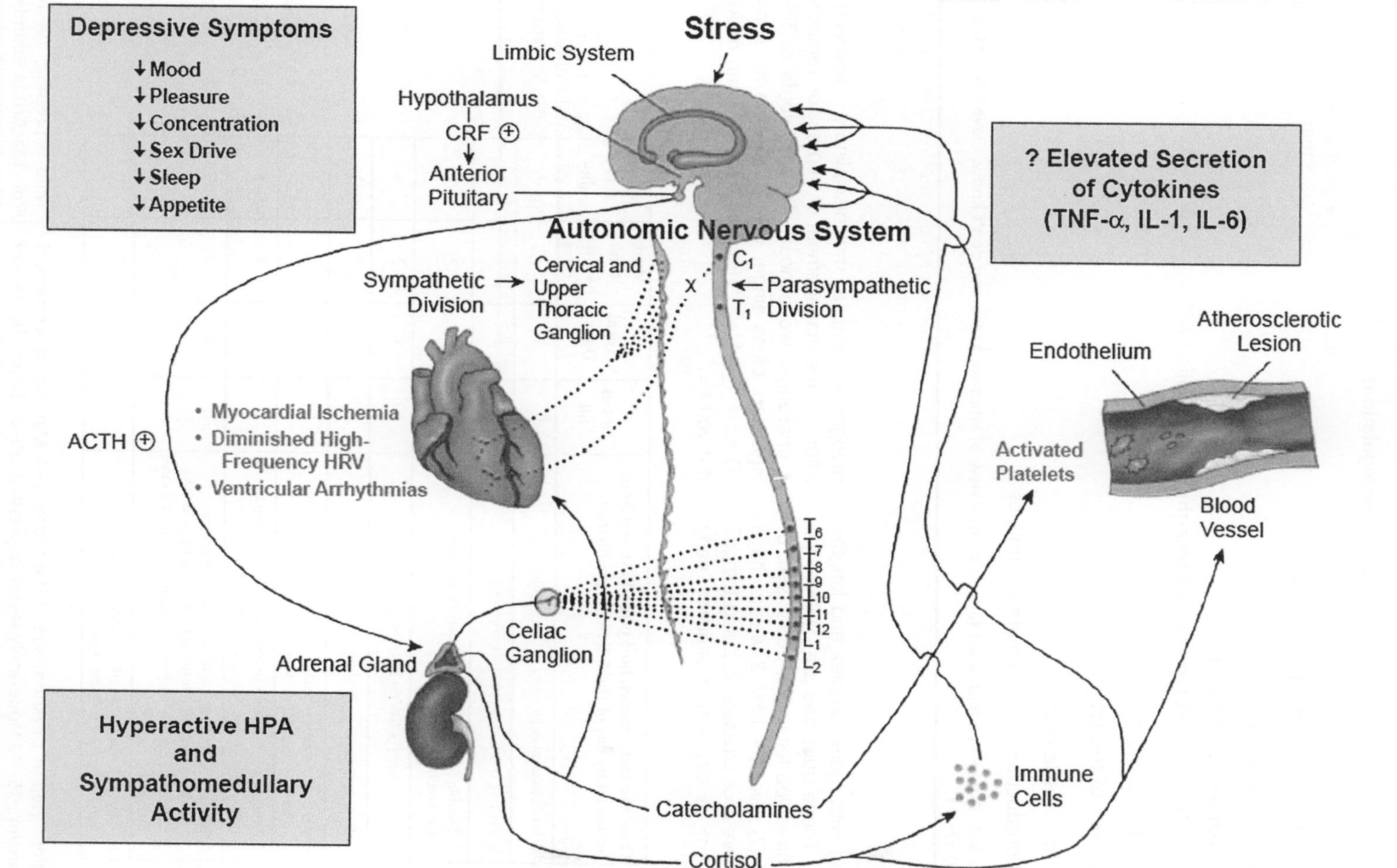

Fig. 2. Hypothetical pathophysiologic alternations associated with depression that likely contribute to increased vulnerability to cardiovascular disease. Autonomic nervous system innervation of the heart via parasympathetic vagus (X) and sympathetic (postganglionic efferents from cervical and upper thoracic paravertebral ganglia) nerves are shown. ACTH, corticotropin; CRF, corticotrophin-releasing factor; HPA, hypothalamic-pituitary-adrenocortical axis; HRV, heart rate variability; HPA, hypothalamic-pituitary-adrenocortical axis; IL-1, interleukin-1; IL-6, interleukin-6; TNF-α, tumor necrosis factor α. (*From* Musselman DL, Evans DL, Nemeroff CB. The relationship of depression to cardiovascular disease: epidemiology, biology, and treatment. Arch Gen Psychiatry 1998;55:580–92; with permission.)

Box 2
Possible psychophysiologic mechanisms for depression in heart failure

High sympathetic tone (cardiovascular autonomic dysregulation)

- Reduced heart rate variability
- Elevated levels of circulating catecholamines

Platelet activation (prothrombotic)

- Dysfunctional serotonin signaling
- Elevated levels of platelet factor 4 and beta-thromboglobulin

Elevated levels of cortisol (atherosclerosis)

- Elevated levels of free fatty acids

Inflammation (atherosclerosis)

- Elevated production of inflammatory cytokines

Data from Silver MA. Depression and heart failure: an overview of what we know and don't know. Cleve Clin J Med 2010;77(Suppl 3):S7–11.

when compared with more complex and lengthy questionnaires. Those questions are (1) Over the past 2 weeks, have you felt down, depressed, or hopeless? and (2) Over the past 2 weeks, have you felt little interest or pleasure in doing things? The management of depression requires early recognition and a multidisciplinary approach. Although the management of depression remains a challenge, we concur with the words of the legendary blues singer Otis Rush from his song "Double Trouble": "Hey, they say you can make it if you try."

Over the last 2 weeks, how often have you been bothered by any of the following problems?	Not at all	Several Days	More than half the days	Nearly every day
1. Little interest or pleasure in doing things	0	1	2	3
2. Feeling down, depressed, or hopeless	0	1	2	3
3. Trouble falling or staying asleep, or sleeping too much	0	1	2	3
4. Feeling tired or having little energy	0	1	2	3
5. Poor appetite or overeating	0	1	2	3
6. Feeling bad about yourself – or that you are a failure or have let yourself or your family down	0	1	2	3
7. Trouble concentrating on things, such as reading the newspaper or watching television	0	1	2	3
8. Moving or speaking so slowly that other people could have noticed. Or the opposite – being so fidgety or restless that you have been moving around a lot more than usual	0	1	2	3
9. Thoughts that you would be better off dead, or of hurting yourself in some way	0	1	2	3

Fig. 3. The Patient Health Questionnaire. Total Score: 1–4 Minimal depression; 5–9 Mild depression; 10–14 Moderate depression; 15–19 Moderately severe depression; 20–27 Severe depression. (*From* MacArthur Foundation Initiative on Depression and Primary Care. PRIME-MD Patient Health Questionnaire. Copyright © 1999, Pfizer Inc; MacArthur Toolkit. Copyright April 2006, 3CM, LLC; with permission. Also Available at: http://www.depression-primarycare.org/.)

Ragavendra R. Baliga, MD, MBA
Division of Cardiovascular Medicine
The Ohio State University Medical Center
Columbus, OH, USA

James B. Young, MD
Division of Medicine
Lerner College of Medicine and Endocrinology &
Metabolism Institute, Cleveland Clinic
Cleveland, OH, USA

E-mail addresses:
Ragavendra.baliga@osumc.edu (R.R. Baliga)
youngj@ccf.org (J.B. Young)

REFERENCES

1. Rutledge T, Reis VA, Linke SE, et al. Depression in heart failure a meta-analytic review of prevalence, intervention effects, and associations with clinical outcomes. J Am Coll Cardiol 2006;48(8):1527–37.
2. Sullivan MD, Levy WC, Crane BA, et al. Usefulness of depression to predict time to combined end point of transplant or death for outpatients with advanced heart failure. Am J Cardiol 2004; 94(12):1577–80.
3. Vaccarino V, Kasl SV, Abramson J, et al. Depressive symptoms and risk of functional decline and death in patients with heart failure. J Am Coll Cardiol 2001;38(1):199–205.
4. Sullivan M, Simon G, Spertus J, et al. Depression-related costs in heart failure care. Arch Intern Med 2002;162(16):1860–6.
5. Lederbogen F, Gilles M, Maras A, et al. Increased platelet aggregability in major depression? Psychiatry Res 2001;102(3):255–61.
6. Serebruany VL, Glassman AH, Malinin AI, et al. Platelet/endothelial biomarkers in depressed patients treated with the selective serotonin reuptake inhibitor sertraline after acute coronary events: the Sertraline AntiDepressant Heart Attack Randomized Trial (SADHART) Platelet Substudy. Circulation 2003;108(8):939–44.
7. Rozanski A, Blumenthal JA, Kaplan J. Impact of psychological factors on the pathogenesis of cardiovascular disease and implications for therapy. Circulation 1999;99(16):2192–217.
8. Rumsfeld JS, Havranek E, Masoudi FA, et al. Depressive symptoms are the strongest predictors of short-term declines in health status in patients with heart failure. J Am Coll Cardiol 2003;42(10): 1811–7.
9. O'Connor CM, Jiang W, Kuchibhatla M, et al. Safety and efficacy of sertraline for depression in patients with heart failure: results of the SADHART-CHF (Sertraline Against Depression and Heart Disease in Chronic Heart Failure) trial. J Am Coll Cardiol 2010; 56(9):692–9.
10. Lichtman JH, Bigger JT Jr, Blumenthal JA, et al. Depression and coronary heart disease: recommendations for screening, referral, and treatment: a science advisory from the American Heart Association Prevention Committee of the Council on Cardiovascular Nursing, Council on Clinical Cardiology, Council on Epidemiology and Prevention, and Interdisciplinary Council on Quality of Care and Outcomes Research: endorsed by the American Psychiatric Association. Circulation 2008;118(17): 1768–75.
11. U.S. Preventive Services Task Force. Screening for depression in adults: U.S. preventive services task force recommendation statement. Ann Intern Med 2009;151(11):784–92.
12. Konstam V, Moser DK, De Jong MJ. Depression and anxiety in heart failure. J Card Fail 2005;11(6): 455–63.
13. Silver MA. Depression and heart failure: an overview of what we know and don't know. Cleve Clin J Med 2010;77(Suppl 3):S7–11.

Preface
Depression and Heart Failure

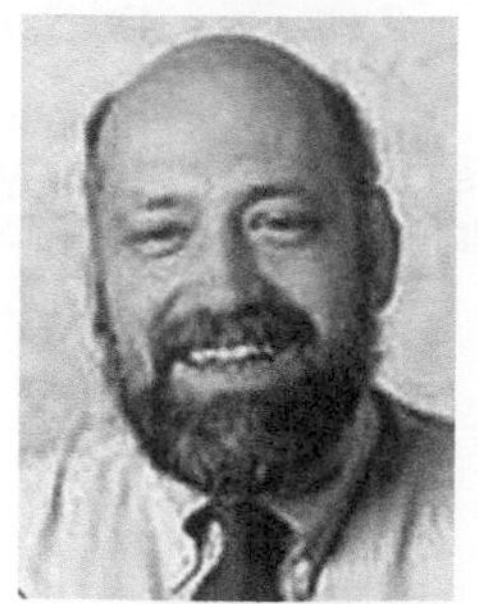
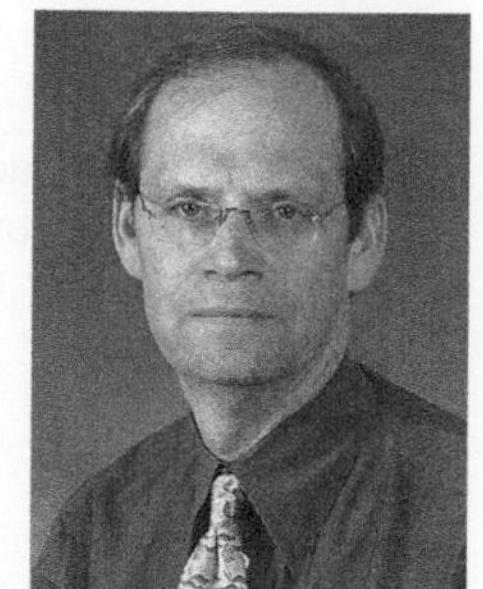

Philip F. Binkley, MD, MPH   Stephen S. Gottlieb, MD
Guest Editors

How important is depression in patients with heart failure? The reviews presented in this issue of *Heart Failure Clinics* should help to elucidate the prevalence and consequences of depression as well as clarify the present state of knowledge about treatment. The aim is to provide a framework for not only proper 2010 clinical care, but also to help frame the questions that need to be answered.

Dr Gnanasekaran starts this issue off by looking at the epidemiology of the problem and quoting a meta-analysis, concluding that the prevalence of depression is 21.6% in patients with heart failure. Dr Freedland and colleagues explore the impact of depression on prognosis, but realize that causation is not clear. More specifically, Drs Kop, Synowski, and Gottlieb focus on how neurohormones and inflammation can influence, and be influenced by, depression.

Since it is also important to look at the impact of patient characteristics, Dr Mehta looks at the specific issues related to women and reports a higher prevalence of depression and worse outcomes. Possible mechanisms are discussed. Meanwhile, Dr Maixner and colleagues discuss the older patient and how comorbidities, cognitive function, and psychosocial issues might affect diagnosis and course.

From their earliest use, implantable cardiac defibrillators were recognized as a source for anxiety and depression in their recipients despite their lifesaving benefits. This important topic is further examined by Drs Freedenberg and colleagues.

The importance of depression in the setting of congestive heart failure demands that depression be detected and accurately diagnosed. Drs Yeager, Saveanu, and Binkley, and colleagues discuss the challenges and methods for implementing depression screening in a heart failure population based on their experience in establishing such a program. Screening for depression is only a first step and does not establish the diagnosis. Drs Saveanu and Mayes discuss the approach required to establish the diagnosis of depression in this population that has numerous heart failure symptoms that may mimic those of depression. Once depression is diagnosed, health care providers must decide whether treatment is warranted, and if so, what kind of therapy should be implemented. Issues involved in these important management decisions are discussed by Drs Echols and Jiang.

Not only does congestive heart failure itself promote the occurrence of depression, but the leading therapies for heart failure may themselves contribute to the incidence or progression of depression. Beta blocker therapy is often cited as contributing to depression, but the evidence for this is carefully reviewed by Dr Verbeek and colleagues.

The editors and authors hope that this issue will further raise the awareness of the significant impact of depression on the course of congestive heart failure and inspire further thought and investigation that will improve the treatment and

Heart Failure Clin 7 (2011) xix–xx
doi:10.1016/j.hfc.2010.09.001

quality of life of our patients with chronic heart failure.

Philip F. Binkley, MD, MPH
The Division of Cardiovascular Medicine
The Ohio State University College of Medicine
The Ohio State University College of Public Health
Columbus, OH, USA

Stephen S. Gottlieb, MD
Cardiomyopathy and Pulmonary
Hypertension Program
University of Maryland
Baltimore, MD, USA

E-mail addresses:
Philip.Binkley@osumc.edu (P.F. Binkley)
sgottlie@medicine.umaryland.edu (S.S. Gottlieb)

Epidemiology of Depression in Heart Failure

Gowrishankar Gnanasekaran, MD, MPH

KEYWORDS

• Epidemiology • Depression • Heart failure • Pathogenesis

Congestive heart failure (CHF) and depression have become increasingly rampant in the growing US population.[1–5] Depression in CHF has been extensively studied recently, because of the high prevalence of the diseases and their tendency to worsen medical prognosis. More recently, there has been an exponential growth of patients with heart failure (HF). According to the National Heart, Lung and Blood Institute, an estimated 4.8 million Americans have CHF and about 400,000 new cases are diagnosed each year. CHF is also the most frequent cause of hospitalization in older adults and has accounted for more than 1 million annual hospital admissions in the past 10 years, resulting in $60 billion in health-care expenses.[6–8] Almost $5 billion of the total cost of HF has been attributed to depression.[7]

Major advances in treatment of HF have prolonged survival, provoking considerable interest in identifying methodologies to improve quality of life (QOL) and functional capacity of patients. QOL encompasses physical, mental, emotional, social, and functional health of the individual. Depression is a major public health problem, which has significant impact on all components of QOL by increasing mortality and frequency of readmissions in patients with HF.[9,10] The World Health Organization report ranked depression as the fourth-most common medical condition, predicting that it is to become the second major disease with disease burden worldwide by 2020. It is estimated to cause more disabilities than many other chronic conditions, including diabetes and osteoarthritis.[11,12] In a multicenter trial of 48,612 patients from 259 hospitals, the investigators reported increased mortality and morbidity associated with patients diagnosed with depression and HF.[13] In their meta-analysis of depression in HF, Rutledge and colleagues[14] have been able to quantify the precise magnitude of increased risk of cardiac events in depressed patients. In addition to CHF, many chronic medical problems have been linked with depression, including diabetes mellitus (DM).[15,16] Fava and colleagues[17] have observed depression to manifest as a life-threatening complication of endocrine diseases, like Cushing and thyroid disease and hyperprolactinemia.

Growing evidence supports this comorbid association, if left unchecked, posing a significant threat to the health of patients. Better understanding of the epidemiology and etiology of depression in HF becomes critically important, providing a better insight in understanding this association to improve QOL and regain function in patients.

EPIDEMIOLOGY

The incidence of depression in HF has been cited by fewer studies than prevalence. In their study of 4538 patients aged 60 years and older who were enrolled in the Systolic Hypertension in the Elderly Program (SHEP), Abramson and colleagues[18] found a covariate-adjusted hazard ratio of 2.82 after adjusting for occurrence of myocardial infarction (MI). They concluded that depression is independently associated with a substantially increased risk of HF among older patients with isolated systolic hypertension.

A study using the Center for Epidemiologic Study Depressive Symptomatology Questionnaire, a

Division of General Internal Medicine & Geriatrics, Department of Internal Medicine, Ohio State University Medical Center, 2050 Kenny Road, Suite 2335, Columbus, OH 43210, USA
E-mail address: gowrishankar.gnanasekaran@osumc.edu

Heart Failure Clin 7 (2011) 1–10
doi:10.1016/j.hfc.2010.08.002
1551-7136/11/$ – see front matter

self-reporting depression questionnaire, assessed emotional support before a hospital admission to be an independent predictor of fatal and nonfatal cardiac events.[19] Apparently, the researchers made the assessment of depression well before the diagnosis of HF, making it difficult to establish a positive correlation between these diseases.

On the other hand, the prevalence of depression in HF has been observed by multiple studies. In their study of 204 outpatients with HF, Sherwood and colleagues[20] reported that symptoms of depression were associated with increased risk of death or hospitalization during a median 3-year follow-up. In their prospective study of 374 hospitalized patients with HF, Jiang and colleagues[21] investigated the prevalence of depression and the significant mortality and morbidity associated in terms of readmission rates. They identified that patients with HF and depression had 13% and 26% mortality at 3 months and 1 year, respectively. Furthermore, depressed patients were twice as likely to be hospitalized compared with nondepressed patients. Jiang and colleagues have used Beck Depression Inventory (BDI) as a tool to assess the severity of depression. In their subgroup analysis on depressive symptoms and long-term mortality, 30% of subjects were found to be depressed and were found to be younger or with much more severe HF as classified by the New York Heart Association (NYHA).

In their study on 155 outpatients with HF, Gottlieb and colleagues[22] examined the influence of race, sex, NYHA classification, and age on QOL and frequency of depression. Almost 50% of the study population, 79% of whom were men and 21%, women, were found to be depressed using the BDI scale. QOL was assessed using the Medical Outcome Study Short Form (SF-36) and the Minnesota Living with Heart Failure Questionnaire. The younger population was found to be more depressed compared with the older; 64% of women were found to be depressed compared with 44% of men. Among men, blacks were observed to be more depressed than whites, and there was no significant difference seen in women based on ethnic classifications. Almost 68% of people had severe HF classified as NYHA 111 or higher, and the rate of depression was almost double in patients with class 111 HF compared with class 11.

In their study of depression and risk of HF in the elderly, Williams and colleagues[23] examined a community sample and reported depression as an independent risk factor of HF, mostly in elderly women. In their report on gender difference in the *depression cardiovascular link*, Naqvi and colleagues[24] identified depression to be twice as high in women as in men.

Freedland and colleagues[2] examined the prevalence of depression in a sample of 682 hospitalized patients with HF and found more than half (55%) at least met the criteria for depression using the BDI scale. The strongest correlates identified were greater functional impairments and younger age.

Koenig[5] found the prevalence of depression to be 36.5% in inpatients aged 60 years and older admitted in a tertiary care hospital. Frasure-Smith and colleagues[25] reported a higher incidence of depression in patients with a recent MI in the previous 1 to 3 weeks, with an ejection fraction (EF) of 35% or less or Kilip class 11 or greater HF.

Havranek and colleagues[3] used the Medical Outcomes Study Depression Tool to identify independent predictors like living alone, alcohol abuse, and financial burden from medical care associated with development of depressive symptoms among outpatients with HF. The incidence of these predictors at 1 year was 16%, 36%, and 69%, respectively. Furthermore, they used the Kansas City Cardiomyopathy Questionnaire and identified patients with worse HF developed significant depressive symptoms at year one.

The Organized Program to Initiate Life Saving Treatment in Hospitalized Patients (OPTIMIZE-HF) evaluated the association of depression with hospital treatments and postdischarge mortality. In their analysis of 48,612 patients from 259 hospitals, depression was found more commonly in the female gender, in whites, and in patients with associated comorbidities of HF, including DM, chronic obstructive pulmonary disease, and anemia. Furthermore, investigators found a significant increase in 60- to 90-day mortality in patients with a history of depression, and these patients were less likely to receive cardiac interventions and referral to outpatient rehabilitation programs.[13] **Fig. 1** shows the Kaplan-Meir curve for postdischarge mortality in patients hospitalized with HF and history of depression.

Rohyans and colleagues[26] analyzed the sociodemographic variables associated with depressive symptoms in patients with HF. They observed that depression was more prevalent in younger patients, women, and patients with more severe HF based on NYHA classification. The researchers used the Personal Health Questionnaire (PHQ 9) for their depression evaluation, whereas many other studies have used BDI as the screening scale. Furthermore, in their regression analysis of elderly patients with HF, they found that patients who had functional impairment

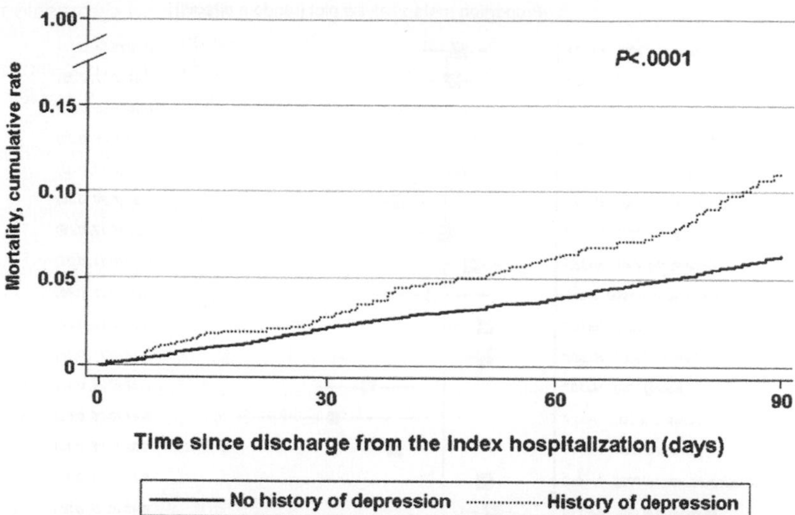

Fig. 1. Kaplan-Meir curve for postdischarge mortality was increased in patients hospitalized with HF and history of depression. (*Reproduced from* Albert NM, Fonarow GC, Abraham WT, et al. Depression and clinical outcomes in heart failure: an OPTIMIZE-HF analysis. Am J Med 2009;122:366; with permission.)

and lacked problem-focused coping mechanisms tended to be more depressed compared with those who did not.

In their study on depressive symptoms with respect to long-term mortality in patients with atrial fibrillation and CHF. Nancy Frasure-Smith and colleagues[25] reported that elevated depressive symptoms significantly predicted cardiovascular (CV) mortality in rate- and rhythm-controlled treatment groups. The covariate-adjusted depression-related increase in CV death was similar to the increase with not taking anticoagulants or being prescribed aldosterone antagonists, important treatment factors for the disease. The Canadian Amiodarone Myocardial Infarction Arrhythmia Trial (CAMIAT) found that depression significantly predicted sudden cardiac death in placebo-treated patients but not in those receiving amiodarone.[27] **Fig. 2** shows the prevalence rates of clinically significant depression among patients with HF in the meta-analytic review of Rutledge and colleagues[14].

Wide heterogeneity has been observed in the reported prevalence of depression in HF across the various studies done, ranging from 11% to 25% for outpatients and 35% to 70% for inpatients. In their meta-analysis of depression in HF, Rutledge and colleagues[14] have examined at least 36 publications and have calculated an overall point estimate prevalence rate of 21.6%. The variation observed can be attributed to several factors, including the assessment methods used in diagnosing depression, the severity of HF, and the different characteristics of the patient population enrolled in these studies. Of these, the different assessment tools of depression and severity of HF seem to have a greater impact on the variations observed. In their systematic review, Delville and colleagues[28] analyzed the most common instruments used for evaluating depression in adults with HF. In the 16 articles that met the inclusion criteria, 6 self-reporting instruments and 2 diagnostic interviews were identified. Depressive symptoms were reported in 14% to 60% of adults with HF. Self-reporting questionnaires provided a higher incidence of depressive symptoms, 21% to 60%, compared with diagnostic interviews, which ranged from 14% to 39%. A possible explanation would be the perception of lower QOL in patients with depression and subsequent reporting of diminished functional status. Based on the NYHA classification, a fourfold increase in depression was observed in patients with class 4 HF compared with class 1 HF. Furthermore, the prevalence of depression in Caucasian patients was found to be 9% to 54% with an aggregate of 25% compared with 7% to 44% with an aggregate of 18.7% in the minority group.

Inconsistencies in the use of depression assessment methodologies in these various studies have been a limiting factor in systematic analysis of the prevalence of these comorbid diseases. Probably, the use of standardized psychiatric measures would make the measurement more equitable in future studies.

Depression is annotated to be a behavioral disease manifesting biologic changes, which makes it constantly change over time. Although these studies provide compelling evidence of increased prevalence of depression in HF, there

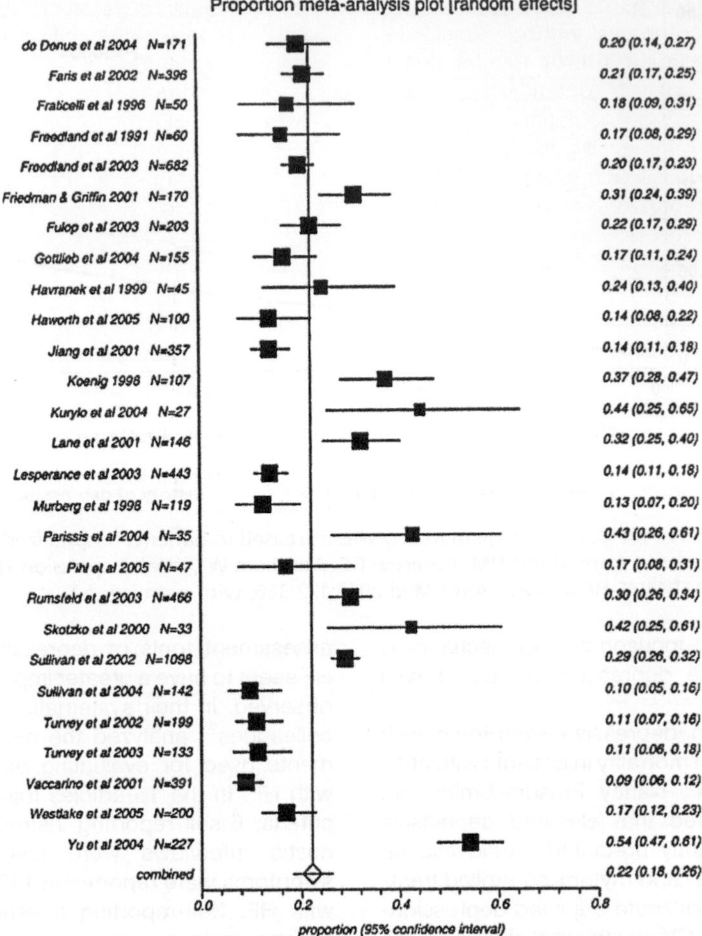

Fig. 2. Shows the prevalence rates of clinically significant depression among patients with HF in the meta-analytic review of Rutledge and colleagues. The prevalence rate widely varied, ranging from 9% to 60% and the aggregated point estimate was 21.5%. (*Reproduced from* Rutledge T, Reis VA, Linke SE, et al. Depression in heart failure: a meta-analytic review of prevalence, intervention effects, and associations with clinical outcomes. J Am Coll Cardiol 2006;48:1527–37; with permission.)

is a lack of information on changes in depression over time and their influence on patients with HF. More outcome studies are necessary to systematically analyze the diseases, taking into consideration the heterogeneity observed. This study tries to draw the attention of future investigators to the further research needed to address this paucity of knowledge. Furthermore, a better understanding on the areas of incidence of depression in HF and associated health-care costs is important.

DEPRESSION IN CHF IN THE ELDERLY

Depression and cardiovascular diseases are among the top 5 chronic disorders leading to disability worldwide in the elderly population.[12] Aging is considered a byproduct of an interaction between genetic, environmental, and lifestyle factors, which predisposes the elderly to multiple vascular abnormalities. Elderly people have heightened levels of oxidative stress and inflammation, which in combination with other abnormalities, such as cellular senescence, can conspire to induce proatherosclerotic changes.[29] In their study of prevalence of CV diseases involving centenarians, Cicconetti and colleagues[30] reported a prevalence of 16.7%, of which 8% was due to HF. Vascular disease enhances functional decline and has a major impact on QOL in the elderly population.[10] In patients with HF, the association of depression has led to poorer QOL, increased hospitalization, and mortality.[31] As regards physical functioning, depressed patients with cardiac disease scored, on average, 77.6% of normal functioning compared with controls.[32] In acutely ill hospitalized older adults, the functional capacity of the patient deteriorates more compared with the rest of population.[33] Koenigh[5] reported a high prevalence of 36.5% of major depression by Diagnostic and Statistical Manual of Mental Disorders fourth edition (DSM-IV) criteria in 107 elderly patients admitted with CHF. There was no difference in mortality reported, but most patients (57.5%) met the criteria for depression. Data from the Hispanic Established Population for the Epidemiologic Study of the Elderly indicated higher death rates in patients with a high level of depressive symptoms and DM.[34] Furthermore, under-recognition of depression in this population has been associated with increased risk of recurrent falls.[34] In a study that used the 2001 to 2003 National Hospital Discharge Survey data sets, the investigators found that ambulatory older adults who were discharged with a primary diagnosis of HF and a secondary diagnosis of depression had a significant increase in nursing home admissions.[35]

Carels[10] study found a positive correlation between depression and QOL indices like physical, emotional, and social support; mood; and coping behaviors in patients with CHF. Chung and colleagues[36] further analyzed the effects of depressive symptoms and anxiety on QOL in patients with CHF and their spouses. QOL was assessed using the Minnesota Living with Heart Failure Questionnaire and the investigators reported that patients and their spouses had poorer QOL with higher depressive symptoms.

Fulop and colleagues[6] analyzed the course of depression and economic consequences in older patients with CHF. Almost 36% of the study population of 203 subjects were found to be depressed using the geriatric depression scale, and 22% were depressed according to the Structured Clinical Interview of the DSM-III–R nonpatient edition. They also found that depressed patients were using more medical resources compared with the nondepressed population.

In their study of major depression and disability in older primary-care patients with HF, Friedman and colleagues[37] examined the association between depression and dependence on activities of daily living and instrumental activities in an elderly population. A progressive increase in prevalence of depression to about 40% was reported in patients with increased dependency on instrumental activities of daily living.

Gottlieb and colleagues[22] reported that for every 10 years more than mean age 64 years, the likelihood of depressive symptoms tends to decrease by 26%. Although their observation is surprising, it would be prudent to understand that subclinical depression is widely prevalent and left underdiagnosed in this population. Recent National Institute of Mental Health studies show that 13% to 27% of elderly patients might have subclinical depression, and most would not meet the diagnostic criteria for major depression using standard screening questionnaires. Furthermore, cognitive capability in the country's elderly population would limit the utility of these screening questionnaires. Using more structured scales for the geriatric population and diagnostic interviews would improve understanding of the epidemic in this age group.

BIOLOGY OF THE EPIDEMIC

Mounting evidence of this perilous association has not prompted significant interventions. Similarity of symptoms, like fatigue, malaise, weight gain, and insomnia, shared by these diseases increases the difficulty of delineating the 2 disease processes. Superficially, depression can be thought of as a somatic outcome of the CV changes that happen in HF. If this is considered a plausible explanation, treatment of HF would have remitted depression and the association would have been nullified effortlessly.

An analogous way to identify the etiology is to understand the biology of the disease processes. Common pathophysiology includes biologic reasons, like neurohumoral activation, sympathoadrenal activation, and hypercoagulability. Psychosocial reasons, including medication noncompliance, lower social support, and concern for medical stigmata, have also been associated with worse outcomes.[38] Gottlieb and colleagues[22] point out that only 7% of patients in their study were taking antidepressants.

Medication noncompliance is a potential mechanism documented to produce adverse outcome in these diseases.[39–41] Studies have shown that medication noncompliance causes 125,000 deaths annually in the United States and leads to 10% of hospital admission and 23% of nursing home admissions.[42] In their study, Casey and colleagues[43] reported elevated levels of depression predicting failure to complete a 12-week phase 2 cardiac rehabilitation program. Furthermore, patients with a history of depression were less likely to receive coronary interventions and cardiac devices or be referred to outpatient disease management programs. Depression tends to produce more noncompliance, which could instigate a vicious cycle of worsening depression and HF.

Grippo and Johnson[44] have hypothesized sympathoadrenal activation as a possible mechanism of this epidemic. Hypersecretion of norepinephrine in unipolar depression has been reported in previous studies.[45–47] Benedict and colleagues[48] found an independent relation of neurohumoral activation and severity of left ventricular (LV) function in a subgroup of patients enrolled in the Studies of Left Ventricular Dysfunction (SOLVD) registry. The 2 central components of stress response are the hypothalamic pituitary adrenocortical axis and sympathoadrenal system. In a depressive state, escalated stress response does not react to the counter-regulatory response, resulting in hyperactivity of the adrenocortical axis and sympathoadrenal axis. This results in increased cortisol levels, which predisposes patients to enhanced CV disease. Depression causes dysregulation of the autonomic nervous control in HF, resulting in increased sympathetic tone, thereby increasing resting heart rate and decreasing heart-rate variability (HRV). Augmented sympathetic tone further increases levels of plasma cortisol, serotonin, rennin, aldosterone, and free radicals that worsen the disease processes. Hypothetical schema of the various pathophysiological changes found in depression and CV diseases are shown in **Fig. 3**.

Elevated levels of inflammatory cytokines have also been proposed as a possible mechanism for worsening depression and HF.[49] The Vesnarinone Multicenter Trial (VEST) revealed that proinflammatory cytokines, like tumor necrosis factor (TNF) and IL-6, and their receptors sTNFR1 and sTNFR2 independently predicted increased mortality in patients with advanced HF.[49] Sliwa and colleagues[50] found that pentoxifylline, a platelet antiagrregant, significantly lowered the cytokine levels and improved LVEF in patients with idiopathic cardiomyopathy. Smith[51] in 1991 postulated the macrophage theory of depression in which he reported excessive secretion of IL-1 and other macrophage products in the pathogenesis of depression. In their meta-analysis, Zorilla and colleagues[52] found an association between major depression and immune activation reminiscent of an acute-phase response. Any acute cardiac event activates the immune system, which

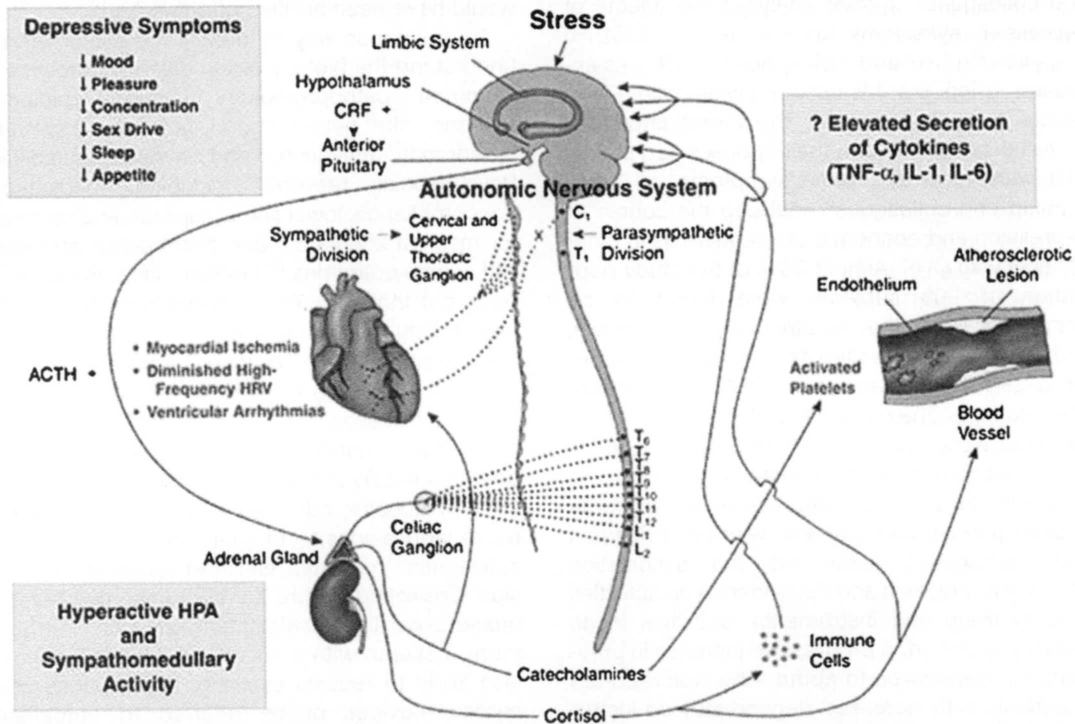

Fig. 3. Hypothetical schema of the various pathophysiological changes found in depression and CV diseases. (*Reproduced from* Musselman DL, Evans DL, Nemeroff CB. The relationship of depression to cardiovascular disease, epidemiology, biology and treatment. Arch Gen Psychiatry 1998;55:580–92; with permission. Copyright ©1998 American Medical Association. All rights reserved.)

triggers the cytokine cascade. The failing heart then becomes the source for production of TNF-α, which secondarily activates the immune system. Decreased tissue perfusion in CHF leads to production of inflammatory cytokines in the systemic tissues, which further accelerates the vicious cycle.

HRV has been studied as another potential mechanism contributing to diminished survival in depressed patients with CV disease. HRV, which is measured as the standard deviation of successive intervals between two successive R waves, has been a valid way of measuring the functioning of the sympathetic, parasympathetic, and rennin-angiotensin mechanism. CV homeostasis is maintained by these nervous systems that alter the heart rate. A higher degree of HRV predicts a better cardiac outcome, and HRV is significantly depressed in patients with severe HF and in depressed patients, which reflects the decreased parasympathetic tone associated with these comorbid diseases.[53]

In their study of 10,294 patients 65 years and older, Markovitz and colleagues[54] were able to propose platelet activation as a possible cause in the proposed link. Platelets contain adrenergic, serotonergic, and dopaminergic receptors. Activation of the α-adrenoreceptors increase the level of catecholamines and initiate platelet response. This results in activation of the arachidonate pathway, causing thrombus formation and vascular damage. Serotonin-induced platelet activation can cause thrombosis and vascular constriction.

Other mechanisms leading to poorer outcomes include the severity of HF noted in depressed patients compared with the nondepressed. One possible explanation would be the deterioration in the cardiopulmonary reserve in patients with severe HF and their diminished perception of QOL. McCaffrey and colleagues[55] have hypothesized a genetic vulnerability in both these diseases. Sociodemographic indicators, like younger age and female sex, and psychological indicators, like comorbid psychiatric disorder, situational stressors, and coping sources, are valid predictors of depression, and better understanding them would add value in better understanding this association.

ANTIDEPRESSANTS IN HF

Little is known about the effectiveness of antidepressant therapy in patients with CHF. Studies have found that 16% to 26% of depressed patients with CHF receive antidepressants.[5,56–60] Three trials have been published so far on the utility of treatment of depression in HF. It is crucial to understand that depression is more than just a somatic reaction to CHF and that prompt evaluation and treatment would be of benefit in terms of mortality and morbidity. The recent Enhancing Recovery in Coronary Heart Disease (ENRICHD) trial, which enrolled 2481 patients hospitalized for MI in the previous 30 days, reported lack of efficacy of nonpharmacologic strategies in treatment of depression in patients who had had an MI. However, a post hoc analysis of participants in the ENRICHD trial found that the use of a selective serotonin reuptake inhibitor (SSRI) was associated with 40% reduction in recurrent MI and death after adjustments for demographic and CV variables.[61] The Montreal Heart Attack Readjustment Trial (M-HART), which randomized 1376 patients who had had an MI to telephone monitoring, found higher cardiac and all-cause mortality, especially in women who had received the nonpharmacologic intervention for depression. The study concluded, cautioning that nonpharmacologic treatment can potentially be harmful to patients who have had a recent MI.[62,63] A possible explanation may be that the intervention reminded the patients of their disease state and increased distress in this population. Pharmacologic treatments for depression are controversial in HF, because of the potential side effects associated with psychiatric medications. Tricyclics affect the cardiac system. SSRIs like sertraline and citalopram are found to be safe in heart disease, because they are the least likely to inhibit the cytochrome P450 enzymes. However, there is no randomized study that is evaluating the safety and efficacy of antidepressants in HF.

The Sertraline Antidepressant Heart Attack Randomization Trial (SADHART) evaluated the use of antidepressants in patients with heart disease and demonstrated that depression can be treated without increasing the complications of CV events in patient with coronary artery disease. The investigators also found a nonsignificant reduction in the composite endpoint of MI or death from coronary heart disease.[64] Whether therapy for depression would improve CV outcome remains undetermined. The ongoing SADHART-HF study will provide important data to address this paucity of knowledge. Morbidity, Mortality and Mood in Depressed Heart Failure patients (MOOD-HF), a large randomized placebo-controlled trial, is investigating the utility of the drug escitalopram, an SSRI, to improve outcomes in depressed patients with CHF of NYHA class II to IV and impaired LV systolic function. The Interpersonal Theory and Citalopram for Depression in Coronary Disease (CREATE) trial is comparing the efficacy and safety of interpersonal therapy and SSRI in the treatment of depression in patients with heart disease. Currently, cognitive behavioral therapy is the only known safe and effective treatment of depression in patients with heart disease.[65] The Myocardial Infarction and Depression Intervention Trial (MIND IT) compared the efficacy of antidepressants like mirtazapine and citalopram (Celexa) to improve cardiac outcomes in an 18-month trial in patients who had had a recent MI and had reported no difference in cardiac prognosis. A post hoc analysis comparing responders to medication with nonresponders to treatment reported that the nonresponse group may be associated with an increased cardiac event rate.[66]

SUMMARY

Increasing evidence supports the occurrence of depression in CHF. The impact of the disease is still under-recognized and standard protocols to address this serious occurrence have not been established. This article intends to refresh our memory on the health-care burden associated with this occurrence. Updated literature on the epidemiology of the disease provides the knowledge and insight needed to understand the complex burden of the disease in terms of mortality, morbidity, health-care costs, and QOL. Accounting for sociodemographic predictors of depression, like female gender; comorbid psychiatric disorders; situational stressors; and coping sources, including social support; play an important role in ameliorating the disease process. The author has found wide heterogeneity in the prevalence of depression in HF across the various studies conducted, partly because of the assessment methods used to diagnose depression. This study directs future research in directions to address these gaps. Use of standardized depression assessment measures that involve a self-reported screening followed by a structured interview would better validate the diagnosis. Furthermore, "elder-friendly" screening tools would add more value in unraveling subclinical depression in our elderly population. A conscientious effort to understand the shared pathophysiology in these diseases highlights the importance of their early recognition to appropriate interventions. Furthermore, this knowledge would lead to identification of potential biologic markers, including markers of systemic inflammation, inflammatory cytokines, and changes in HRV, for early interventions.

Future studies need to be conducted to investigate the utility of treatments for depression in reducing CV mortality and their safety profile. Early detection and treatment is important to improving QOL. Depression is associated with poor medication compliance, and interventional efforts should target a broad range of clinical outcomes to effectively assess potential benefits. This becomes increasingly important in our elderly population in whom drug-drug interaction and medication compliance is a challenge. Health-care provider knowledge and awareness of this association is warranted and becomes crucially important to give patients and caregivers the necessary tools and methods to develop better coping strategies during distress.

REFERENCES

1. Aimonino N, Tibaldi V, Barale S, et al. Depressive symptoms and quality of life in elderly patients with exacerbation of chronic obstructive pulmonary disease or cardiac heart failure: preliminary data of a randomized controlled trial. Arch Gerontol Geriatr 2007;44(Suppl 1):7.
2. Freedland KE, Rich MW, Skala JA, et al. Prevalence of depression in hospitalized patients with congestive heart failure. Psychosom Med 2003;65:119.
3. Havranek EP, Ware MG, Lowes BD. Prevalence of depression in congestive heart failure. Am J Cardiol 1999;84:348.
4. Holzapfel N, Muller-Tasch T, Wild B, et al. Depression profile in patients with and without chronic heart failure. J Affect Disord 2008;105:53.
5. Koenig HG. Depression in hospitalized older patients with congestive heart failure. Gen Hosp Psychiatry 1998;20:29.
6. Fulop G, Strain JJ, Stettin G. Congestive heart failure and depression in older adults: clinical course and health services use 6 months after hospitalization. Psychosomatics 2003;44:367.
7. Sullivan M, Simon G, Spertus J, et al. Depression-related costs in heart failure care. Arch Intern Med 2002;162:1860.
8. Unutzer J, Schoenbaum M, Katon WJ, et al. Health-care costs associated with depression in medically Ill fee-for-service medicare participants. J Am Geriatr Soc 2009;57:506.
9. Bekelman DB, Dy SM, Becker DM, et al. Spiritual well-being and depression in patients with heart failure. J Gen Intern Med 2007;22:470.
10. Carels RA. The association between disease severity, functional status, depression and daily quality of life in congestive heart failure patients. Qual Life Res 2004;13:63.
11. Egede LE. Major depression in individuals with chronic medical disorders: prevalence, correlates and association with health resource utilization, lost productivity and functional disability. Gen Hosp Psychiatry 2007;29:409.

12. Lopez AD, Mathers CD. Measuring the global burden of disease and epidemiological transitions: 2002–2030. Ann Trop Med Parasitol 2006;100:481.
13. Albert NM, Fonarow GC, Abraham WT, et al. Depression and clinical outcomes in heart failure: an OPTIMIZE-HF analysis. Am J Med 2009;122:366.
14. Rutledge T, Reis VA, Linke SE, et al. Depression in heart failure a meta-analytic review of prevalence, intervention effects, and associations with clinical outcomes. J Am Coll Cardiol 2006;48:1527.
15. Aujla N, Abrams KR, Davies MJ, et al. The prevalence of depression in white-European and South-asian people with impaired glucose regulation and screen-detected type 2 diabetes mellitus. PLoS One 2009;4:e7755.
16. Ell K, Katon W, Cabassa LJ, et al. Depression and diabetes among low-income Hispanics: design elements of a socioculturally adapted collaborative care model randomized controlled trial. Int J Psychiatry Med 2009;39:113.
17. Fava GA, Sonino N, Morphy MA. Major depression associated with endocrine disease. Psychiatr Dev 1987;5:321.
18. Abramson J, Berger A, Krumholz HM, et al. Depression and risk of heart failure among older persons with isolated systolic hypertension. Arch Intern Med 2001;161:1725.
19. Krumholz HM, Butler J, Miller J, et al. Prognostic importance of emotional support for elderly patients hospitalized with heart failure. Circulation 1998;97:958.
20. Sherwood A, Blumenthal JA, Trivedi R, et al. Relationship of depression to death or hospitalization in patients with heart failure. Arch Intern Med 2007; 167:367.
21. Jiang W, Kuchibhatla M, Clary GL, et al. Relationship between depressive symptoms and long-term mortality in patients with heart failure. Am Heart J 2007;154:102.
22. Gottlieb SS, Khatta M, Friedmann E, et al. The influence of age, gender, and race on the prevalence of depression in heart failure patients. J Am Coll Cardiol 2004;43:1542.
23. Williams SA, Kasl SV, Heiat A, et al. Depression and risk of heart failure among the elderly: a prospective community-based study. Psychosom Med 2002;64:6.
24. Naqvi TZ, Naqvi SS, Merz CN. Gender differences in the link between depression and cardiovascular disease. Psychosom Med 2005;67(Suppl 1):S15.
25. Frasure-Smith N, Lesperance F, Habra M, et al. Elevated depression symptoms predict long-term cardiovascular mortality in patients with atrial fibrillation and heart failure. Circulation 2009;120:134.
26. Rohyans LM, Pressler SJ. Depressive symptoms and heart failure: examining the sociodemographic variables. Clin Nurse Spec 2009;23:138.
27. Cairns JA, Connolly SJ, Roberts R, et al. Canadian Amiodarone Myocardial Infarction Arrhythmia Trial (CAMIAT): rationale and protocol. CAMIAT Investigators. Am J Cardiol 1993;72:87F.
28. Delville CL, McDougall G. A systematic review of depression in adults with heart failure: instruments and incidence. Issues Ment Health Nurs 2008;29: 1002.
29. Paradies G, Petrosillo G, Paradies V, et al. Oxidative stress, mitochondrial bioenergetics and cardiolipin in aging. Free Radic Biol Med 2010;48(10): 1286–95.
30. Cicconetti P, Tafaro L, Tedeschi G, et al. [Cardiovascular risk factors and diseases in centenarians]. Recenti Prog Med 2001;92:731 [in Italian].
31. Guallar-Castillon P, Magarinos-Losada MM, Montoto-Otero C, et al. [Prevalence of depression and associated medical and psychosocial factors in elderly hospitalized patients with heart failure in Spain]. Rev Esp Cardiol 2006;59:770 [in Spanish].
32. Cassano P, Fava M. Depression and public health: an overview. J Psychosom Res 2002;53:849.
33. Mallery LH, MacDonald EA, Hubley-Kozey CL, et al. The feasibility of performing resistance exercise with acutely ill hospitalized older adults. BMC Geriatr 2003;3:3.
34. Black SA, Markides KS. Depressive symptoms and mortality in older Mexican Americans. Ann Epidemiol 1999;9:45.
35. Ahmed A, Ali M, Lefante CM, et al. Geriatric heart failure, depression, and nursing home admission: an observational study using propensity score analysis. Am J Geriatr Psychiatry 2006;14:867.
36. Chung ML, Moser DK, Lennie TA, et al. The effects of depressive symptoms and anxiety on quality of life in patients with heart failure and their spouses: testing dyadic dynamics using Actor-Partner Interdependence Model. J Psychosom Res 2009;67:29.
37. Friedman B, Lyness JM, Delavan RL, et al. Major depression and disability in older primary care patients with heart failure. J Geriatr Psychiatry Neurol 2008;21:111.
38. Johansson P, Dahlstrom U, Brostrom A. Consequences and predictors of depression in patients with chronic heart failure: implications for nursing care and future research. Prog Cardiovasc Nurs 2006;21:202.
39. Bagchi AD, Esposito D, Kim M, et al. Utilization of, and adherence to, drug therapy among medicaid beneficiaries with congestive heart failure. Clin Ther 2007;29:1771.
40. Hauptman PJ. Medication adherence in heart failure. Heart Fail Rev 2008;13:99.
41. van der Wal MH, Jaarsma T. Adherence in heart failure in the elderly: problem and possible solutions. Int J Cardiol 2008;125:203.

42. Smith DL. Compliance packaging: a patient education tool. Am Pharm 1989;NS29:42.
43. Casey E, Hughes JW, Waechter D, et al. Depression predicts failure to complete phase-II cardiac rehabilitation. J Behav Med 2008;31:421.
44. Grippo AJ, Johnson AK. Stress, depression and cardiovascular dysregulation: a review of neurobiological mechanisms and the integration of research from preclinical disease models. Stress 2009;12:1.
45. Haenisch B, Linsel K, Bruss M, et al. Association of major depression with rare functional variants in norepinephrine transporter and serotonin1A receptor genes. Am J Med Genet B Neuropsychiatr Genet 2009;150B:1013.
46. Potter WZ, Manji HK. Catecholamines in depression: an update. Clin Chem 1994;40:279.
47. Sahoo M, Subho C. Cortisol hypersecretion in unipolar major depression with melancholic and psychotic features: dopaminergic, noradrenergic and thyroid correlates. Psychoneuroendocrinology 2007;32:210 [author reply 211].
48. Benedict CR, Johnstone DE, Weiner DH, et al. Relation of neurohumoral activation to clinical variables and degree of ventricular dysfunction: a report from the Registry of Studies of Left Ventricular Dysfunction. SOLVD Investigators. J Am Coll Cardiol 1994;23:1410.
49. Deswal A, Petersen NJ, Feldman AM, et al. Cytokines and cytokine receptors in advanced heart failure: an analysis of the cytokine database from the Vesnarinone trial (VEST). Circulation 2001;103:2055.
50. Sliwa K, Skudicky D, Candy G, et al. Randomised investigation of effects of pentoxifylline on left-ventricular performance in idiopathic dilated cardiomyopathy. Lancet 1998;351:1091.
51. Smith RS. The macrophage theory of depression. Med Hypotheses 1991;35:298.
52. Zorrilla EP, Luborsky L, McKay JR, et al. The relationship of depression and stressors to immunological assays: a meta-analytic review. Brain Behav Immun 2001;15:199.
53. Catipovic-Veselica K, Galic A, Jelic K, et al. Relation between major and minor depression and heart rate, heart-rate variability, and clinical characteristics of patients with acute coronary syndrome. Psychol Rep 2007;100:1245.
54. Markovitz JH, Shuster JL, Chitwood WS, et al. Platelet activation in depression and effects of sertraline treatment: An open-label study. Am J Psychiatry 2000;157:1006.
55. McCaffery JM, Frasure-Smith N, Dube MP, et al. Common genetic vulnerability to depressive symptoms and coronary artery disease: a review and development of candidate genes related to inflammation and serotonin. Psychosom Med 2006;68:187.
56. Alexopoulos GS, Streim J, Carpenter D, et al. Using antipsychotic agents in older patients. J Clin Psychiatry 2004;65(Suppl 2):5.
57. Conn DK, Goldman Z. Pattern of use of antidepressants in long-term care facilities for the elderly. J Geriatr Psychiatry Neurol 1992;5:228.
58. Koenig HG. Physician attitudes toward treatment of depression in older medical inpatients. Aging Ment Health 2007;11:197.
59. O'Connor CM, Jiang W, Kuchibhatla M, et al. Antidepressant use, depression, and survival in patients with heart failure. Arch Intern Med 2008; 168:2232.
60. Parissis J, Fountoulaki K, Paraskevaidis I, et al. Sertraline for the treatment of depression in coronary artery disease and heart failure. Expert Opin Pharmacother 2007;8:1529.
61. Jaffe AS, Krumholz HM, Catellier DJ, et al. Prediction of medical morbidity and mortality after acute myocardial infarction in patients at increased psychosocial risk in the Enhancing Recovery in Coronary Heart Disease Patients (ENRICHD) study. Am Heart J 2006;152:126.
62. Frasure-Smith N. The montreal heart attack readjustment trial. J Cardiopulm Rehabil 1995;15:103.
63. Frasure-Smith N, Lesperance F, Gravel G, et al. Long-term survival differences among low-anxious, high-anxious and repressive copers enrolled in the Montreal heart attack readjustment trial. Psychosom Med 2002;64:571.
64. Shapiro PA, Lesperance F, Frasure-Smith N, et al. An open-label preliminary trial of sertraline for treatment of major depression after acute myocardial infarction (the SADHAT Trial). Sertraline Anti-Depressant Heart Attack Trial. Am Heart J 1999;137:1100.
65. Shapiro PA. Treatment of depression in patients with congestive heart failure. Heart Fail Rev 2009;14:7.
66. de Jonge P, Honig A, van Melle JP, et al. Nonresponse to treatment for depression following myocardial infarction: association with subsequent cardiac events. Am J Psychiatry 2007;164:1371.

Effect of Depression on Prognosis in Heart Failure

Kenneth E. Freedland, PhD[a,*], Robert M. Carney, PhD[a], Michael W. Rich, MD[b,c]

KEYWORDS

• Depression • Major depressive disorder • Heart failure
• Prognosis • Mortality

Depression is a common comorbid condition in patients with heart failure (HF), and it is associated with a poor prognosis. Whether the prognosis of HF can be improved by treating depression has not yet been established, but depression nevertheless deserves clinical attention. This article discusses the definition and measurement of depression in patients with HF, research on the relationship between depression and HF outcomes, some candidate mechanisms that may help to explain this relationship, and the status of depression as a risk factor for adverse outcomes in HF. It concludes by considering the implications of these issues for further research and for the assessment and treatment of depression in HF.

DEFINITIONS AND MEASURES OF DEPRESSION IN HEART FAILURE

The prognostic importance of depression depends on how it is defined and measured. In the American Psychiatric Association's Diagnostic and Statistical Manual of Mental Disorders (DSM-IV-TR),[1] a major depressive episode is defined as the presence of a particular constellation of depressive symptoms (**Box 1**). In the course of an individual's lifetime, there may be only a single episode of major depression (MD), or there may be recurrent episodes. The first (or only) episode may occur in childhood, adolescence, or adulthood, and, for any given episode, the duration may vary from as little as a few weeks to a few years or even longer. The durations of interepisode intervals are highly variable as well. Consequently, major depressive disorder (MDD) can follow different lifetime courses in different individuals.

The criteria for an episode of minor depression (md) are the same as for an MD episode, except that there are only 2 to 4 symptoms rather than 5 to 9. When MD episodes resolve, they usually do so gradually. Consequently, an individual who had 7 or 8 symptoms during a MD episode may have only 3 or 4 symptoms when the episode is in partial remission. If a cross-sectional assessment of depression is performed at this time, without regard to the history of the episode or whether there is a past history of MD episodes, then a major depressive episode in partial remission may be misdiagnosed as an episode of md.

This work was supported in part by grant nos R01MH051419 and R01HL091918 from the National Institutes of Health.
Disclosures: Dr Carney or a member of his family is a stockholder in Pfizer Inc, Forest Laboratories, and Johnson & Johnson, Inc. Dr Rich has a small research grant from Astellas Pharma US. Dr Freedland has nothing to disclose.
[a] Department of Psychiatry, Behavioral Medicine Center, Washington University School of Medicine, 4320 Forest Park Avenue, Suite 301, St Louis, MO 63108, USA
[b] Division of Cardiology, Washington University School of Medicine, 660 South Euclid Avenue, Box 8086, St Louis, MO 63110, USA
[c] Cardiac Rapid Evaluation Unit, Barnes-Jewish Hospital, St Louis, MO, USA
* Corresponding author.
E-mail address: freedlak@bmc.wustl.edu

Heart Failure Clin 7 (2011) 11–21
doi:10.1016/j.hfc.2010.08.003
1551-7136/11/$ – see front matter

Box 1
DSM-IV-TR criteria for major depressive episodes

- At least 5 of the following 9 symptoms persist for at least 2 weeks and represent a change from the individual's previous level of functioning:

  Depressed mood (eg, feels sad, down, blue)

  Loss of interest or pleasure in most or all usual activities

  Significant change in appetite or weight, whether decreased or increased

  Insomnia or hypersomnia (excessive sleepiness)

  Agitation (restlessness, excessive motor activity) or psychomotor retardation (slowing of movements or speech)

  Fatigue or loss of energy

  Feelings of worthlessness or excessive guilt

  Inability to concentrate, think clearly, or make decisions

  Suicidal ideation, wishes to die, or thoughts of being better off dead
- Depressed mood and loss of interest or pleasure are cardinal symptoms of MD; at least 1 of these symptoms must be present
- The depressive symptoms are associated with significant impairment in 1 or more important areas of functioning (eg, social, occupational, recreational)
- The symptoms are not solely the direct, physiologic effects of a medical condition (eg, an endocrine disorder), a medication, or substance abuse

As discussed later, severe depression may have worse prognostic implications in heart failure than milder forms of depression. Thus, when evaluating patients with heart failure, care should be taken to avoid misdiagnosing an episode of MD in partial remission as an episode of md. However, this is difficult because many patients are unable to provide accurate details about symptoms that have already abated.

Because the lifetime course of MDD is highly variable, some patients experience their first depressive episode after the onset of chronic heart failure. When this occurs, the onset of depression may occur soon after, or long after, the onset of heart failure. In other cases, the first episode of depression may have occurred years, or even decades, before the onset of heart failure, as well as before the onset of HF precursors such as hypertension or coronary heart disease. Furthermore, some patients have multiple episodes of depression long before they develop heart failure. If comorbid MD were simply a psychological reaction to heart failure, it would be tempting to dismiss its apparent prognostic implications as epiphenomenal. Clearly, the temporal relationship between these conditions is far too complex to assume that depression is always, or even usually, an emotional reaction to heart failure.

In clinical settings, many patients are diagnosed as having MD without regard to whether they meet the DSM-IV-TR criteria. According to a recent survey, most nonpsychiatrist physicians, and even a substantial minority of psychiatrists, do not use the DSM-IV criteria when diagnosing MDD.[2] As a result, some patients with md, or with no recognized depressive disorder, are misdiagnosed as having MD. This misdiagnosis is usually avoided in research studies by following the DSM-IV-TR criteria and using a standardized interview such as the Depression Interview and Structured Hamilton (DISH)[3] to ensure that all of the criterion symptoms of MDD are carefully assessed.

However, depression can also be defined by self-report questionnaires such as the Beck Depression Inventory (BDI),[4] or a new version of this instrument, the BDI-II.[5,6] Total scores on instruments such as the BDI are often used to measure the severity of depressive symptoms, and standard cutoff scores such as 10 on the BDI or 14 on the BDI-II are often used to define depression or clinically significant depression. When administered to patients with carefully diagnosed depressive disorders, the scores on such measures reflect the severity of depression. In contrast, when they are administered to patients who have not had a diagnostic evaluation, increased scores may or may not indicate the presence of a depressive disorder. In patients with heart failure, many of whom have multiple medical comorbidities, endorsement of symptoms such as fatigue or insomnia may indicate depression, but these symptoms may also be caused, at least in part, by medical illness or its treatment. Consequently, it is important to exercise caution in interpreting nonspecific symptoms such as fatigue when evaluating the prognostic importance of depression in patients with heart failure.

DEPRESSION AS A PREDICTOR OF MORTALITY IN HEART FAILURE

In the first prospective study of MD as a predictor of mortality in heart failure, Freedland and colleagues[7] enrolled 60 patients who were 70 years or older at the time of hospital admission for heart failure. Seventeen percent of the patients met criteria for a major depressive episode, according to a standardized diagnostic interview. Vital status was determined 1 year after the index hospitalization, with no patients lost to follow-up. During follow-up, 50% of the patients with depression died, compared with 29% of the patients without depression. This study provided the first evidence that MD may have adverse prognostic implications in patients hospitalized for heart failure. When the investigators sought to replicate this finding in a larger (n = 682) sample of hospitalized patients with heart failure, they found that MD was an independent predictor of survival over 1 year, after adjusting for left ventricular ejection fraction (LVEF) and other covariables.[8]

Subsequent research has confirmed that depression increases the risk of mortality in patients with heart failure. The studies that have been conducted to date are heterogeneous with respect to the medical and demographic characteristics of the samples, the measures used to assess depression, the duration of follow-up, and the potential confounders that were included in the statistical models. Despite these differences, most of the published evidence shows that the presence of depression alters the risk of mortality and other adverse outcomes in heart failure.

One of the earliest prospective studies was conducted in Norway. In this study,[9] 119 clinically stable outpatients with symptomatic HF (71% men, mean age 66 ± 10 years) were recruited from a cardiology practice and followed for 2 years. Most of the patients were in New York Heart Association (NYHA) class II (41%) or III (46%) heart failure at enrollment. Depression was measured by the Zung[10] Depression Scale. Twenty (17%) of the patients died during a 2-year follow-up period. A Cox proportional hazards regression analysis was conducted to model the effect of depression on survival, adjusting for gender, age, and, as an index of the severity of heart failure, the prohormone of atrial natriuretic factor (pro-ANF). In this model, the hazard ratio (HR) for a 1-point increase on the Zung scale was 1.08 (P = .002). The participants also completed several other questionnaires assessing heart failure–related emotional distress, quality of life, and perceived health. A factor analysis of the scores on these questionnaires and the Zung scale yielded 2 factors, depressed mood and subjective health. When these factors were entered into a Cox regression model along with the same covariates as before, depressed mood emerged as an even stronger inverse predictor of 2-year survival (HR, 1.90; P = .002). This study provided the first evidence that depression increases the risk of mortality among outpatients with heart failure.

Murberg and Furze[11] subsequently published a 6-year follow-up of this cohort. They found that depression at baseline continued to predict mortality during this period (risk ratio [RR] per point on the Zung scale, 1.05; 95% confidence interval [CI], 1.00–1.08; P = .02), after adjustment for gender, age, and pro-ANP, as well as for the personality trait of neuroticism. The strength of the association was smaller than the investigators had reported in their earlier 2-year follow-up study, but it was still detectable years after the index hospitalization and the baseline assessment of depression.

Koenig[12] enrolled a consecutive sample of 107 older (age ≥60 years) patients with heart failure who were hospitalized at a university teaching hospital. The National Institute of Mental Health Diagnostic Interview Schedule (DIS)[13] was administered to diagnose MD at baseline, and md was identified by a combination of criterion symptoms and scores on 2 different depression scales, the Center for Epidemiologic Studies - Depression (CES-D)[14] scale and the 17-item Hamilton Rating Scale for Depression (HAM-D).[15] Thirty-nine (36%) of the patients had MD at baseline, 23 (22%) had md, and 45 (42%) had no depressive disorder. During a median 46-week follow-up, 28% of the patients with MD, 30% of those with md, and 20% of those with no depression died. Although a higher proportion of participants who were depressed than who were not depressed died during the follow-up, the difference was not statistically significant in this small sample.

A larger study by Vaccarino and colleagues[16] was the first to examine the effect of depression on a composite outcome of functional decline or death. A cohort of 391 patients (49% women), who were at least 50 years old on hospital admission for decompensated heart failure, were assessed for depression and followed prospectively for 6 months. The 15-item short form of the Geriatric Depression Scale (GDS)[17] was used to assess depression at baseline. Functional decline was defined as an increase in the number of limitations in activities of daily living (ADLs) between baseline and 6 months, as assessed by the Katz ADL scale.[18] In a series of multivariable models, GDS scores were adjusted for demographic factors, medical history, baseline functional status, clinical characteristics at enrollment (systolic blood pressure, serum creatinine, heart rate) and LVEF. Twenty-nine percent of the patients had an ejection fraction of 55% or higher at baseline. Functional decline or death occurred in 159 (41%) of the participants, and the event rate increased as the level of depression increased (nondepressed, 31%; mildly depressed, 34%; moderately depressed, 49%; severely depressed, 60%; $P = .001$). In the fully adjusted model, the rates corresponded to RRs of 1.00 (referent), 1.10, 1.39, and 1.82, respectively ($P = .004$). Unlike the mildly and moderately depressed group, the CI around the RR did not include 1.00 in the severe group, indicating that this group was clearly at high risk of functional decline or death.

When Vaccarino and colleagues decomposed the outcome, they found that increasing levels of depression were significantly associated in univariate analyses with functional decline ($P = .004$) based on event rates of 22%, 22%, 34%, and 46% in the nondepressed and mildly, moderately, and severely depressed groups, respectively, and with death from any cause ($P = .02$), based on event rates of 11%, 16%, 22%, and 26%. The association with functional decline persisted in the fully adjusted model (RR, 1.00, 1.15, 1.65, and 2.16; $P = .01$), but the association with death was not statistically significant (RR, 1.00, 1.07, 1.25, and 1.68; $P = .27$). Because functional decline often precedes death in chronic heart failure, it is possible that the multivariable association with death would have been significant if the follow-up had been extended to 1 year. Nevertheless, this study replicated earlier findings that depression has prognostic importance in elderly patients who have been hospitalized with heart failure, but it did so with a different measure of depression and a composite outcome that had not been examined in previous studies.

Jiang and colleagues[19] were the first to publish a study of the prognostic value of depression in patients hospitalized with heart failure that was not restricted to elderly participants. They screened a series of patients who were at least 18 years old at admission and who had an LVEF of 35% or less and/or were in heart failure that was NYHA class II or higher. Patients who scored 10 or higher on the BDI were asked to undergo a modified version of the DIS interview to identify MD. The outcomes included all-cause mortality and rehospitalization 3 months and 1 year after baseline. Of 357 patients who completed the BDI, 126 (35%) scored at or more than the cutoff score. One hundred (79%) of these patients completed the DIS, and 46 met criteria for MD. Patients who scored 10 or higher on the BDI but who did not have MD according to the DIS were classified as having mild depression. The ages (mean $\pm$ standard deviation) of the nondepressed, mild depression, and MD groups were 64 $\pm$ 13, 63 $\pm$ 13, and 63 $\pm$ 13 years, respectively. Thus, most of the participants were at least 60 years old, despite younger patients being eligible.

The mortalities were 6%, 7%, and 13% at 3 months in the nondepressed, mild depression, and MD groups, respectively, and 14%, 11%, and 26% at 1 year. Readmission rates were 37%, 43%, and 52% at 3 months, and 52%, 56%, and 80% at 1 year. In univariate analyses, MD predicted mortality at 1 year (odds ratio [OR], 2.23; 95% CI, 1.04–4.77), $P = .04$), but not at 3 months, and md did not predict mortality at either point. The association with 1-year mortality was no longer significant after adjustment for age, NYHA class, baseline LVEF, and cause of heart failure. In contrast, MD was a significant predictor of rehospitalization within 3 months (OR, 1.90; 95% CI, 1.00–3.59; $P = .04$) and 1 year (OR, 3.07; 95% CI, 1.41–6.66; $P = .005$), and the 1-year effect persisted after multivariable adjustment (OR, 2.57; 95% CI, 1.16–5.68; $P = .02$). The results provided only equivocal evidence that MD increases the risk of 1-year mortality in patients hospitalized with heart failure, but it yielded clear evidence that patients with MD are more likely than their nondepressed counterparts to be rehospitalized.

In a secondary analysis of data from the same cohort, Hedayati and colleagues[20] stratified the sample according to the presence or absence of chronic kidney disease (CKD). They reported that MD was more prevalent among patients with (22%) than without (13%) severe CKD, as was depression defined by a BDI score of 10 or higher (55% vs 13%). After adjustment for age and severe CKD, MD remained an independent predictor of 1-year mortality compared with mild depression (OR, 3.13; 95% CI, 1.02–9.26), although not when compared with the nondepressed reference group (OR, 2.07; 95% CI, 0.93–4.63). Overall, these findings suggest that MD may have prognostic importance in heart failure, including patients with severe CKD.

Most of the studies in this area have been based on samples with diverse heart failure causes. A study from the United Kingdom was the first to focus exclusively on patients with nonischemic heart failure. Based on hospital records and a clinical echocardiography database, Faris and colleagues[21] retrospectively identified 396 consecutive adult patients (mean age 53 $\pm$ 15 years; 74% men) at a tertiary cardiac care hospital in London with a principal discharge diagnosis of heart failure caused by nonischemic dilated cardiomyopathy. Unlike the preceding studies, the retrospective design of this study precluded the use of standardized depression questionnaires or interviews. Instead, patients were classified as clinically depressed if a diagnosis of depression was listed in their medical record. At enrollment, 33% of the patients were in NYHA class I heart failure, 37% in class II, 20% in class III, and 10% in class IV. Eighty-three (21%) of the patients were classified as depressed.

The duration of follow-up varied considerably (mean 48 ± 35 months; range 3–84 months). During follow-up, there were 83 deaths (21% mortality), and 15 (4%) of the patients underwent heart transplantation. There were 660 hospital readmissions; rehospitalizations occurred at a rate of 1.7 per patient year on average. Clinical depression predicted mortality in both an unadjusted model (HR, 2.1; 95% CI, 1.4–3.2; *P* = .0005) and after multivariable adjustment (HR, 3.0; 95% CI, 1.4–6.6; *P* = .004). It also predicted hospital readmissions in both univariate (*P* = .01) and multivariable (*P* = .03) models.

Sullivan and colleagues[22] were the first to examine depression in relation to the combined endpoint of heart transplantation or death in outpatients with advanced heart failure. They recruited a consecutive series of 142 patients (age 53 ± 10 years; 78% men; mean NYHA class 2.7 ± 0.7) from a heart failure/pretransplant specialty clinic at a university teaching hospital. A structured interview based on the DSM-IV criteria for mood disorders, the Primary Care Evaluation of Mental Disorders (PRIME-MD)[23] was administered to identify MD and md. The 24-item version of the HAM-D and the 20-item Symptom Checklist (SCL-20) depression scale[24] were used to assess the severity of depression, and extensive data were collected at baseline to document the severity of heart failure and other medical conditions. The cohort was followed with regularly scheduled contacts for a mean of 3 years ± 7 months. During this period, 15 (11%) of the patients died and 24 (17%) received a heart transplant. Thirteen of the deaths were from cardiovascular causes, and 2 were from cancer.

In a univariate Cox regression analysis, having any depression diagnosis at baseline (whether MD, md, or dysthymia, which is a chronic, mild form of depression) significantly increased the hazard of the primary combined endpoint (HR, 2.54; 95% CI, 1.16–5.55; *P* = .02). This effect persisted (HR, 2.41; 95% CI, 1.24–4.68; *P*<.01) after multivariable adjustment for age, serum sodium, NYHA class, systolic blood pressure, and a geriatric version of the Cumulative Illness Rating Scale.[25] Although the study was underpowered to examine mortality and transplantation as separate endpoints, the investigators did so in exploratory univariate analyses. Depression diagnosis did not have a significant effect in the time-to-death analysis (HR, 1.65; 95% CI, 0.51–5.28; *P* = .40), but it did in the transplant analysis (HR, 3.29; 95% CI, 1.31–8.27; *P* = .01). These effects were specific to depression diagnosis; neither the HAM-D nor the SCL-20 predicted any of these outcomes. In additional multivariable analyses, the investigators found that patients with a depression diagnoses had a higher number of HF-related hospitalizations during the first year of follow-up (1.5 ± 1.8 vs 0.6 ± 1.4; *P* = .04), as well as more HF clinic visits (2.4 ± 1.7 vs 1.7 ± 1.8; *P* = .04). Taken together, the findings from this study suggest that depression may increase the likelihood of rehospitalization and heart transplantation, but they do not provide evidence that depression increases the risk of mortality.

A European study by Jünger and colleagues[26] was the first to use the Hospital Anxiety and Depression Scale (HADS)[27] in a study of heart failure mortality. The HADS omits somatic symptoms of depression such as fatigue, which presumably makes it a more specific measure of comorbid depression in medically ill patients compared with other depression scales. In this study, 209 outpatients (age 54 ± 10 years; 86% male), with stable NYHA class I to III heart failure were enrolled and followed for an average of approximately 2 years. The endpoint was all-cause mortality, and observations were censored at the time of heart transplantation if it occurred. Forty-five patients died during the follow-up period. Depression was a significant predictor of survival in a univariate Cox regression analysis (HR, 1.09; 95% CI, 1.02–1.17; *P* = .007), and remained significant (HR, 1.08; 95% CI, 1.01–1.15; *P* = .02) after adjustment for LVEF and peak oxygen consumption (V_{O_2}) obtained from cardiopulmonary exercise testing.

In a secondary analysis, the investigators explored whether the mortality risk associated with depression is stable over time. To the contrary, they found that the risk increases with time. During the first 6 months of observation, the HR for depression, as defined by a score of 6 or higher on the HADS Depression Scale, was 1.0 (95% CI, 0.44–2.39; *P* = .95). It increased steadily in each subsequent 6-month period, reaching a peak at 30 months (HR, 8.22; 95% CI, 2.62–25.84; *P*<.001). Prior studies had suggested that, even if depression is assessed at a single and perhaps arbitrary point in the course of heart failure, it can have a durable influence on survival. This study went beyond these findings to show that the risk from depression may increase with time.

As noted earlier, most studies have not focused on patients with a particular heart failure cause.

A study by Rumsfeld and colleagues[28] was the first to examine the prognostic importance of depression in patients with an acute myocardial infarction (MI) complicated by heart failure. The prognostic value of comorbid depression in acute MI was already well established[29] when this study was published, but Rumsfeld and colleagues[28] went beyond the existing literature to study the subset of patients whose acute MIs are complicated by HF. The findings were based on a planned substudy of the Epleronone Post-Acute Myocardial Infarction Heart Failure Efficacy and Survival Study (EPHESUS). This study used another self-reported depression scale, the Medical Outcomes Study Depression (MOS-D) questionnaire.[30] Of 634 patients included in this analysis, 143 (23%) scored more than the depression cutoff on the MOS-D at baseline. The primary outcome was all-cause mortality in a mean follow-up period of 16 months, and cardiovascular death or hospitalization was examined as a composite endpoint. In univariate analyses, the patients with depression had a significantly higher all-cause mortality than the patients without depression (29% vs 18%, $P = .004$), as well as a higher rate of cardiovascular death or rehospitalization (42% vs 33%, $P = .02$). These relationships remained significant in multivariable regression models after adjustment for a large set of demographic, cardiac, other medical, and treatment variables, including for all-cause mortality (HR, 1.78; 95% CI, 1.11–2.63; $P = .01$) and for cardiovascular death or rehospitalization (HR, 1.41; 95% CI, 1.03–1.93; $P = .03$). The results were consistent across several subgroups defined by demographic and medical characteristics, although there was a trend toward a higher depression-associated risk of mortality among patients with a prior history of MI.

A study by Sherwood and colleagues[31] was one of the first to prospectively examine whether depression predicts death or rehospitalization in heart failure when taking the effects of antidepressant medications into account. It was also one of the first studies of depression in HF to use N-terminal pro-brain natriuretic peptide (NT-proBNP) as a marker of the severity of heart failure. In this study, 204 outpatients with heart failure and an LVEF of 40% or less completed the BDI at enrollment. Participants were followed for a mean of 3 years, and none were lost to follow-up. During this period, 54 (26%) of the patients died and 126 (62%) were hospitalized at least once; 98 (48%) were hospitalized at least once for cardiovascular reasons. In a Cox regression model adjusting for age, HF cause, LVEF, and NT-proBNP, both the baseline BDI score (HR, 1.06; 95% CI, 1.03–1.09; $P<.001$) and antidepressant medications at baseline (HR, 1.75; 95% CI, 1.14–2.68; $P = .01$) were independent predictors of the primary combined endpoint of death or cardiovascular rehospitalization. In a secondary model of time to death or all-cause hospitalization, the BDI effect was identical to that found in the primary model, but the effect of antidepressant medication weakened slightly (HR, 1.57; 95% CI, 1.06–2.34; $P = .02$). The magnitude of the effects of depression and antidepressants in relation to all-cause mortality were similar to those found in the primary model, but they were not statistically significant. These data show that depression is associated with a worse HF prognosis even among patients receiving antidepressant medications.

A more recent and larger study by O'Conner and colleagues[32] sought to clarify whether the apparent prognostic value of depression in HF is attributable to the use of antidepressants, or whether it is better explained by depression per se. They enrolled 1006 hospitalized patients with clinically diagnosed HF who were in NYHA class II or higher, who had an LVEF of 35% or lower, or both. The participants completed the BDI during the index hospitalization. Use of antidepressants at the index hospitalization was determined from inpatient pharmacy records and hospital discharge summaries. One hundred and sixty-two (16%) of the patients were taking an antidepressant at enrollment. One-hundred and twenty-nine (80%) of them were taking a selective serotonin reuptake inhibitor (SSRI) alone; 8 (5%) were taking an SSRI in combination with a tricyclic antidepressant (TCA); and 24 (15%) were taking a TCA alone or other antidepressants. Thirteen percent of the patients without depression were taking an antidepressant medication. In comparison, 25% of the patients who scored 10 or higher on the BDI were taking an antidepressant, and the proportion increased along with the severity of depression such that 34% of those with a BDI score of 19 or higher were on an antidepressant. Patients taking an antidepressant were more likely to be white and married.

The mean duration of follow-up was 2.7 ± 2.0 years (median, 2.2 years). During this period, 429 patients died, including 161 (53%) who were depressed at baseline and 268 (38%) who scored in the nondepressed range on the BDI. Among patients who were not taking an antidepressant at baseline, 42% died; in contrast, death occurred in 44% of the patients who were taking an SSRI only, 55% of those who were taking a TCA, and 62% of those who were taking other antidepressants. In univariate analyses, both depression as defined by a BDI score of 10 or higher

(HR, 1.39; 95% CI, 1.12–1.74; P = .003) and any type of antidepressant use (HR, 1.32; 95% CI, 1.03–1.69; P = .03) predicted shorter survival. When adjusted for demographic factors, baseline LVEF, NYHA class, and HF cause, antidepressant use was no longer a significant predictor of shorter survival (HR, 1.24; 95% CI, 0.94–1.64; P = .13) but depression remained significant (HR, 1.33; 95% CI, 1.07–1.66; P = .01). When the analysis was restricted to SSRI antidepressants, depression continued to predict shorter survival in both univariate and multivariable models, but SSRIs did not predict outcomes in either model. These findings helped to allay concerns about potential adverse effects of antidepressants in patients with HF, and pointed to the need for controlled clinical trials to evaluate the safety and efficacy of these agents in patients with heart failure and comorbid depression.

In most of the preceding studies, the multivariable models adjusted for gender as a potential confounder. However, none of them examined whether the effects of depression on HF prognosis differ between men and women. This question was addressed by a study conducted in German by Faller and colleagues.[33] The investigators enrolled a consecutive series of 231 patients (age 64 ± 13 years; 29% women) presenting with heart failure (25% in NYHA class I, 44% in class II, 25% in class III, and 6% in class IV), without restrictions as to cause and with no exclusion criteria except refusal to participate. Depression was assessed with the PHQ-9,[34] a well-established depression screening tool that has the advantage of providing both a total severity score and an algorithm to identify probable cases of DSM-IV MD or md.

Cox proportional hazards regression was used to model survival for a median follow-up period of 2.7 years. None of the participants were lost to follow-up, and 59 (26%) of the patients died. In the overall sample, probable MD predicted shorter survival both in a univariate analysis (HR, 3.3; 95% CI, 1.8–6.1; P<.001) as well as in a multivariable analysis adjusting for sex, age, cause, NYHA class, LVEF, and the presence or absence of systolic dysfunction (HR, 2.4; 95% CI, 1.3–4.6; P<.01). Probable md did not have a significant effect on survival. The gender subgroup analyses were limited by small sample sizes (only 12 women and 19 men had probable MD). Nevertheless, probable MD had a strong effect on survival among women (adjusted HR, 4.5; 95% CI, 1.3–15.8; P = .02). The hazard ratio was smaller and statistically nonsignificant in men (adjusted HR, 2.1; 95% CI, 0.9–4.6; P = .08). However, this study was not adequately powered to definitively determine whether gender moderates the effect of depression on survival in HF, and it did not formally test for a depression-by-gender interaction, but it did suggest that depression may have worse prognostic implications in women than in men.

Given the multiplicity of depression measures that have been used in HF research, it would be useful to know whether they differ with respect to their ability to predict adverse outcomes if administered to the same patients. In one of the first studies to address this question, Parissis and colleagues[35] administered both the Zung Depression Scale and the BDI to 155 hospitalized patients with heart failure (83% male; age, 65 ± 12 years; 9%, 33%, 51%, and 17% in NYHA class I, II, II, and IV, respectively). The patients were followed for 6 months, during which time 61 (39%) were either rehospitalized or died, and 10 (16%) died. In univariate logistic regression analyses, the Zung scale predicted death or rehospitalization (OR, 1.06; 95% CI, 1.03–1.10; P<.001), but the BDI did not. The Zung scale remained a significant predictor of rehospitalization or death (OR, 1.07; 95% CI, 1.01–1.14; P = .03) after multivariable adjustment for NYHA class, BNP, and 6-minute walk test performance. Thus, in this particular study, the Zung scale predicted clinical outcomes of HF but the BDI did not. It is not clear why the BDI predicted clinical outcomes in previous studies but not in this one.

Some of the most recent research has involved larger samples than were enrolled in many of the earlier studies. Macchia and colleagues[36] linked hospital discharge records, medication prescription databases, and vital statistics from 6 local health districts in Italy to identify 48,117 patients with heart failure. It was not possible to assess depression directly, so the investigators defined depressed cases as patients who were exposed to antidepressant medications during the 12 months preceding the index date. These cases were subclassified as occasionally exposed if at least 1 antidepressant prescription was filled during the preindex year (n = 3328; 6.9%), and as chronically exposed if 3 or more prescriptions were filled (n = 1632; 3.4%). The patients with depression were slightly older (median age, 79 years) than the patients without depression (78 years), and they were more likely to be female (68% vs 58%). Patients were followed for up to 1 year or until the occurrence of all-cause mortality, nonfatal cardiovascular events, hospitalization for HF, or hospitalization for any reason. The effects of depression on these outcomes were analyzed in Cox regression models, adjusting for age, sex, and medical comorbidities, as well as an antidepressant treatment propensity score to reduce the potential for residual confounding. Depression was associated with a higher risk of all-cause mortality (HR, 1.20; 95% CI, 1.08–1.33; P = .0006) and a composite cardiovascular endpoint including MI, stroke, and transient ischemic attack (HR, 1.23; 95% CI, 1.13–1.34; P<.0001). Depression did not predict higher rates of rehospitalization for HF or for any cause. Despite its large size, these findings must be interpreted with caution because use of antidepressants is only a proxy for depression, and it misclassifies patients who are depressed but not on an antidepressant. Nevertheless, the study provides additional support for the adverse prognostic effect of depression in patients with heart failure.

Albert and colleagues[37] conducted a 60- to 90-day follow-up of a sample of 5791 elderly patients (mean age 73 ± 14 years) from among 48,612 participants in the Organized Program to Initiate Lifesaving Treatment in Hospitalized Patients with Heart Failure (OPTIMIZE-HF) registry. Approximately 14% of the sample were classified as depressed from hospital records. Sixty percent of the patients with depression were women, compared with 51% of the patients without depression. Depression predicted all-cause mortality in both unadjusted (HR, 1.36; 95% CI, 1.04–1.79; P = .03) and adjusted models (HR, 1.46; 95% CI, 1.05–2.03; P = .03).

Using data from the Coordinating study evaluating Outcomes of Advising and Counseling in HF patients (COACH) multicenter randomized trial in the Netherlands, Lesman-Leegte and colleagues[38] studied 958 patients in NYHA class II to IV heart failure (37% women, age 71 ± 11 years, 51% in class II HF and 49% in class III or IV) who completed the CES-D depression questionnaire at baseline. Based on a CES-D score of 16 or higher, 377 (39%) of the patients had depression, and 200 (21%) were classified as having severe depression based on a CES-D score of 24 or higher. The patients were followed for 18 months, during which time 40% of the patients reached the primary composite endpoint of HF readmission or death; 26% survived the follow-up but with at least 1 HF readmission, and 27% of the patients died.

In a univariate analysis, depression predicted the primary composite endpoint (HR per 10-point increase on the CES-D, 1.10; 95% CI, 1.01–1.20; P = .04), and this remained significant after multivariable adjustment for age, sex, and BNP (HR, 1.13; 95% CI, 1.02–1.26; P = .02). In secondary analyses, depression also predicted HF readmission (adjusted HR, 1.17; 95% CI, 1.02–1.33; P = .02) and mortality (adjusted HR, 1.17; 95% CI, 1.03–1.34; P = .02). Post hoc analyses suggested that the risk of HF readmission or death increases in linear fashion along with the severity of depression.

Frasure-Smith and colleagues[39] recently published the first study of the prognostic importance of depression in patients with both HF and atrial fibrillation (AF). Their sample consisted of 974 participants (18% women, age 66 ± 11 years) in the AF-CHF trial, which compared rate-control versus rhythm-control strategies for AF. Three-hundred and twelve (32%) of the participants were classified as depressed because of a BDI-II score of 14 or higher. The participants were followed for a mean of 39 ± 18 months, during which time there were 302 all-cause deaths. Of these, 246 were judged to be cardiovascular deaths, and 111 of those were presumed to be arrhythmic. The dichotomous BDI-II classification predicted cardiovascular deaths in both an unadjusted model (HR, 1.59; 95% CI, 1.24–2.05; P<.001) and in a model adjusted for demographic and medical covariates (HR, 1.57; 95% CI, 1.20–2.07; P = .001). It was an even stronger predictor of arrhythmic deaths (univariate HR, 1.82; 95% CI, 1.25–2.65; P = .002; adjusted HR, 1.69; 95% CI, 1.13–2.53; P = .01) The continuous BDI-II scores were also significant predictors of these outcomes, and both the dichotomous and continuous BDI-II scores predicted all-cause mortality as well. Furthermore, a secondary analysis suggested that patients who are both depressed and unmarried may comprise a group at especially high risk of cardiovascular mortality.

In addition to the findings summarized earlier, several other studies have investigated the effect of depression on heart failure outcomes.[40–44] Despite many differences among these studies, they all add to the growing evidence that depression does have independent prognostic value in heart failure.

CAUSAL MODELS AND CANDIDATE MECHANISMS

Numerous studies have investigated biobehavioral mechanisms that may help to explain the well-documented effects of depression on cardiovascular morbidity and mortality in patients with coronary heart disease (CHD).[45] There has been much less research on mechanisms that may account for the adverse prognostic effects of depression in heart failure, but there is substantial overlap between the candidate mechanisms in CHD and CHF.[46]

The search for mechanisms implies that depression is a causal risk factor for adverse outcomes in heart failure, not merely a risk marker. However, the causal status of depression in HF is unknown. There have been NO well-designed, adequately powered trials to determine whether treating depression can improve medical outcomes in heart failure. It is possible, although unlikely, that, when depression is observed in patients with heart failure, it is simply a byproduct of HF (or its treatment) rather than a comorbid condition in its own right. If so, the increased risks associated with depression should be attributed to the depression-inducing aspects of the heart failure rather than to depression per se. As discussed earlier, the lifetime courses of heart disease and depression are too complex and vary too much across individuals to dismiss the latter as a direct consequence of the former. In addition, studies that have examined relationships among depression, heart failure, and outcomes have not provided any compelling evidence that the apparent adverse effects of depression are better explained by associated characteristics of heart failure.[12,47] It is also possible that depression and heart failure could share genetic substrates that could explain why these disorders are so highly coprevalent, but, as yet, there is little empirical basis for speculation about this.

If depression does complicate heart failure in ways that increase the risk of death or other adverse medical outcomes, then both behavioral and biologic mechanisms must be considered. In many different patient populations, depression has been identified as a strong predictor of noncompliance with prescribed medications,[48] physical inactivity,[49] and smoking.[50] In patients with heart failure, depression has been identified as one of the most important barriers to effective HF self-care.[51]

In addition to these behavioral pathways, some of the physiologic concomitants of depression might have adverse effects on the course and outcome of HF. For example, depression is associated with sleep apnea syndromes[52] and with low heart rate variability (HRV),[53] a marker of sympathetic-parasympathetic imbalance that may predispose to arrhythmias and ischemia. Both sleep apnea[54] and low HRV[55] have adverse prognostic implications in HF. Depression may worsen these and other physiologic risk markers in heart failure.

IMPLICATIONS FOR RESEARCH AND TREATMENT

Depression is an independent risk marker for mortality, hospitalization, and other adverse medical outcomes in heart failure. However, the studies that have been reviewed herein are heterogeneous with respect to the composition of the samples, their design and methodological rigor, the methods used to assess depression, the potential confounders for which the models were adjusted, and the duration of follow-up. A systematic review and meta-analysis is needed to evaluate the effects of these factors on the predictive value of depression in patients with heart failure.

Whether depression is a causal risk factor, or merely a risk marker, for mortality and other adverse outcomes in heart failure has not been determined. Research on the mechanistic connections between depression and heart failure outcomes is at an early stage, and it lags behind similar research on depression in CHD. There have been no large randomized controlled trials designed to determine whether treatment of depression can reduce medical morbidity and mortality in heart failure; there have been few trials of treatments for comorbid depression per se in heart failure. The largest antidepressant trial to date, SADHART-CHF, recently concluded with no difference in depression outcomes between patients with heart failure treated with sertraline compared with patients treated with a placebo.[56]

Our research group recently conducted a randomized, controlled pilot study of cognitive behavior therapy (CBT) for outpatients with heart failure. The results suggested that CBT may be an efficacious treatment of depression in these patients,[57] and they were sufficiently promising to warrant replication and extension. In an ongoing randomized trial, we are combining CBT for depression with an intervention to enhance self-care in heart failure. It is possible that this sort of combined approach could affect multiple behavioral and physiologic mechanisms, and thereby improve the prognosis of patients with depression. Additional research is needed to test other psychotherapeutic interventions, other antidepressant medications, and other intervention strategies such as preference-based, stepped, or collaborative care for comorbid depression in heart failure. Although it is not yet known whether any form of depression treatment can affect cardiac outcomes, MD deserves clinical attention in patients with heart failure, just as it does in other patient populations.

REFERENCES

1. American Psychiatric Association, Task Force on DSM-IV. Diagnostic and statistical manual of mental disorders (DSM-IV-TR). Washington, DC: American Psychiatric Association; 2000.

2. Zimmerman M, Galione J. Psychiatrists' and nonpsychiatrist physicians' reported use of the DSM-IV criteria for major depressive disorder. J Clin Psychiatry 2010;71(3):235–8.
3. Freedland KE, Skala JA, Carney RM, et al. The Depression Interview and Structured Hamilton (DISH): rationale, development, characteristics, and clinical validity. Psychosom Med 2002;64(6): 897–905.
4. Beck AT, Ward CH, Mendelson M, et al. An inventory for measuring depression. Arch Gen Psychiatry 1961;4:561–71.
5. Beck AT, Steer RA, Ball R, et al. Comparison of beck depression inventories -IA and -II in psychiatric outpatients. J Pers Assess 1996;67(3):588–97.
6. Steer RA, Brown GK, Beck AT, et al. Mean Beck Depression Inventory-II scores by severity of major depressive episode. Psychol Rep 2001;88(3 Pt 2): 1075–6.
7. Freedland KE, Carney RM, Rich MW, et al. Depression in elderly patients with congestive heart failure. J Geriatr Psychiatry 1991;24:59–71.
8. Freedland KE, Carney RM, Davila-Roman VG, et al. Major depression and survival in congestive heart failure. Psychosom Med 1998;60:118.
9. Murberg TA, Bru E, Svebak S, et al. Depressed mood and subjective health symptoms as predictors of mortality in patients with congestive heart failure: a two-years follow-up study. Int J Psychiatry Med 1999;29(3):311–26.
10. Zung WW. A self-rating depression scale. Arch Gen Psychiatry 1965;12:63–70.
11. Murberg TA, Furze G. Depressive symptoms and mortality in patients with congestive heart failure: a six-year follow-up study. Med Sci Monit 2004; 10(12):CR643–8.
12. Koenig HG. Depression in hospitalized older patients with congestive heart failure. Gen Hosp Psychiatry 1998;20(1):29–43.
13. Robins LN, Helzer JE, Croughan J, et al. National Institute of Mental Health Diagnostic Interview Schedule. Its history, characteristics, and validity. Arch Gen Psychiatry 1981;38(4):381–9.
14. Radloff L. The CES-D scale: a self-report depression scale for research in the general population. Appl Psychol Meas 1977;1:385–90.
15. Hamilton M. Development of a rating scale for primary depressive illness. Br J Soc Clin Psychol 1967;6:278–96.
16. Vaccarino V, Kasl SV, Abramson J, et al. Depressive symptoms and risk of functional decline and death in patients with heart failure. J Am Coll Cardiol 2001;38(1):199–205.
17. Yesavage JA, Brink TL, Rose TL, et al. Development and validation of a geriatric depression screening scale: a preliminary report. J Psychiatr Res 1982; 17(1):37–49.
18. Katz S, Downs TD, Cash HR, et al. Progress in development of the index of ADL. Gerontologist 1970;10(1):20–30.
19. Jiang W, Alexander J, Christopher E, et al. Relationship of depression to increased risk of mortality and rehospitalization in patients with congestive heart failure. Arch Intern Med 2001;161(15):1849–56.
20. Hedayati SS, Jiang W, O'Connor CM, et al. The association between depression and chronic kidney disease and mortality among patients hospitalized with congestive heart failure. Am J Kidney Dis 2004;44(2):207–15.
21. Faris R, Purcell H, Henein MY, et al. Clinical depression is common and significantly associated with reduced survival in patients with non-ischaemic heart failure. Eur J Heart Fail 2002;4(4):541–51.
22. Sullivan MD, Levy WC, Crane BA, et al. Usefulness of depression to predict time to combined end point of transplant or death for outpatients with advanced heart failure. Am J Cardiol 2004; 94(12):1577–80.
23. Spitzer RL, Williams JB, Kroenke K, et al. Utility of a new procedure for diagnosing mental disorders in primary care. The PRIME-MD 1000 study. JAMA 1994;272(22):1749–56.
24. Derogatis LR. Symptom checklist-90-R administration, scoring, and procedures manual. Minneapolis (MN): National Computer Systems; 1994.
25. Miller MD, Paradis CF, Houck PR, et al. Rating chronic medical illness burden in geropsychiatric practice and research: application of the Cumulative Illness Rating Scale. Psychiatry Res 1992;41(3):237–48.
26. Jünger J, Schellberg D, Muller-Tasch T, et al. Depression increasingly predicts mortality in the course of congestive heart failure. Eur J Heart Fail 2005;7(2):261–7.
27. Zigmond AS, Snaith RP. The Hospital Anxiety and Depression Scale. Acta Psychiatr Scand 1983; 67(6):361–70.
28. Rumsfeld JS, Jones PG, Whooley MA, et al. Depression predicts mortality and hospitalization in patients with myocardial infarction complicated by heart failure. Am Heart J 2005;150(5):961–7.
29. Frasure-Smith N, Lesperance F, Talajic M. Depression following myocardial infarction. Impact on 6-month survival. JAMA 1993;270(15):1819–25.
30. Burnam MA, Wells KB, Leake B, et al. Development of a brief screening instrument for detecting depressive disorders. Med Care 1988;26(8):775–89.
31. Sherwood A, Blumenthal JA, Trivedi R, et al. Relationship of depression to death or hospitalization in patients with heart failure. Arch Intern Med 2007; 167(4):367–73.
32. O'Connor CM, Jiang W, Kuchibhatla M, et al. Antidepressant use, depression, and survival in patients with heart failure. Arch Intern Med 2008;168(20): 2232–7.

33. Faller H, Stork S, Schowalter M, et al. Depression and survival in chronic heart failure: does gender play a role? Eur J Heart Fail 2007;9(10):1018–23.
34. Kroenke K, Spitzer RL, Williams JB. The PHQ-9: validity of a brief depression severity measure. J Gen Intern Med 2001;16(9):606–13.
35. Parissis JT, Nikolaou M, Farmakis D, et al. Clinical and prognostic implications of self-rating depression scales and plasma B-type natriuretic peptide in hospitalised patients with chronic heart failure. Heart 2008;94(5):585–9.
36. Macchia A, Monte S, Pellegrini F, et al. Depression worsens outcomes in elderly patients with heart failure: an analysis of 48,117 patients in a community setting. Eur J Heart Fail 2008;10(7):714–21.
37. Albert NM, Fonarow GC, Abraham WT, et al. Depression and clinical outcomes in heart failure: an OPTIMIZE-HF analysis. Am J Med 2009;122(4):366–73.
38. Lesman-Leegte I, van Veldhuisen DJ, Hillege HL, et al. Depressive symptoms and outcomes in patients with heart failure: data from the COACH study. Eur J Heart Fail 2009;11(12):1202–7.
39. Frasure-Smith N, Lesperance F, Habra M, et al. Elevated depression symptoms predict long-term cardiovascular mortality in patients with atrial fibrillation and heart failure. Circulation 2009;120(2):134–40, 3p.
40. Friedmann E, Thomas SA, Liu F, et al. Relationship of depression, anxiety, and social isolation to chronic heart failure outpatient mortality. Am Heart J 2006;152(5):940–8.
41. Johansson P, Dahlstrom U, Alehagen U. Depressive symptoms and six-year cardiovascular mortality in elderly patients with and without heart failure. Scand Cardiovasc J 2007;41(5):299–307.
42. Okonkwo OC, Sui X, Ahmed A. Disease-specific depression and outcomes in chronic heart failure: a propensity score analysis. Compr Ther 2007;33(2):65–70.
43. Rozzini R, Sabatini T, Frisoni GB, et al. Depression and major outcomes in older patients with heart failure. Arch Intern Med 2002;162(3):362–4.
44. Tousoulis D, Antoniades C, Drolias A, et al. Selective serotonin reuptake inhibitors modify the effect of beta-blockers on long-term survival of patients with end-stage heart failure and major depression. J Card Fail 2008;14(6):456–64.
45. Skala JA, Freedland KE, Carney RM. Coronary heart disease and depression: a review of recent mechanistic research. Can J Psychiatry 2006;51(12):738–45.
46. Parissis JT, Fountoulaki K, Paraskevaidis I, et al. Depression in chronic heart failure: novel pathophysiological mechanisms and therapeutic approaches. Expert Opin Investig Drugs 2005;14(5):567–77.
47. Koenig HG, Johnson JL, Peterson BL. Major depression and physical illness trajectories in heart failure and pulmonary disease. J Nerv Ment Dis 2006;194(12):909–16.
48. DiMatteo MR, Lepper HS, Croghan TW. Depression is a risk factor for noncompliance with medical treatment: meta-analysis of the effects of anxiety and depression on patient adherence. Arch Intern Med 2000;160(14):2101–7.
49. Teychenne M, Ball K, Salmon J. Physical activity and likelihood of depression in adults: a review. Prev Med 2008;46(5):397–411.
50. Freedland KE, Carney RM, Skala JA. Depression and smoking in coronary heart disease. Psychosom Med 2005;67(Suppl 1):S42–6.
51. Riegel B, Moser DK, Anker SD, et al. State of the science: promoting self-care in persons with heart failure: a scientific statement from the American Heart Association. Circulation 2009;120(12):1141–63.
52. Carney RM, Howells WB, Freedland KE, et al. Depression and obstructive sleep apnea in patients with coronary heart disease. Psychosom Med 2006;68(3):443–8.
53. Carney RM, Freedland KE. Depression and heart rate variability in patients with coronary heart disease. Cleve Clin J Med 2009;76(Suppl 2):S13–7.
54. Parish JM, Somers VK. Obstructive sleep apnea and cardiovascular disease. Mayo Clin Proc 2004;79(8):1036–46.
55. Sandercock GR, Brodie DA. The role of heart rate variability in prognosis for different modes of death in chronic heart failure. Pacing Clin Electrophysiol 2006;29(8):892–904.
56. Coletta AP, Clark AL, Cleland JG. Clinical trials update from the Heart Failure Society of America and the American Heart Association meetings in 2008: SADHART-CHF, COMPARE, MOMENTUM, thyroid hormone analogue study, HF-ACTION, I-PRESERVE, beta-interferon study, BACH, and ATHENA. Eur J Heart Fail 2009;11(2):214–9.
57. Freedland KE, Skala JA, Carney RM. Treatment of depression and anxiety in heart failure: a randomized, controlled pilot study. Proceedings of the 27th annual meeting of the Society of Behavioral Medicine 2006;27:91.

Depression in Heart Failure: Biobehavioral Mechanisms

Willem J. Kop, PhD[a,b,*], Stephen J. Synowski, PhD[a], Stephen S. Gottlieb, MD[a]

KEYWORDS

- Depression • Heart failure • Biobehavioral mechanisms
- Cardiovascular • disease

Depression is associated with an increased risk of adverse cardiovascular disease (CVD)[1–5] and heart failure progression.[6–11] The largest published meta-analysis to date provides a review of 54 observational studies (combined N = 146,538), and indicates that depression is consistently predictive of new-onset (incident) cardiac events in individuals free of CVD, as well as recurrent events in patients with a known diagnosis of CVD.[1] The magnitude of the CVD risk associated with depression is approximately comparable to that of traditional risk factors, such as hypercholesterolemia and hypertension.[12–14] The American Heart Association published a Scientific Advisory in 2008 recommending systematic detection and treatment for depression in patients with CVD, including screening; subsequent referral for comprehensive evaluation for depression diagnosis and management; and monitoring for adherence, treatment safety, and efficacy.[15,16]

Depression is the most common and well-documented psychological factor associated with heart failure (HF) progression.[6,17] Clinical major depressive disorder and subthreshold depressive symptoms are associated with a greater than 2-fold risk for several adverse outcomes, including mortality,[7–11] hospitalizations,[7,10,18] increased health care costs,[19] and functional decline.[8,20] This article provides a selective review of the consequences of depression in HF relevant to patient risk stratification and quality of life, and reviews the biological and behavioral (biobehavioral) mechanisms by which depression may lead to poor HF outcomes.

PATHOPHYSIOLOGICAL PROCESSES AND CLINICAL CHARACTERISTICS OF HF AS RELATED TO DEPRESSION

The etiology of depression in HF is influenced by 3 broad components that frequently accompany both conditions (**Table 1**): (1) symptomatology (eg, fatigue, sleep problems)[21] (2) behavioral characteristics (eg, reduced physical activity); and (3) shared biological processes, such as neurohormonal dysregulation and inflammation. Of the 9 defining characteristics of depression, 4 overlap with the symptoms of HF (see **Table 1**). Biobehavioral processes in HF (particularly reduced physical activity,[21–24] neurohormonal dysregulation,[25–31] and inflammation[31–42]) may not only increase the risk of HF progression but also new-onset, recurrent, or sustained depression in patients with HF. Furthermore, depression may by itself further adversely affect these biological processes (see later discussion), potentially resulting in a vicious

Funding sources: The research reported in this article was supported in part by grant number R0–1 HL079376 from the National Heart, Lung, and Blood Institute (WJK).

[a] Division of Cardiology, Department of Medicine, University of Maryland School of Medicine, 22 South Greene Street, HSF II/S012C, Baltimore, MD 21201, USA

[b] Department of Medical Psychology and Neuropsychology, Center of Research on Psychology in Somatic diseases (CoRPS), PO Box 90153, 5000 LE Tilburg, The Netherlands

* Corresponding author. Division of Cardiology, Department of Medicine, University of Maryland School of Medicine, 22 South Greene Street, HSF II/S012C, Baltimore, MD 21201.

E-mail address: w.j.kop@uvt.nl

Heart Failure Clin 7 (2011) 23–38
doi:10.1016/j.hfc.2010.08.011
1551-7136/11/$ – see front matter

Table 1
Unique (left and right columns) and common (middle column) characteristics of heart failure and depression

	Heart Failure	Both Heart Failure and Depression	Depression
Symptoms & signs	Dyspnea Congestion Fluid retention Exercise intolerance	Fatigue/lack of energy[a] Weight changes[a] Insomnia or hypersomnia[a] Diminished ability to concentrate or think (cognitive impairments)[a]	Depressed mood[a] Diminished pleasure in activities (anhedonia)[a] Psychomotor retardation/ agitation[a] Feelings of worthlessness/ guilt[a] Recurrent thoughts of death[a] Irritability Social withdrawal Anxiety Sexual dysfunction
Behavioral factors		Reduced physical activity	Medication nonadherence Smoking Alcohol consumption Illicit drug use ↓ Health care seeking Reduced information sharing with health care providers
Biological processes	Impaired LVEF[b] Underlying CVD[b] Natriuretic peptides	Neurohormones (NE, E, HPA, RAAS) Autonomic nervous system dysregulation Inflammation (IL-6, CRP, TNFa)	

Abbreviations: CRP, C-reactive protein; E, epinephrine; HPA, hypothalamic-pituitary adrenal; NE, norepinephrine; RAAS, renin-angiotensin-aldosterone system; TNF, tumor necrosis factor.
[a] Diagnostic criteria for depression indicates symptoms of depression per DSM-IV criteria.
[b] Present in a subset of patients with HF.

cycle leading to increased depression and exaggerated HF progression. In addition, comorbid conditions in HF, such as anemia and kidney failure, may result in symptoms consistent with depression, particularly fatigue. Little is known about which biobehavioral processes are bidirectionally associated with both depression and HF and which processes display unique independent associations. Because of the common characteristics of HF and depression, it is not always possible to disentangle cause-effect relationships between depression and HF severity in predicting adverse HF progression.

It has been argued that depressive symptoms in HF are secondary to the severity of underlying disease or the pharmacologic treatment of HF or CVD. However, there is little support for this notion because poor left ventricular (LV) pump function, angiographically documented coronary artery disease severity, and inducibility of ischemia are minimally associated with depressive symptoms.[12,13] Evidence of a relationship between depression and subclinical CVD severity is also inconsistent when examining noninvasive indices, such as carotid intima-media thickness and coronary calcification.[43–45] One study reported that patients with poor cardiac pump function (ie, left ventricular ejection fraction [LVEF] < 30%) are at risk for developing future depressive symptoms,[46] but the magnitude of cross-sectional associations has been minima across multiple studies. In addition to echocardiographic measures of cardiac structure and function, natriuretic peptides and other biomarkers are increasingly used as additional diagnostic tools in HF risk stratification and management. Studies on the associations between depression and natriuretic peptides have been mixed with positive,[47–49] but more commonly negative[11,50–52] findings. Other aspects of HF biology, such as myocardial fibrosis, may be adversely affected by depression.[53] Cardiac medications, such as beta-adrenergic blocking agents, may play a role in the onset and sustained presence of depressive symptoms in HF, but there is little empirical support for what has been referred to as the *beta-blocker blues*.[54,55] The high prevalence of depression in HF is therefore not likely to be an artifact of underlying cardiac dysfunction, CVD, or pharmacotherapy, but may in part be a consequence of common symptoms and shared pathophysiological processes (see **Table 1**).

The etiology of depression in HF entails more than the common features of both conditions as outlined in **Table 1** and includes: (1) genetic vulnerability factors, (2) central nervous system abnormalities, (3) socio-environmental experiences associated with psychological distress, (4) cognitive vulnerability factors and coping resources, and (5) psychological reactions to HF and other disease-related challenges. Common genetic factors have been identified for both depression and CVD, and 20% of variability in depressive symptoms and CVD is purportedly attributable to common genetic factors.[56] Genetic variation related to neurohormones and neurotransmitters, such as serotonin, as well as inflammation may be associated with both depression and HF, but this requires further empirical validation. Recent evidence indicates that depression in HF may be associated with brain perfusion defects in the medial temporal region.[57] Significant regional cerebral blood flow reductions were found in the left anterior parahippocampal gyrus and hippocampus, and the right posterior hippocampus and parahippocampal gyrus among patients with HF with major depressive disorder relative to both nondepressed patients with HF and healthy controls.[57] Brain imaging studies may be helpful in identifying which aspects of depression are likely to be directly related to HF biology and which ones are not.

Regarding psychosocial precipitants of depression in HF, the diathesis-stress model proposes that depression develops when cumulative stressors exceed the individual's vulnerability threshold.[58] *Sustained* adverse socio-environmental factors increase the risk of new-onset depression in HF. For example, living alone, medical care-related economic burden, alcohol abuse, and poor quality of life are predictors of depression in HF (7.9% developed depression in 1 year for those without these factors, and these percentages were markedly higher in case of 1, 2, or greater than 2 of these factors [15.5%, 36.2%, and 69.2%, respectively]).[59] These observations are consistent with the well-documented protective effects of social support and social networks for both depression and CVD.[60–62] Some evidence suggests that spirituality may act as a buffer for developing depression, which may be cultural specific.[63,64] Cognitive vulnerability factors and negative attributional styles may predispose individuals to develop depression.[65–68] Individuals who are depressed are more likely to engage in self-blame for their problems as compared with nondepressed controls.[69] In addition to these chronic psychosocial factors, major *life events* and high expressed emotion can trigger the onset and recurrence of depression.[70,71] Such life events often, but not necessarily, involve the loss of a cherished person, object, or situation. Depressed individuals appraise life events and health-related adversities as more unpleasant and stressful compared with control participants.[72,73] Thus, psychological reactions to psychologically distressing circumstances, including life-threatening and debilitating disease, may lead to depression in HF. Active coping resources,[62,74] engagement in pleasant activities, and behavioral activation[75] may reduce the risk of developing depression in HF.

Prevalence of Depression and Heart Failure

The primary definition of depression used in this review is based on the *Diagnostic and Statistical Manual of Mental Disorders* (Fourth Edition; DSM-IV) criteria for major depressive disorder.[76] The prevalence of depression in patients with HF ranges from 15% to 40%,[7–10,18–20,77–79] which is higher than prevalence rates observed in patients with CVD without HF (10%–25%)[19] or the general population (2%–9%).[3,80] In a meta-analysis published in 2006, major depressive disorder in HF was present in 21.5% (interview-based diagnosis 19.3%, questionnaire-based clinically significant depressive symptoms in 33.6%).[6] Observations from the Enhancing Recovery in Coronary Heart Disease trial indicate that the presence of HF among subjects after myocardial infarction is associated with increased depression,[81] supporting the additive effects of coronary artery disease and HF for depression. Subthreshold depressive symptoms, as assessed by self-report questionnaires, are common in HF, with up to 77.5% of individuals scoring higher than the normative cut-off values for depression.[82,83]

The presence and severity of depression is highest at the time of acute HF exacerbations,[77] and is related to functional HF severity.[19,82] However, there is no evidence for higher depression rates among inpatients versus outpatients.[6] As shown in **Fig. 1**, HF severity by New York Heart Association (NYHA) class IV is associated with more prevalent depression compared with class I (42% vs 11%).[6] HF symptomatology may result in inflated levels of the somatic components of depression, particularly fatigue.[55,82,84,85] Research from the

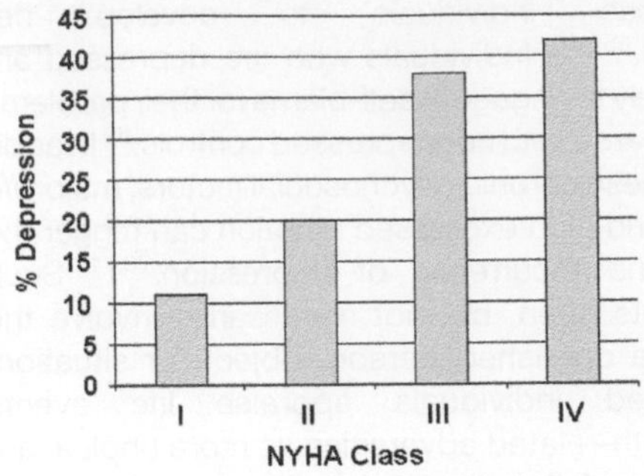

Fig. 1. Association between functional heart failure severity based on New York Heart Association classification index and severity of depression. (*Data from* Rutledge T, Reis VA, Linke SE, et al. Depression in heart failure a meta-analytic review of prevalence, intervention effects, and associations with clinical outcomes. J Am Coll Cardiol 2006;48(8):1527–37.)

authors' group suggests that depression is associated with elevated self-reported HF symptoms, thereby potentially leading to inaccuracies of HF diagnosis because of underestimated physical function.[86]

Very little is known about the prevalence and predictive value of depression in patients with HF with preserved ejection fraction (HF-PEF, or diastolic HF). Systolic HF is commonly associated with worse symptoms and prognosis compared with HF-PEF. To provide preliminary data regarding this issue, the authors examined data from a recently published study on the relationship between depression and fibrosis markers in HF and age- and sex-matched controls (with and without traditional CVD risk factors) from the Cardiovascular Health Study.[53] As shown in **Fig. 2**, the presence (ie, CES-D10 ≥ 8) and severity of depression was elevated in subjects with HF versus controls, but no differences were found between systolic HF versus HF-PEF.

A diagnosis of HF by itself (ie, a history of HF with minimal symptoms: NHYA class I) is commonly not associated with markedly increased levels of depression. However, concurrent symptoms and limitations promote the presence of depression (see **Fig. 1**). Poor cardiac pump function or underlying CVD are not likely causes of depression in HF (see previous discussion). It is not known whether the increased prevalence of depression in symptomatic HF reflects the burden of disease,

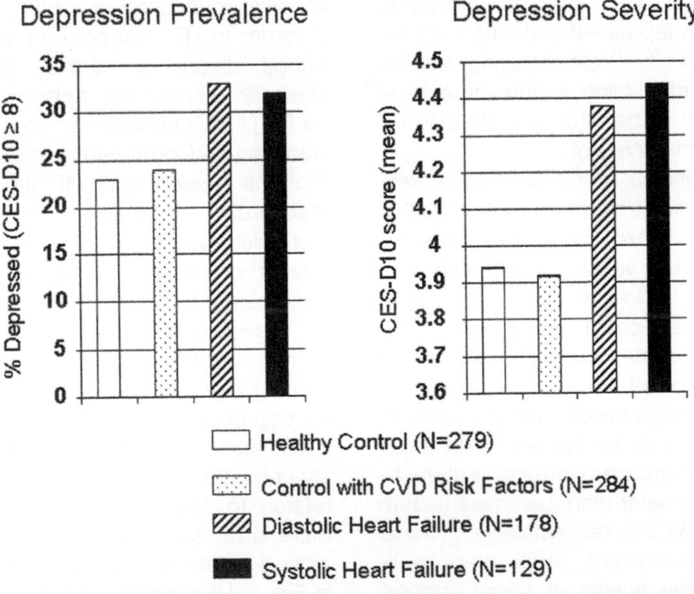

Fig. 2. The prevalence (*left panel*) and severity (*right panel*) of depression as related to heart failure status, using a case-control design. Presence of depression was defined as a score greater than or equal to 8 on the 10-item Centers for Epidemiologic Studies Depression scale. Systolic HF was defined as a positive history of HF with impaired ejection fraction (LVEF <55%) and diastolic HF (HF-PEF) as LVEF greater than or equal to 55%. (*Data from* Kop WJ, Kuhl EA, Barasch E, et al. Association between depressive symptoms and fibrosis markers: the Cardiovascular Health Study. Brain Behav Immun 2010;24(2):229–35.)

increased biological correlates of functionally severe HF (eg, neurohormonal dysregulation and inflammation), or patients' knowledge and psychological reaction to the fact that functionally severe HF is associated with poor prognosis.

Predictive Value of Depression for Adverse Heart Failure Outcomes

Among patients with HF, depression is associated with a greater than 2-fold risk for mortality,[7–10] hospitalization,[7,10,18] increased health care costs,[19] and functional decline.[8,20] Meta-analysis of 8 longitudinal studies examining mortality and secondary HF outcomes revealed an aggregated risk ratio of 2.1 (95% CI = 1.7–2.6; range 1.7 to 3.0) associated with depression in HF[6] (see also XXX and colleagues in this volume of Heart Failure Clinics). Subsequent studies have further confirmed the adverse long-term HF outcomes associated with depression,[11] and these adverse consequences are also observed in mental disorders other than depression.[17] Some evidence suggests that the effects of depression on hospitalizations and mortality become stronger with longer (>6 months) follow-up duration.[19] The somatic components of depression (eg, fatigue, sleep problems) appear to be better predictors of mortality in patients with HF compared with cognitive-affective symptoms (eg, depressed mood).[87] Further research is needed to determine whether this differential effect reflects functional HF severity or somatic depressive symptoms *per se*.

Large-scale epidemiologic studies have also shown that depression is predictive of elevated risk for incident HF.[88,89] These associations tend to be less strong than the mortality risk among clinical HF populations, which is in part explained by the longer follow-up needed to yield sufficient numbers of incident HF endpoints.

Depression and Quality of Life in Heart Failure

Health-related quality of life (HR-QOL) reflects the impact of health issues on an individual's satisfaction with life and ability to meet physical and emotional needs. Measures of QOL can be reliably obtained using self-report questionnaires, including general QOL measures[90,91] and HF-specific measures.[92,93] QOL assessments are useful in describing how illness interferes with patients' conditions of daily living. In chronic diseases, such as HF, functional disease indicators (6-minute walk test and NYHA class) have been used as additional measures of patients' QOL. These functional measures are more strongly related to health-related QOL than the typical objective measures of clinical HF status and outcomes (eg, LVEF and natriuretic peptides).[94,95] Quality of life is of particular importance because of its clinical implications in terms of patient-reported outcomes and its prognostic value for HF progression.[96–100] The predictive value of QOL is not explained by objective HF severity indices, but the independence of QOL from depression requires further investigation.

Depression is a significant predictor of poor QOL in patients with HF,[20,101,102] and some evidence suggests that these associations may be stronger in women than in men.[103] Research from the authors' group[50] and others[101,102] has shown that depressed mood is more robustly associated with poor QOL as compared with standard objective indicators of CVD and HF severity.[104] Based on the HF-ACTION (A Controlled Trial Investigating Outcomes of Exercise Training) study, a large randomized trial of aerobic exercise training in subjects with systolic HF, the authors found that objective assessments of disease severity (LVEF and B-type natriuretic peptide) were not related to Beck Depression Inventory (BDI) depression scores, and peak oxygen consumption was only slightly related to depression scores. Exercise stress testing duration, NYHA class, 6-minute walk distance, and peak respiratory exchange ratio were independently associated with depression scores.[50]

A reverse pattern has also been documented, such that poor QOL predicts depressive symptoms during 1-year follow-up.[59] Research from patients with left ventricular assist devices indicates that marked reductions of severe HF (NYHA class IV) following device placement is accompanied by substantial improvements in QOL,[105] but the potential mediating role of depression in these circumstances has not been studied in detail. A conceptual model, partially derived from other publications in this field,[94,106] is presented in **Fig. 3**. We postulate that HR-QOL in HF is strongly related to psychosocial factors, even in the absence of depression, and that health perceptions play a primary role in QOL (see **Fig. 2**A). Thus, measures of HF outcomes are variably associated with depression, such that more subjective measures are more strongly correlated with depression than objective disease measures, such as LVEF and natriuretic peptides (see **Fig. 2**B). It is likely that poor functional status and depression are mutually reinforcing phenomena, both affecting HR-QOL, and that longitudinal assessments are needed to disentangle cause-effect relationships.

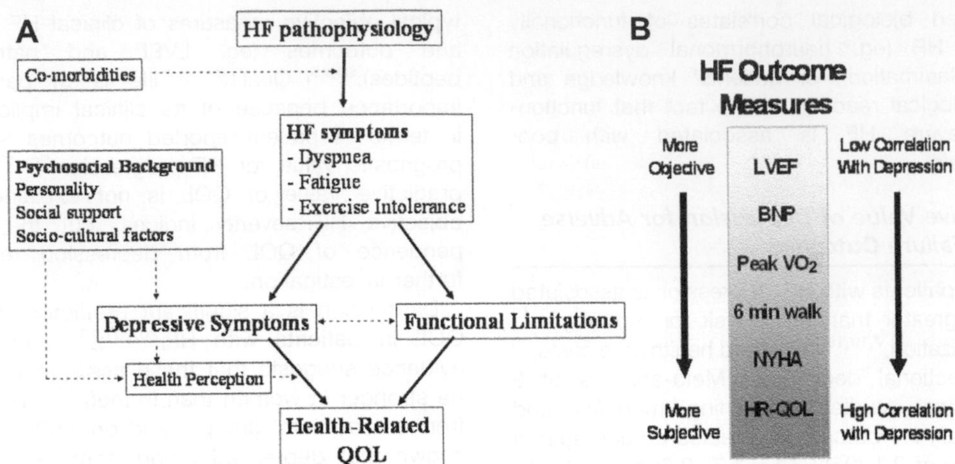

Fig. 3. Conceptual model of the relationship between depression and cardiac disease severity as related to quality of life in patients with heart failure. (*A*) The severity of HF pathophysiology and HF-related comorbidities are primary determinants of HF symptoms. Typical symptoms of HF influence depressive symptoms and functional limitations. Depressive symptoms and functional limitations are inter-related phenomena and both lead to impaired health-related quality of life. Psychosocial background factors may further promote the onset of depression and affect quality of life via altered health perceptions. (*B*) Outcome measures in heart failure range from objective indices, such as left ventricular ejection fraction (EF) and natriuretic peptides (BNP), to functional measures (peak VO_2 max and 6-minute walk test), to measures that are based on subjective reports (NYHA class and HR-QOL). Evidence indicates that depression is substantially associated with subjective HF outcomes; whereas, objective HF outcomes measures are not strongly related to depression. (*Partially derived from* Rector TS. A conceptual model of quality of life in relation to heart failure. J Card Fail 2005;11(3):173–6; and Heo S, Moser DK, Riegel B, et al. Testing a published model of health-related quality of life in heart failure. J Card Fail 2005;11(5):372–9.)

Association between neurohormones and autonomic nervous system dysregulation with depression: relevance to heart failure progression

Increased sympathetic nervous system activity, including elevated catecholamine levels, as well as reduced feedback control of the hypothalamic-pituitary adrenal (HPA) axis are well documented in depression (for general reviews see[107–110]; specific to CVD[12,111–114]). Norepinephrine (NE) and epinephrine (E) are also elevated in HF[115–120] with NE having significant predictive power for adverse HF prognosis.[25–31] Patients with decompensated HF show increased plasma NE and E; whereas, patients with chronic, stable HF usually display increased plasma NE without substantial changes in E.[117] Increased release and turnover of NE combined with decreased efficiency of cardiac NE storage and reuptake both contribute to elevated cardiac adrenergic drive in HF.[116,121] In contrast to consistently elevated plasma NE levels in HF, myocardial NE levels are often reduced, although not necessarily at early stages of HF.[122]

HPA dysregulation in depression may play an additional role in HF progression.[123] Cortisol and aldosterone levels independently predict mortality in HF.[124,125] In addition, and consistent with the role of HPA dysregulation in HF, mineralocorticoid receptor blockade with spironolactone (a nonspecific aldosterone receptor antagonist) is effective in reducing total mortality and incident HF in patients with systolic LV dysfunction.[123,126] Many studies have demonstrated increased HPA activity among depressed individuals, as indicated by elevated levels of corticotropin releasing factor (CRF), reduced adrenocorticotropin responses to CRF, and increased cortisol levels. Corticotropin (ACTH) is the primary trigger of cortisol release and adrenocortical aldosterone.[127,128] The pathophysiology of hypercortisolemia in depression may therefore be influenced in part by altered mineralocorticoid receptor function.[110,129] Although cortisol has antagonistic properties for mineralocorticoid receptors under usual physiologic conditions, cortisol may be an agonist in conditions of tissue damage or oxidative stress, similar to aldosterone.[125] Mineralocorticoid blockade leads to cortisol elevations,[129] which may be of particular relevance in depressed patients with HF. Cortisol also plays an important role in acute life-threatening conditions[130] (eg, stroke[131]), which may further increase the risk of depression-related adverse outcomes in HF.

Neurohormonal activation in HF also includes the renin-angiotensin-aldosterone system (RAAS).[132–135]

NE and RAAS markers are independent predictors of HF outcome, and that their correlation is generally low (r <0.15).[31] Circulating RAAS markers are integral to HF and its effector hormones (angiotensin II and aldosterone) promote collagen deposition and fibrosis, as well as cardiac remodeling.[132,136] Although the RAAS and HPA systems are interrelated,[128,137] the evidence for elevated RAAS hormones in depression is sparse.

Autonomic nervous system dysregulation is commonly observed in HF, particularly sympathetic nervous system activation or parasympathetic withdrawal. Autonomic dysregulation also predicts HF progression.[138] Prior cross-sectional studies using heart rate variability analysis have shown that depression is associated with indices of autonomic dysfunction.[139–141] It is not known whether elevated catecholamines, HPA-axis, and RAAS hormone levels combined with autonomic nervous system dysregulation as observed in both depression and HF display additive or synergistic effects on clinical HF progression.

Inflammation and depression: relevance to heart failure progression

Depression is associated with increased levels of circulating cytokines and elevated acute phase proteins.[142–145] As shown in **Table 1**, the inflammatory correlates of depression[142–146] and the inflammation-related correlates and predictors of HF outcomes[32–40] display considerable overlap (ie, elevated interleukin [IL]-6, tumor necrosis factor [TNF]α, and C-reactive protein [CRP]).[147–149] Inflammatory processes may therefore play an important role in the pathophysiological pathways accounting for increased risk of HF progression among depressed individuals.[148,149] Other immune system parameters associated with depression include lower albumin levels, higher numbers of circulating neutrophils and monocytes, and reduced numbers of lymphocytes.[142] In addition to numeric measures of immune parameters, depression is also associated with reduced natural killer cell activity and lower lymphocyte proliferative response to mitogen stimulation.[142,150] Indicators of partial immune activation in depression are probably mediated by the effects of glucocorticoids on the immune system[145,151,152] that may vary with the clinical characteristics of the depressive disorder.[108] Increased inflammation markers associated with depression and negative affect have been observed in cross-sectional studies in subjects with cardiovascular disorders, including hypertension,[135] coronary artery disease,[153] myocardial infarction,[137] and HF[51,154] (for reviews see[142,147–149]).

A shift in the Th1/Th2 ratio may play a role in the association between depressive symptoms and HF progression. This notion is supported in part by a small study in 18 subjects with HF, showing that higher depression scores were associated with a prospective increase in incidence of cardiac related hospitalizations and/or death ($P = .04$), which coincided with a lower interferon [IFN]-γ/IL-10 ratio expressed by CD4 + T cells in patients with elevated depressive symptom scores at baseline and a prospective increased incidence of cardiac related hospitalization or death over a two-year period.[51] Other research indicates that patients with HF with the Type D (distressed) personality have elevated levels of TNFα (4.8 $\pm$ 0.9 vs 2.5 $\pm$ 0.2 pg/mL, $P = .003$), sTNFR1 (1814 $\pm$ 314 vs 1134 $\pm$ 78 pg/mL, $P = .014$), and sTNFR2 (2465 $\pm$ 243 vs 1874 $\pm$ 118 pg/mL, $P = .019$).[154]

In addition to efferent central nervous system effects on the immune system, a reverse relationship has also been documented, such that inflammatory processes cause central nervous system responses via both humoral and neural pathways. These central nervous system changes may induce depressive symptoms,[155] although the exact mechanism accounting for these associations requires further research.[156,157] Administration of proinflammatory cytokines (eg, TNFα) results in elevated extracellular cerebral serotonin[158] as well as depressed mood, increased sleep, and general malaise.[157] Among patients treated for melanoma, depression develops in response to TNFα administration, primarily among individuals who display an initial HPA response to TNFα. This depressive mood response can be reduced by pretreatment with paroxetine.[159] Peripheral cytokines may stimulate the nucleus tractus solitarius, via afferent projections of the vagus nerve, to activate specific brain regions, including the hypothalamus and the paraventricular nucleus.[157] Fatigue and other depressive symptoms could be secondary to central nervous system responses to inflammation processes, referred to as "sickness behavior."[155,156,160] These findings indicate that depression in HF is bidirectionally associated with inflammation and that both factors may contribute to HF progression.

CONCLUDING REMARKS AND FUTURE DIRECTIONS

This article provides evidence that depression is common in patients with HF (approximately 1 in 5 patients)[6–10,18–20,77–79] and associated with a greater than 2-fold risk for subsequent mortality[6–11] and HF-related clinical endpoints.[18–20]

Depression may adversely affect HF progression by exacerbating common biological processes and increasing adverse health behaviors, such as medication nonadherence[74] and substance abuse, as well as reducing optimal seeking of adequate health care and effective communications with health care providers. Depression is minimally related to objective disease severity measures in HF (eg, LVEF and natriuretic peptides), more strongly with functional measures (eg, 6-minute walk test), significantly with health care professional-assessed functional status (eg, NYHA class), and even stronger with patient-reported HF status (eg, HR-QOL). It is therefore important to provide screening, referral, and treatment for depression in patients with HF. The 2008 science advisory from the American Heart Association is consistent with these clinical and epidemiologic findings.[15] Variability among studies, potential biases, and incomplete adjustments for covariates have been raised as concerns in attributing adverse causal effects to depression[1,16] However, screening for depression in HF is important because of the immediate adverse impact of depression on QOL and health behaviors relevant to the clinical care of HF, as well as the consistent findings showing adverse prognosis in individual with HF and depression across many studies even when using a range of assessment tools. Screening for depressive mood disorders and related psychological conditions can only be useful if treatment contingencies are available, including access to mental health professionals and adequate reimbursement options.[16] Further standardization of assessment and referral strategies as well as improved treatments for depression in HF are warranted.

HF stage and severity should be considered in the evaluation and treatment of depression. Depression is more common in functionally severe HF (particularly NYHA Class III and IV; see **Fig. 1**). Detection and treatment of depression is of particular importance in this subgroup. Because adverse events occur frequently in a short time in these patients with HF, depression intervention should first and foremost target immediate reductions of depressive symptoms to lower this risk factor for short-term adverse HF outcome. In addition, recent developments in the treatment of severe HF (eg, by left ventricular assist devices) as well as referrals for heart transplantation require further investigation of the predictive value and treatment of depression in these conditions.[161] Optimal interventions would address a spectrum of biobehavioral mechanisms that positively affect depressive symptoms as well as physical activity and other health behaviors, particularly those with beneficial effects on neurohormonal and inflammation processes.

More than 30% of depressed patients with HF do not show remission of depression over time[19] because of insufficient use of antidepressant medications and lack of referral to mental health professionals.[19,162–164] Research-based intervention studies suggest that pharmacotherapy, psychotherapy, and exercise can be effective in the treatment of depression in patients with HF. Antidepressive interventions result in significant reduction in depression (Cohen's $d = 0.4$)[6] and improved QOL (see elsewhere in this issue), but no single treatment option shows superiority over other interventions. Gottlieb and colleagues conducted the first published double-blind randomized trial on selective serotonin-norepinephrine reuptake inhibitors (SSRIs) in depressed patients with HF[165] and found that 12-weeks controlled-release paroxetine improved depression and quality of life in 14 actively treated patients versus 14 placebo controls (recovery rates of 69% vs 23%; $P = .024$). The Sertraline Against Depression and Heart Disease in Chronic Heart Failure study examined the effects of sertraline in HF (N = 469). No beneficial effects of sertraline over a nurse-based nonpharmacologic control intervention were observed in depression and quality of life.[166–168] Nonpharmacologic psychological treatment (8 weekly mindfulness meditation, coping skills training, and support group sessions) resulted in lower depression and anxiety scores (p-values <0.05) and improved quality of life ($P = .03$), but no beneficial effects were found for death or HF rehospitalizations.[169]

The main challenge for research and clinical implementation of depression intervention in patients with HF is that antidepressant treatments have not resulted in consistently significant reductions in cardiac events (mortality and rehospitalizations).[166,169] These negative findings are in contrast to the well-documented risk of depression for HF progression, and the generally positive effects of antidepressive interventions on quality of life. A similar pattern of results has been found in other CVD populations. If modification of a risk factor (ie, depression) does not result in changes in the outcome of interest (ie, HF progression), then the risk indicator may merely be a disease marker or a consequence of a common causal factor. As outlined in **Table 1**, this concern is of particular importance in HF. Post-hoc analyses in patients with CVD suggest that patients who remain depressed or get worse during treatment are at higher risk of adverse events; whereas, patients who improve display lower event rates.[170–172] Most evidence suggests that cognitive behavioral therapy and stress reduction as well as pharmacotherapy are beneficial in reducing depression in patients with HF, although the magnitude of improvement has generally been modest. Thus, it is possible that residual depression is partially a consequence of an underlying HF-related biological condition that predicts HF progression. In a large percentage of patients with HF, psychological or pharmacologic interventions do not reduce depression to a sufficiently low level to result in improved HF prognosis (ie, residual levels of depression often remain higher than the cutoff for elevated risk). It may therefore be important to aggressively treat depression in patients with HF[170] and adjust treatment strategies in a timely manner if treatment is not successful.

More attention is needed to identify individuals with a primarily somatic presentation of depression and other states of energy depletion that are not directly related to HF.[87] These conditions will be missed when screening is based on mood or anhedonia only. Because of the overlap in symptoms of depression and HF (eg, fatigue), establishing differential diagnosis and treatment plans are challenging. The somatic components of depression may have different neuro-immunologic concomitants than typical depression (for reviews see[12,162,173]), and fatigue and exhaustion remain significant predictors of adverse cardiovascular health outcomes, even after adjustment for typical depression.[85] Whether intervention strategies should be specifically directed to somatic depressive symptoms versus typical cognitive-affective depressive symptoms in HF requires further investigation.

Depression is associated with a wide range of other psychosocial factors, including avoidant coping; small social networks and low social support; anxiety; and personality traits, such as neuroticism and type D.[174,175] In addition, adverse health behaviors are inter-related and inadequate adherence to multiple healthy life style behaviors is common.[176,177] Patients with depression are less likely to follow recommendations to reduce cardiac risk during recovery from a myocardial infarction.[178] Interventions need to be tailored to patients' specific needs, including sociocultural aspects, age, and psychosocial background factors.[179] Novel interventions include breathing therapy, vagal and other biofeedback techniques, methods derived from complementary medicine, among others. As multiple aspects of depression in HF overlap with HF-related disease processes, it may not be feasible to fully eradicate depression in HF. Thus, in addition to minimizing depressive symptoms, interventions that target active coping, positive thinking, and optimal health behaviors may be of particular relevance in patients with HF with subthreshold depressive symptoms. Issues related to implementation and long-term efficacy of such nontraditional interventions require further research in diverse HF populations, and reimbursement for these types of therapies needs further attention.

In conclusion, depression is common in HF and associated with poor prognosis. Depression often remains undetected because of its partial overlap with HF-related symptoms and the incorrect assumption that some level of depression is a normal psychological reaction to cardiac disease. Determination of the pathways by which depression affects HF progression is important to identify potential targets for novel interventions. Biobehavioral mechanisms accounting for the elevated risk of mortality and HF progression associated with depression include adverse health behaviors, particularly physical inactivity, medication nonadherence, poor dietary control, and smoking, as well as altered biological variables, including neurohormones, autonomic nervous system dysregulation, and inflammation. Behavioral and pharmacologic interventions have had variable success in reducing depression in HF and antidepressive intervention have not consistently resulted in a better HF or CVD prognosis. It will therefore be important to further our understanding of the etiologic factors involved in depression in HF, determine biobehavioral pathways involved in the association between depression and adverse HF outcomes,[180,181] and develop integrative treatments. Novel interventions would advance toward further reductions in depression, promote health behaviors, and positively affect the biology of HF with the long-term goal of improving patients' quality of life and reducing risk of clinical HF progression.

REFERENCES

1. Nicholson A, Kuper H, Hemingway H. Depression as an aetiologic and prognostic factor in coronary heart disease: a meta-analysis of 6362 events among 146 538 participants in 54 observational studies. Eur Heart J 2006;27(23):2763–74.
2. Rozanski A, Blumenthal JA, Kaplan J. Impact of psychological factors on the pathogenesis of cardiovascular disease and implications for therapy. Circulation 1999;99(16):2192–217.
3. Wulsin LR, Singal BM. Do depressive symptoms increase the risk for the onset of coronary disease? A systematic quantitative review. Psychosom Med 2003;65(2):201–10.
4. Penninx BW, Beekman AT, Honig A, et al. Depression and cardiac mortality: results from

a community-based longitudinal study. Arch Gen Psychiatry 2001;58(3):221–7.

5. Lesperance F, Frasure-Smith N, Talajic M, et al. Five-year risk of cardiac mortality in relation to initial severity and one-year changes in depression symptoms after myocardial infarction. Circulation 2002;105(9):1049–53.
6. Rutledge T, Reis VA, Linke SE, et al. Depression in heart failure a meta-analytic review of prevalence, intervention effects, and associations with clinical outcomes. J Am Coll Cardiol 2006;48(8):1527–37.
7. Jiang W, Alexander J, Christopher E, et al. Relationship of depression to increased risk of mortality and rehospitalization in patients with congestive heart failure. Arch Intern Med 2001;161(15): 1849–56.
8. Vaccarino V, Kasl SV, Abramson J, et al. Depressive symptoms and risk of functional decline and death in patients with heart failure. J Am Coll Cardiol 2001; 38(1):199–205.
9. Murberg TA, Bru E, Svebak S, et al. Depressed mood and subjective health symptoms as predictors of mortality in patients with congestive heart failure: a two-years follow-up study. Int J Psychiatry Med 1999;29(3):311–26.
10. Faris R, Purcell H, Henein MY, et al. Clinical depression is common and significantly associated with reduced survival in patients with non-ischaemic heart failure. Eur J Heart Fail 2002; 4(4):541–51.
11. Sherwood A, Blumenthal JA, Trivedi R, et al. Relationship of depression to death or hospitalization in patients with heart failure. Arch Intern Med 2007;167(4):367–73.
12. Kop WJ. Chronic and acute psychological risk factors for clinical manifestations of coronary artery disease. Psychosom Med 1999;61(4):476–87.
13. Carney RM, Freedland KE, Rich MW, et al. Depression as a risk factor for cardiac events in established coronary heart disease: a review of possible mechanisms. Ann Behav Med 1995;17(2):142–9.
14. Frasure-Smith N, Lesperance F, Talajic M. Depression and 18-month prognosis after myocardial infarction. Circulation 1995;91(4):999–1005.
15. Lichtman JH, Bigger JT Jr, Blumenthal JA, et al. Depression and coronary heart disease: recommendations for screening, referral, and treatment: a science advisory from the American Heart Association prevention committee of the council on cardiovascular nursing, council on clinical cardiology, council on epidemiology and prevention, and interdisciplinary council on quality of care and outcomes research: endorsed by the American psychiatric association. Circulation 2008; 118(17):1768–75.
16. Ziegelstein RC, Thombs BD, Coyne JC, et al. Routine screening for depression in patients with coronary heart disease never mind. J Am Coll Cardiol 2009;54(10):886–90.
17. Rathore SS, Wang Y, Druss BG, et al. Mental disorders, quality of care, and outcomes among older patients hospitalized with heart failure: an analysis of the national heart failure project. Arch Gen Psychiatry 2008;65(12):1402–8.
18. Rozzini R, Sabatini T, Frisoni GB, et al. Depression and major outcomes in older patients with heart failure. Arch Intern Med 2002;162(3):362–4.
19. Koenig HG. Depression in hospitalized older patients with congestive heart failure. Gen Hosp Psychiatry 1998;20(1):29–43.
20. Rumsfeld JS, Havranek E, Masoudi FA, et al. Depressive symptoms are the strongest predictors of short-term declines in health status in patients with heart failure. J Am Coll Cardiol 2003;42(10): 1811–7.
21. Pina IL, Apstein CS, Balady GJ, et al. Exercise and heart failure: a statement from the american heart association committee on exercise, rehabilitation, and prevention. Circulation 2003;107(8): 1210–25.
22. Marcus BH, Williams DM, Dubbert PM, et al. Physical activity intervention studies: what we know and what we need to know: a scientific statement from the American Heart Association council on nutrition, physical activity, and metabolism (subcommittee on physical activity); council on cardiovascular disease in the young; and the interdisciplinary working group on quality of care and outcomes research. Circulation 2006;114(24): 2739–52.
23. Riegel B, Moser DK, Anker SD, et al. State of the science: promoting self-care in persons with heart failure: a scientific statement from the American Heart Association. Circulation 2009;120(12): 1141–63.
24. Zuluaga MC, Guallar-Castillon P, Rodriguez-Pascual C, et al. Mechanisms of the association between depressive symptoms and long-term mortality in heart failure. Am Heart J 2010;159(2): 231–7.
25. Cohn JN, Levine TB, Olivari MT, et al. Plasma norepinephrine as a guide to prognosis in patients with chronic congestive heart failure. N Engl J Med 1984;311(13):819–23.
26. Isnard R, Pousset F, Chafirovskaia O, et al. Combination of B-type natriuretic peptide and peak oxygen consumption improves risk stratification in outpatients with chronic heart failure. Am Heart J 2003;146(4):729–35.
27. Anand IS, Fisher LD, Chiang YT, et al. Changes in brain natriuretic peptide and norepinephrine over time and mortality and morbidity in the valsartan heart failure trial (Val-HeFT). Circulation 2003; 107(9):1278–83.

28. Benedict CR, Francis GS, Shelton B, et al. Effect of long-term enalapril therapy on neurohormones in patients with left ventricular dysfunction. SOLVD Investigators. Am J Cardiol 1995;75(16):1151–7.
29. Anker SD. Catecholamine levels and treatment in chronic heart failure. Eur Heart J 1998;(19 Suppl F):F56–61.
30. Packer M, Lee WH, Kessler PD, et al. Role of neurohormonal mechanisms in determining survival in patients with severe chronic heart failure. Circulation 1987;75(5 Pt 2):IV80–92.
31. Francis GS, Cohn JN, Johnson G, et al. Plasma norepinephrine, plasma renin activity, and congestive heart failure. Relations to survival and the effects of therapy in V-HeFT II. The V-HeFT VA cooperative studies group. Circulation 1993;87(Suppl 6):VI40–8.
32. Cesari M, Penninx BW, Newman AB, et al. Inflammatory markers and onset of cardiovascular events: results from the health ABC study. Circulation 2003;108(19):2317–22.
33. Kapadia SR. Cytokines and heart failure. Cardiol Rev 1999;7(4):196–206.
34. Blum A, Miller H. Pathophysiological role of cytokines in congestive heart failure. Annu Rev Med 2001;52:15–27.
35. Maeda K, Tsutamoto T, Wada A, et al. High levels of plasma brain natriuretic peptide and interleukin-6 after optimized treatment for heart failure are independent risk factors for morbidity and mortality in patients with congestive heart failure. J Am Coll Cardiol 2000;36(5):1587–93.
36. Orus J, Roig E, Perez-Villa F, et al. Prognostic value of serum cytokines in patients with congestive heart failure. J Heart Lung Transplant 2000;19(5):419–25.
37. Deswal A, Petersen NJ, Feldman AM, et al. Cytokines and cytokine receptors in advanced heart failure: an analysis of the cytokine database from the vesnarinone trial (VEST). Circulation 2001;103(16). 2055–2059.
38. Rauchhaus M, Doehner W, Francis DP, et al. Plasma cytokine parameters and mortality in patients with chronic heart failure. Circulation 2000;102(25):3060–7.
39. Kell R, Haunstetter A, Dengler TJ, et al. Do cytokines enable risk stratification to be improved in NYHA functional class III patients? comparison with other potential predictors of prognosis. Eur Heart J 2002;23(1):70–8.
40. Nicoletti A, Heudes D, Mandet C, et al. Inflammatory cells and myocardial fibrosis: spatial and temporal distribution in renovascular hypertensive rats. Cardiovasc Res 1996;32(6):1096–107.
41. Funder JW. Steroids, hypertension and cardiac fibrosis. Blood Press Suppl 1995;2:39–42.
42. York KM, Hassan M, Sheps DS. Psychobiology of depression/distress in congestive heart failure. Heart Fail Rev 2009;14(1):35–50.
43. Elovainio M, Keltikangas-Jarvinen L, Kivimaki M, et al. Depressive symptoms and carotid artery intima-media thickness in young adults: the cardiovascular risk in young finns study. Psychosom Med 2005;67(4):561–7.
44. Kop WJ, Berman DS, Gransar H, et al. Social network and coronary artery calcification in asymptomatic individuals. Psychosom Med 2005;67(3):343–52.
45. Agatisa PK, Matthews KA, Bromberger JT, et al. Coronary and aortic calcification in women with a history of major depression. Arch Intern Med 2005;165(11):1229–36.
46. van Melle JP, de JP, Ormel J, et al. Relationship between left ventricular dysfunction and depression following myocardial infarction: data from the MIND-IT. Eur Heart J 2005;26(24):2650–6.
47. Parissis JT, Nikolaou M, Farmakis D, et al. Clinical and prognostic implications of self-rating depression scales and plasma B-type natriuretic peptide in hospitalised patients with chronic heart failure. Heart 2008;94(5):585–9.
48. Parissis JT, Papadopoulos C, Nikolaou M, et al. Effects of levosimendan on quality of life and emotional stress in advanced heart failure patients. Cardiovasc Drugs Ther 2007;21(4):263–8.
49. Parissis JT, Farmakis D, Nikolaou M, et al. Plasma B-type natriuretic peptide and anti-inflammatory cytokine interleukin-10 levels predict adverse clinical outcome in chronic heart failure patients with depressive symptoms: a 1-year follow-up study. Eur J Heart Fail 2009;11(10):967–72.
50. Gottlieb SS, Kop WJ, Ellis SJ, et al. Relation of depression to severity of illness in heart failure (from Heart Failure And a controlled trial investigating outcomes of exercise training [HF-ACTION]). Am J Cardiol 2009;103(9):1285–9.
51. Redwine LS, Mills PJ, Hong S, et al. Cardiac-related hospitalization and/or death associated with immune dysregulation and symptoms of depression in heart failure patients. Psychosom Med 2007;69(1):23–9.
52. Feola M, Rosso GL, Peano M, et al. Correlation between cognitive impairment and prognostic parameters in patients with congestive heart failure. Arch Med Res 2007;38(2):234–9.
53. Kop WJ, Kuhl EA, Barasch E, et al. Association between depressive symptoms and fibrosis markers: the cardiovascular health study. Brain Behav Immun 2010;24(2):229–35.
54. Ko DT, Hebert PR, Coffey CS, et al. Beta-blocker therapy and symptoms of depression, fatigue, and sexual dysfunction. JAMA 2002;288(3):351–7.

55. Kop WJ, Appels A, Mendes de Leon CF, et al. The relationship between severity of coronary artery disease and vital exhaustion. J Psychosom Res 1996;40:397–405.
56. McCaffery JM, Frasure-Smith N, Dube MP, et al. Common genetic vulnerability to depressive symptoms and coronary artery disease: a review and development of candidate genes related to inflammation and serotonin. Psychosom Med 2006;68(2): 187–200.
57. Alves TC, Rays J, Fraguas R Jr, et al. Association between major depressive symptoms in heart failure and impaired regional cerebral blood flow in the medial temporal region: a study using 99m Tc-HMPAO single photon emission computerized tomography (SPECT). Psychol Med 2006;36(5): 597–608.
58. Monroe SM, Simons AD. Diathesis-stress theories in the context of life stress research: implications for the depressive disorders. Psychol Bull 1991; 110(3):406–25.
59. Havranek EP, Spertus JA, Masoudi FA, et al. Predictors of the onset of depressive symptoms in patients with heart failure. J Am Coll Cardiol 2004;44(12):2333–8.
60. Knox SS, Uvnas-Moberg K. Social isolation and cardiovascular disease: an atherosclerotic pathway? Psychoneuroendocrinology 1998;23(8): 877–90.
61. Frasure-Smith N, Lesperance F, Gravel G, et al. Social support, depression, and mortality during the first year after myocardial infarction. Circulation 2000;101(16):1919–24.
62. MacMahon KM, Lip GY. Psychological factors in heart failure: a review of the literature. Arch Intern Med 2002;162(5):509–16.
63. Gusick GM. The contribution of depression and spirituality to symptom burden in chronic heart failure. Arch Psychiatr Nurs 2008;22(1):53–5.
64. Bekelman DB, Dy SM, Becker DM, et al. Spiritual well-being and depression in patients with heart failure. J Gen Intern Med 2007;22(4):470–7.
65. Kwon P, Laurenceau JP. A longitudinal study of the hopelessness theory of depression: testing the diathesis-stress model within a differential reactivity and exposure framework. J Clin Psychol 2002; 58(10):1305–21.
66. Anderson CA, Miller RS, Riger AL, et al. Behavioral and characterological attributional styles as predictors of depression and loneliness: review, refinement, and test. J Pers Soc Psychol 1994; 66(3):549–58.
67. Sweeney PD, Anderson K, Bailey S. Attributional style in depression: a meta-analytic review. J Pers Soc Psychol 1986;50(5):974–91.
68. Davidson KW, Rieckmann N, Lesperance F. Psychological theories of depression: potential application for the prevention of acute coronary syndrome recurrence. Psychosom Med 2004; 66(2):165–73.
69. Beekman AT, Deeg DJ, van TT, et al. Major and minor depression in later life: a study of prevalence and risk factors. J Affect Disord 1995;36(1-2): 65–75.
70. Hooley JM, Orley J, Teasdale JD. Levels of expressed emotion and relapse in depressed patients. Br J Psychiatry 1986;148:642–7.
71. Kessler RC. The effects of stressful life events on depression. Annu Rev Psychol 1997;48:191–214.
72. Beck AT, Rush AJ, Shaw BF, et al. Cognitive therapy of depression. New York: Guilford Press; 1979.
73. Cohen LH, Gunthert KC, Butler AC, et al. Daily affective reactivity as a prospective predictor of depressive symptoms. J Pers 2005;73(6):1687–713.
74. Wu JR, Moser DK, Chung ML, et al. Predictors of medication adherence using a multidimensional adherence model in patients with heart failure. J Card Fail 2008;14(7):603–14.
75. Sturmey P. Behavioral activation is an evidence-based treatment for depression. Behav Modif 2009;33(6):818–29.
76. American Psychiatric Association. Diagnostic and statistical manual of mental disorders. 4th edition. Washington, DC: American Psychiatric Association; 1994.
77. Fulop G, Strain JJ, Stettin G. Congestive heart failure and depression in older adults: clinical course and health services use 6 months after hospitalization. Psychosomatics 2003;44(5):367–73.
78. Svarstad BL, Chewning BA, Sleath BL, et al. The brief medication questionnaire: a tool for screening patient adherence and barriers to adherence. Patient Educ Couns 1999;37(2):113–24.
79. Havranek EP, Ware MG, Lowes BD. Prevalence of depression in congestive heart failure. Am J Cardiol 1999;84(3):348–50, A9.
80. Blazer D, Woodbury M, Hughes DC, et al. A statistical analysis of the classification of depression in a mixed community and clinical sample. J Affect Disord 1989;16(1):11–20.
81. Powell LH, Catellier D, Freedland KE, et al. Depression and heart failure in patients with a new myocardial infarction. Am Heart J 2005;149(5):851–5.
82. Freedland KE, Rich MW, Skala JA, et al. Prevalence of depression in hospitalized patients with congestive heart failure. Psychosom Med 2003;65(1): 119–28.
83. Thomas SA, Friedmann E, Khatta M, et al. Depression in patients with heart failure: physiologic effects, incidence, and relation to mortality. AACN Clin Issues 2003;14(1):3–12.
84. Freedland KE, Skala JA, Carney RM, et al. The Depression Interview and Structured Hamilton

(DISH): rationale, development, characteristics, and clinical validity. Psychosom Med 2002;64(6): 897–905.
85. Appels A, Kop WJ, Schouten E. The nature of the depressive symptomatology preceding myocardial infarction. Behav Med 2000;26(2):86–9.
86. Skotzko CE, Krichten C, Zietowski G, et al. Depression is common and precludes accurate assessment of functional status in elderly patients with congestive heart failure. J Card Fail 2000;6(4): 300–5.
87. Schiffer AA, Pelle AJ, Smith OR, et al. Somatic versus cognitive symptoms of depression as predictors of all-cause mortality and health status in chronic heart failure. J Clin Psychiatry 2009; 70(12):1667–73.
88. Abramson J, Berger A, Krumholz HM, et al. Depression and risk of heart failure among older persons with isolated systolic hypertension. Arch Intern Med 2001;161(14):1725–30.
89. Williams SA, Kasl SV, Heiat A, et al. Depression and risk of heart failure among the elderly: a prospective community-based study. Psychosom Med 2002; 64(1):6–12.
90. Flynn KE, Lin L, Ellis SJ, et al. Outcomes, health policy, and managed care: relationships between patient-reported outcome measures and clinical measures in outpatients with heart failure. Am Heart J 2009;158 (Suppl 4):S64–71.
91. Ware JE, Sherbourne CD. The MOS 36-item short-form health survey (SF-36). I. Conceptual framework and item selection. Med Care 1992;30(6): 473–83.
92. Green CP, Porter CB, Bresnahan DR, et al. Development and evaluation of the kansas city cardiomyopathy questionnaire: a new health status measure for heart failure. J Am Coll Cardiol 2000; 35(5):1245–55.
93. Rector TS, Kubo SH, Cohn JN. Validity of the Minnesota living with heart failure questionnaire as a measure of therapeutic response to enalapril or placebo. Am J Cardiol 1993;71(12):1106–7.
94. Rector TS. A conceptual model of quality of life in relation to heart failure. J Card Fail 2005;11(3): 173–6.
95. Grigioni F, Carigi S, Grandi S, et al. Distance between patients' subjective perceptions and objectively evaluated disease severity in chronic heart failure. Psychother Psychosom 2003;72(3): 166–70.
96. Mommersteeg PM, Denollet J, Spertus JA, et al. Health status as a risk factor in cardiovascular disease: a systematic review of current evidence. Am Heart J 2009;157(2):208–18.
97. Spertus JA. Evolving applications for patient-centered health status measures. Circulation 2008;118(20):2103–10.
98. Kosiborod M, Soto GE, Jones PG, et al. Identifying heart failure patients at high risk for near-term cardiovascular events with serial health status assessments. Circulation 2007;115(15). 1975–81.
99. Heidenreich PA, Spertus JA, Jones PG, et al. Health status identifies heart failure outpatients at risk for hospitalization or death. J Am Coll Cardiol 2006;47(4):752–6.
100. Sullivan MD, Levy WC, Russo JE, et al. Summary health status measures in advanced heart failure: relationship to clinical variables and outcome. J Card Fail 2007;13(7):560–8.
101. Muller-Tasch T, Peters-Klimm F, Schellberg D, et al. Depression is a major determinant of quality of life in patients with chronic systolic heart failure in general practice. J Card Fail 2007;13(10):818–24.
102. Faller H, Stork S, Schuler M, et al. Depression and disease severity as predictors of health-related quality of life in patients with chronic heart failure—a structural equation modeling approach. J Card Fail 2009;15(4):286–92.
103. Luttik ML, Lesman-Leegte I, Jaarsma T. Quality of life and depressive symptoms in heart failure patients and their partners: the impact of role and gender. J Card Fail 2009;15(7):580–5.
104. Ruo B, Rumsfeld JS, Hlatky MA, et al. Depressive symptoms and health-related quality of life: the Heart and Soul Study. JAMA 2003;290(2): 215–21.
105. Rogers JG, Aaronson KD, Boyle AJ, et al. Continuous flow left ventricular assist device improves functional capacity and quality of life of advanced heart failure patients. J Am Coll Cardiol 2010; 55(17):1826–34.
106. Heo S, Moser DK, Riegel B, et al. Testing a published model of health-related quality of life in heart failure. J Card Fail 2005;11(5):372–9.
107. Wong ML, Kling MA, Munson PJ, et al. Pronounced and sustained central hypernoradrenergic function in major depression with melancholic features: relation to hypercortisolism and corticotropin-releasing hormone. Proc Natl Acad Sci U S A 2000;97(1): 325–30.
108. Gold PW, Goodwin FK, Chrousos GP. Clinical and biochemical manifestations of depression. Relation to the neurobiology of stress (2) [published erratum appears in N Engl J Med 1988 Nov 24;319(21): 1428]. N Engl J Med 1988;319(7):413–20.
109. Gold PW, Goodwin FK, Chrousos GP. Clinical and biochemical manifestations of depression. Relation to the neurobiology of stress (1). N Engl J Med 1988;319(6):348–53.
110. De Kloet ER, Vreugdenhil E, Oitzl MS, et al. Brain corticosteroid receptor balance in health and disease. Endocr Rev 1998;19(3):269–301.
111. Musselman DL, Evans DL, Nemeroff CB. The relationship of depression to cardiovascular

disease: epidemiology, biology, and treatment. Arch Gen Psychiatry 1998;55(7):580–92.
112. Carney RM, Freedland KE, Miller GE, et al. Depression as a risk factor for cardiac mortality and morbidity: a review of potential mechanisms. J Psychosom Res 2002;53(4):897–902.
113. Lesperance F, Frasure-Smith N. Depression in patients with cardiac disease: a practical review. J Psychosom Res 2000;48(4-5):379–91.
114. Glassman AH, Shapiro PA. Depression and the course of coronary artery disease. Am J Psychiatry 1998;155(1):4–11.
115. Eisenhofer G, Friberg P, Rundqvist B, et al. Cardiac sympathetic nerve function in congestive heart failure. Circulation 1996;93(9):1667–76.
116. Goldstein DS. Plasma norepinephrine as an indicator of sympathetic neural activity in clinical cardiology. Am J Cardiol 1981;48(6):1147–54.
117. Francis GS, Benedict C, Johnstone DE, et al. Comparison of neuroendocrine activation in patients with left ventricular dysfunction with and without congestive heart failure. A substudy of the studies of left ventricular dysfunction (SOLVD). Circulation 1990;82(5):1724–9.
118. Ceconi C, Curello S, Ferrari R. Catecholamines: the cardiovascular and neuroendocrine system. Eur Heart J 1998;19(Suppl F):F2–6.
119. Esler M, Kaye D, Lambert G, et al. Adrenergic nervous system in heart failure. Am J Cardiol 1997;80(11A):7L–14L.
120. Parmley WW. Neuroendocrine changes in heart failure and their clinical relevance. Clin Cardiol 1995;18(8):440–5.
121. Ferrari R, Ceconi C, Curello S, et al. The neuroendocrine and sympathetic nervous system in congestive heart failure. Eur Heart J 1998; 19(Suppl F):F45–51.
122. Pierpont GL, Francis GS, DeMaster EG, et al. Heterogeneous myocardial catecholamine concentrations in patients with congestive heart failure. Am J Cardiol 1987;60(4):316–21.
123. Pitt B, Stier CT Jr, Rajagopalan S. Mineralocorticoid receptor blockade: new insights into the mechanism of action in patients with cardiovascular disease. J Renin Angiotensin Aldosterone Syst 2003;4(3):164–8.
124. Guder G, Bauersachs J, Frantz S, et al. Complementary and incremental mortality risk prediction by cortisol and aldosterone in chronic heart failure. Circulation 2007;115(13):1754–61.
125. Yamaji M, Tsutamoto T, Kawahara C, et al. Serum cortisol as a useful predictor of cardiac events in patients with chronic heart failure: the impact of oxidative stress. Circ Heart Fail 2009;2(6): 608–15.
126. Brown NJ. Eplerenone: cardiovascular protection. Circulation 2003;107(19):2512–8.
127. Whitworth JA, Butty J, Saines D, et al. The effects of ACTH on the renin-aldosterone system in normotensive man. Clin Exp Hypertens A 1985;7(10):1361–76.
128. Murck H, Held K, Ziegenbein M, et al. The Renin-Angiotensin-Aldosterone system in patients with depression compared to controls - a sleep endocrine study. BMC Psychiatry 2003;3(1):15.
129. Young EA, Lopez JF, Murphy-Weinberg V, et al. Mineralocorticoid receptor function in major depression. Arch Gen Psychiatry 2003;60(1):24–8.
130. Giugliano GR, Giugliano RP, Gibson CM, et al. Meta-analysis of corticosteroid treatment in acute myocardial infarction. Am J Cardiol 2003;91(9): 1055–9.
131. Christensen H, Boysen G, Johannesen HH. Serum-cortisol reflects severity and mortality in acute stroke. J Neurol Sci 2004;217(2):175–80.
132. Weber KT. Aldosterone in congestive heart failure. N Engl J Med 2001;345(23):1689–97.
133. Rousseau MF, Gurne O, Duprez D, et al. Beneficial neurohormonal profile of spironolactone in severe congestive heart failure: results from the RALES neurohormonal substudy. J Am Coll Cardiol 2002; 40(9):1596–601.
134. Kereiakes DJ, Kleiman NS, Ambrose JA, et al. Randomized, double-blind, placebo-controlled dose ranging study of Tirofiban (MK-383) platelet IIb/IIIa blockade in high risk patients undergoing coronary angioplasty. J Am Coll Cardiol 1996;27: 536–42.
135. Fagard R, Staessen J, Amery A. Exercise blood pressure and target organ damage in essential hypertension. J Hum Hypertens 1991;5:69–75.
136. Weber KT, Gerling IC, Kiani MF, et al. Aldosteronism in heart failure: a proinflammatory/fibrogenic cardiac phenotype. search for biomarkers and potential drug targets. Curr Drug Targets 2003; 4(6):505–16.
137. Altamura AC, Morganti A. Plasma renin activity in depressed patients treated with increasing doses of lithium carbonate. Psychopharmacologia 1975; 45(2):171–5.
138. Sandercock GR, Brodie DA. The role of heart rate variability in prognosis for different modes of death in chronic heart failure. Pacing Clin Electrophysiol 2006;29(8):892–904.
139. Carney RM, Howells WB, Blumenthal JA, et al. Heart rate turbulence, depression, and survival after acute myocardial infarction. Psychosom Med 2007;69(1):4–9.
140. Glassman AH, Bigger JT, Gaffney M, et al. Heart rate variability in acute coronary syndrome patients with major depression: influence of sertraline and mood improvement. Arch Gen Psychiatry 2007; 64(9):1025–31.
141. van Zyl LT, Hasegawa T, Nagata K. Effects of antidepressant treatment on heart rate variability in

major depression: a quantitative review. Biopsychosoc Med 2008;2:12.
142. Herbert TB, Cohen S. Depression and immunity: a meta-analytic review. Psychol Bull 1993;113(3): 472–86.
143. Miller GE, Stetler CA, Carney RM, et al. Clinical depression and inflammatory risk markers for coronary heart disease. Am J Cardiol 2002;90(12):1279–83.
144. Miller GE, Freedland KE, Duntley S, et al. Relation of depressive symptoms to C-reactive protein and pathogen burden (cytomegalovirus, herpes simplex virus, Epstein-Barr virus) in patients with earlier acute coronary syndromes. Am J Cardiol 2005;95(3):317–21.
145. Suarez EC, Lewis JG, Krishnan RR, et al. Enhanced expression of cytokines and chemokines by blood monocytes to in vitro lipopolysaccharide stimulation are associated with hostility and severity of depressive symptoms in healthy women. Psychoneuroendocrinology 2004;29(9):1119–28.
146. Kop WJ, Gottdiener JS, Tangen CM, et al. Inflammation and coagulation factors in persons > 65 years of age with symptoms of depression but without evidence of myocardial ischemia. Am J Cardiol 2002;89(4):419–24.
147. Kop WJ. The integration of cardiovascular behavioral medicine and psychoneuroimmunology: new developments based on converging research fields. Brain Behav Immun 2003;17(4):233–7.
148. Pasic J, Levy WC, Sullivan MD. Cytokines in depression and heart failure. Psychosom Med 2003;65(2):181–93.
149. Kop WJ, Gottdiener JS. The role of immune system parameters in the relationship between depression and coronary artery disease. Psychosom Med 2005;67(Suppl 1):537–41.
150. Weisse CS. Depression and immunocompetence: a review of the literature. Psychol Bull 1992; 111(3):475–89.
151. Maes M. Evidence for an immune response in major depression: a review and hypothesis. Prog Neuropsychopharmacol Biol Psychiatry 1995; 19(1):11–38.
152. DeRijk RH, Petrides J, Deuster P, et al. Changes in corticosteroid sensitivity of peripheral blood lymphocytes after strenuous exercise in humans. J Clin Endocrinol Metab 1996;81(1):228–35.
153. Appels A, Bar FW, Bar J, et al. Inflammation, depressive symptomatology, and coronary artery disease. Psychosom Med 2000;62(5):601–5.
154. Denollet J, Conraads VM, Brutsaert DL, et al. Cytokines and immune activation in systolic heart failure: the role of Type D personality. Brain Behav Immun 2003;17(4):304–9.
155. Goodkin K, Appels A. Behavioral-neuroendocrine-immunologic interactions in myocardial infarction. Med Hypotheses 1997;48(3):209–14.
156. Dantzer R, Kelley KW. Stress and immunity: an integrated view of relationships between the brain and the immune system. Life Sci 1989;44(26): 1995–2008.
157. Maier SF, Watkins LR. Cytokines for psychologists: implications of bidirectional immune-to-brain communication for understanding behavior, mood, and cognition. Psychol Rev 1998;105(1): 83–107.
158. Capuron L, Ravaud A, Miller AH, et al. Baseline mood and psychosocial characteristics of patients developing depressive symptoms during interleukin-2 and/or interferon-alpha cancer therapy. Brain Behav Immun 2004;18(3):205–13.
159. Musselman DL, Lawson DH, Gumnick JF, et al. Paroxetine for the prevention of depression induced by high-dose interferon alfa. N Engl J Med 2001; 344(13):961–6.
160. White PD. The relationship between infection and fatigue. J Psychosom Res 1997;43(4):345–50.
161. Kop WJ. Role of psychological factors in the clinical course of heart transplant patients. J Heart Lung Transplant 2010;29(3):257–60.
162. Kop WJ, Ader DN. Assessment and treatment of depression in coronary artery disease patients. Ital Heart J 2001;2(12):890–4.
163. Moser DK. Psychosocial factors and their association with clinical outcomes in patients with heart failure: why clinicians do not seem to care. Eur J Cardiovasc Nurs 2002;1(3):183–8.
164. Artinian NT, Artinian CG, Saunders MM. Identifying and treating depression in patients with heart failure. J Cardiovasc Nurs 2004;19(Suppl 6): S47–56.
165. Gottlieb SS, Kop WJ, Thomas SA, et al. A double-blind placebo-controlled pilot study of controlled-release paroxetine on depression and quality of life in chronic heart failure. Am Heart J 2007; 153(5):868–73.
166. O'Connor CM, Jiang W, Kuchibhatla M, et al. Safety and efficacy of sertraline for depression in patients with heart failure: results of the SADHART-CHF (Sertraline Against Depression and Heart Disease in Chronic Heart Failure) trial. J Am Coll Cardiol 2010;56(9):692–9.
167. Jiang W, O'Connor C, Silva SG, et al. Safety and efficacy of sertraline for depression in patients with CHF (SADHART-CHF): a randomized, double-blind, placebo-controlled trial of sertraline for major depression with congestive heart failure. Am Heart J 2008;156(3):437–44.
168. Fraguas R, da Silva Telles RM, Alves TC, et al. A double-blind, placebo-controlled treatment trial of citalopram for major depressive disorder in older patients with heart failure: the relevance of the placebo effect and psychological symptoms. Contemp Clin Trials 2009;30(3):205–11.

169. Sullivan MJ, Wood L, Terry J, et al. The support, education, and research in chronic heart failure study (SEARCH): a mindfulness-based psychoeducational intervention improves depression and clinical symptoms in patients with chronic heart failure. Am Heart J 2009; 157(1):84–90.

170. Glassman AH, Bigger JT Jr, Gaffney M. Psychiatric characteristics associated with long-term mortality among 361 patients having an acute coronary syndrome and major depression: seven-year follow-up of SADHART participants. Arch Gen Psychiatry 2009;66(9):1022–9.

171. Carney RM, Blumenthal JA, Freedland KE, et al. Depression and late mortality after myocardial infarction in the enhancing recovery in coronary heart disease (ENRICHD) study. Psychosom Med 2004;66(4):466–74.

172. de Jonge P, Honig A, van Melle JP, et al. Nonresponse to treatment for depression following myocardial infarction: association with subsequent cardiac events. Am J Psychiatry 2007;164(9):1371–8.

173. Appels A. Depression and coronary heart disease: observations and questions. J Psychosom Res 1997;43(5):443–52.

174. Trivedi RB, Blumenthal JA, O'Connor C, et al. Coping styles in heart failure patients with depressive symptoms. J Psychosom Res 2009;67(4): 339–46.

175. Pelle AJ, van den Broek KC, Szabo B, et al. The relationship between type d personality and chronic heart failure is not confounded by disease severity as assessed by BNP. Int J Cardiol 2009. [Epub ahead of print].

176. Evangelista L, Doering LV, Dracup K, et al. Compliance behaviors of elderly patients with advanced heart failure. J Cardiovasc Nurs 2003;18(3): 197–206.

177. Woo J. Relationships among diet, physical activity and other lifestyle factors and debilitating diseases in the elderly. Eur J Clin Nutr 2000;54(Suppl 3): S143–7.

178. Ziegelstein RC, Fauerbach JA, Stevens SS, et al. Patients with depression are less likely to follow recommendations to reduce cardiac risk during recovery from a myocardial infarction. Arch Intern Med 2000;160(12):1818–23.

179. Lavie CJ, Milani RV. Adverse psychological and coronary risk profiles in young patients with coronary artery disease and benefits of formal cardiac rehabilitation. Arch Intern Med 2006;166(17):1878–83.

180. Joynt KE, Whellan DJ, O'Connor CM. Why is depression bad for the failing heart? a review of the mechanistic relationship between depression and heart failure. J Card Fail 2004;10(3):258–71.

181. Konstam V, Moser DK, De Jong MJ. Depression and anxiety in heart failure. J Card Fail 2005; 11(6):455–63.

Cardiovascular Disease and Depression in Women

Laxmi S. Mehta, MD

KEYWORDS

• Women • Depression • Cardiovascular disease
• Outcomes • Treatment

The interplay between the mind and heart has been frequently referenced in literature since ancient times. This connection is often eluded to and accepted as an everyday phenomenon, however not until recent decades has it been scientifically examined. Several studies have demonstrated increased development of coronary heart disease (CHD)[1] and CHD mortality[2,3] in patients suffering from depression. Recently, cardiovascular and psychiatry specialists have promoted the need to increase awareness of the prevalence, screening for, and treatment of depression in cardiac patients. Previously it was felt that depressive symptoms following a cardiac event were normal and would eventually resolve or "normalize" for the patient. Now we know that not to be true. In fact, depression may have been present before the event or as a result of adaptation to the event. Depression has been shown to be present in 20% of patients after myocardial infarction (MI).[4] Subsequent risk of a cardiac event in depressed patients is 2 to 5 times that of nondepressed patients.[5,6] Interestingly, women suffer from depression more often than men and have worse cardiovascular outcomes.

PREVALENCE OF DEPRESSION

Depression has been shown to be 2 times more prevalent in women compared with men,[7] beginning as early as the adolescent years in women.[8] Psychological and physiologic components may account for some of the gender differences. We also know from cancer data that chronic disease states affect the prevalence of depression. Meta-analysis of data on cancer patients has shown that up to 46% meet the study criteria for depression.[9] Data from the National Health Interview Study demonstrated patients with various forms of cardiovascular disease (CVD) also have a high burden of psychological distress.[10]

The Women's Health Initiative (WHI) provides data regarding the largest group of postmenopausal females in the United States who had baseline screening for depression and were prospectively followed for cardiovascular outcomes. Approximately 16% of the women reported depressive symptoms on the baseline survey. Risk factors for CVD were significantly related to depression. Overweight smokers had 1.56 times the risk of current depression when compared with nonsmokers who were not overweight. Baseline depression was a significant predictor of cardiovascular death in subjects without a prior history of CVD (relative risk [RR] 1.58; 95% confidence interval [CI] 1.19–2.10). Baseline depressive symptoms were associated with stroke in those with a prior history of CVD (RR 1.55; 95% CI 1.21–1.98).[2] These data provide valuable information regarding depression and its association with cardiovascular death and stroke in women; however, large-scale randomized trials

The author has nothing to disclose.
Division of Cardiovascular Medicine, Department of Internal Medicine, The Ohio State University, Suite 200 DHLRI, 473 West 12th Avenue, Columbus, OH 43210, USA
E-mail address: Laxmi.Mehta@osumc.edu

Heart Failure Clin 7 (2011) 39–45
doi:10.1016/j.hfc.2010.08.005
1551-7136/11/$ – see front matter

are necessary to determine whether pharmacologic or nonpharmacologic treatment will affect CVD risk.

DEPRESSION: POTENTIAL RISK FACTORS FOR CVD

Several different pathophysiologic mechanisms have been proposed to elucidate potential links between depression and CVD. Potential mechanisms include hypothalamic-pituitary-adrenal axis dysfunction,[11] increased catecholamines, low heart rate variability,[12] increased inflammatory markers (C-reactive protein [CRP], fibrinogen levels, interleukin [IL]-6),[13,14] impaired vascular function,[15] and enhanced platelet function.[16] Additionally, adverse behaviors in depressed patients, such as poor diet, medication noncompliance, tobacco use, and physical inactivity, may also contribute to the development of cardiovascular disease.

The Women's Ischemia Syndrome Evaluation (WISE) study measured CRP and IL-6 in 559 women who were undergoing a coronary angiogram for evaluation of chest pain or myocardial ischemia. Women with depression had significantly higher levels of CRP and IL-6 compared with women without depression ($P = .0008$); similar findings were seen in patients with possible depression, suggesting depression is associated with inflammation. Depression, but not possible depression, was a predictor of cardiovascular disease. In addition, depression and inflammatory markers were both independent predictors of cardiac outcomes (hospital stays for nonfatal MI, stroke, congestive heart failure, and cardiac mortality) at 6-year follow-up.[17]

Increase in QT dispersion,[18] reduced heart rate variability,[12] and increased sympathetic nervous system activation[19] may be possible mechanisms for ventricular arrhythmias in patients with depression. Previous studies have shown the association of clinical depression with out-of-hospital cardiac arrest[20] and depressive symptoms with ventricular arrhythmias in patients with implantable defibrillators.[21] In 2009, Whang and colleagues[22] assessed the association of depression and risk of sudden cardiac death (SCD), fatal CHD, and nonfatal MI in 63,469 women without baseline history of CHD from the Nurses' Health Study. Depression symptoms were strongly associated with fatal CHD events, even after adjustment for cardiac risk factors. Antidepressant use was also associated with SCD (hazard ratio [HR] 3.34; 95% CI 2.03–5.50), suggesting that proarrhythmic effects from antidepressant medications may be playing a role.

Several studies have shown that depression can predict CVD in men[23] and in both genders,[24,25] but the studies did not examine women separately. Ferketich and colleagues[1] were one of the first to report the effect of depression on CHD risk in women, using data from the National Health and Nutrition Examination Study (NHANES I). A baseline interview and serial follow-up were obtained in 5007 women and 2886 men. This group demonstrated that gender differences exist in the effect of depression on CHD risk. Women with depression had a higher rate of nonfatal CHD events but this was not seen for fatal CHD events, whereas in men, depression was associated with both nonfatal and fatal CHD events.

There is a paucity of data regarding depression and subclinical atherosclerosis. Women with a history of recurrent major depression have an increased risk of coronary and aortic calcification. Middle-aged women with recurrent depression were shown to have 2 to 3 times more likely higher burden of coronary and aortic calcification compared with women with no depression or a single episode of depression.[26] Stewart and colleagues[27] presented data from the Pittsburgh Healthy Heart Project, which followed older men and women for the development of subclinical atherosclerosis. Serial carotid intima-media thickness assessment using B-mode ultrasonography was performed at baseline and at 3-year follow-up. All patients were screened for depressive symptoms, anxiety, and anger/hostility. Patients with higher depressive symptoms were found to have increased change in their carotid intima-media thickness even after controlling for demographic and cardiovascular factors and medication use, whereas there was no change in those patients with anxiety and anger/hostility. These data suggest that depression may play a role in development of early atherosclerosis; however, gender differences were not reported. The Cardiovascular Risk in Young Finns Study examined the association of depressive symptoms and subclinical atherosclerosis in 410 men and 716 women. Depression was assessed at 3 different time intervals but carotid artery intima-media thickness was checked only at follow-up. Men with higher depressive scores were found to have higher carotid intima-media thickness than those with low to moderate scores; however, there was no association found in women. Therefore, it is suggested that there is a link between depressive symptoms and preclinical atherosclerosis in men, but this relationship was not seen in women. Women in this study were young and may have been protected by their youth, as atherosclerosis tends to occur at a later age in women than men, partly because of the protective effects of estrogen.[28] Studies that include women of older age are needed to further assess the association of depression and subclinical atherosclerosis.

One key question is whether depression precedes CVD or is a result of CVD. Depression is associated with prevalence and outcomes of CVD; however, it is unclear if it is truly a risk factor. Depression and CVD may be correlates in numerous studies, yet association does not necessarily prove causation.[29]

DEPRESSION IN WOMEN WITH CVD

CVD is the number 1 killer of women in developed countries. Women have worse cardiovascular outcomes compared with men, are more likely to die post-MI, and are less likely to be offered standard treatment or comply with treatment plans compared with their male counterparts. Women who have had an MI cope with the ramifications of the disease differently. Women often have conflicting roles that hinder caring for themselves as well as lower social support and quality of life compared with men.

Numerous epidemiologic studies of patients who have had an MI have shown the association of depression with increased mortality. In patients who have had an MI, major depression is a significant predictor of early mortality, as early as 6 months.[30] Frasure-Smith and colleagues[31] sought to assess the impact of depression on 5-year survival rates, taking into account gender differences. Secondary analyses of 2 different trials were performed using 896 patients (283 women) who received usual care and survived to discharge. In women, the cardiac death rate was 8.3% in depressed patients and 2.7% in nondepressed patients; similar findings were seen in men (7.0% vs 2.4%). In women and men, in-hospital depression post-MI is a significant predictor of cardiac mortality at 1 year (women: odds ratio [OR] 3.29; 95% CI 1.02–10.59; men: OR 3.05, 95% CI 1.29–7.17). Lespérance and colleagues[32] have also shown that the degree of depression severity at time of MI hospitalization, as opposed to measurements at 1 year, is more closely associated with 5-year survival rates.

Younger women are known to suffer disproportionately higher incidence of depression, but in patients with acute MI it is unclear if this holds true. Between 2003 and 2004, 2988 patients with acute MI (814 women) were enrolled in the Prospective Registry Evaluating Outcomes after Myocardial Infarction: Events and Recovery (PREMIER) study. All patients were screened during the hospitalization for depression using the Primary Care Evaluation of Mental Disorders Brief Patient Health Questionnaire (PHQ), in which a score of 10 or higher was considered positive for depression. The prevalence of depression in this study cohort was 22% in men 60 years or younger, 15% in men older than 60 years, 40% in women 60 years or younger and 21% in women older than age 60 years. Higher PHQ scores were seen in younger patients than older ones (6.4 vs 5.0; $P<.001$), and in women than in men (6.8 vs 5.2; $P<.001$). Younger women had the highest PHQ scores, significantly higher odds ratio for depression than any other group. The risk of depression in young women is 3 times that of older men.[33] More recent data from the PREMIER study demonstrated that women have a higher prevalence of depressive symptoms than men (29% vs 18.8%, $P<.001$), but it has only modest impact on the higher rates of angina and rehospitalization in women. Fewer than 20% of patients with depressive symptoms were actually discharged on antidepressants.[34] Given the higher depression rates and cardiovascular events in young women, more studies are needed to understand mechanisms and treatment of depression in women as well as implications of treatment on outcomes.

Using data from the National Health Information Survey, Ferketich and Binkley[10] demonstrated a high incidence of psychological distress in participants with heart disease. The prevalence of psychological distress varied with the different forms of CVD. Prevalence of psychological distress among the American adults older than 40 years was estimated to be 2.8%. Participants with CHD had the lowest prevalence of psychological distress (4.1%), which was followed by those with MI (6.4%). Participants with congestive heart failure had the highest prevalence of psychological distress (10%). Depression has an impact on quality of life in patients with heart failure. Gottlieb and colleagues[35] studied 155 outpatients with stable NYHA functional class II, III, and IV heart failure and an ejection fraction of less than 40%. Forty-eight percent of the patients of who were screened with 2 different screening questionnaires were considered depressed based on their scores. This study demonstrated in patients with heart failure, men were less likely to be depressed compared with women (44% vs 64%) and depressed patients were more likely to be younger than the nondepressed patients. In addition, the treatment of depression with either pharmacologic or nonpharmacologic methods was shown to improve the quality of life in patients with heart failure.

Depressed patients are more likely to be noncompliant with their cardiac medications, including aspirin; however, it has been shown that improvement in depressive symptoms was associated with increased cardiac medication adherence.[36] In the Heart and Soul Study, patients with stable CHD in the ambulatory setting were prospectively followed for psychosocial factors and health outcomes. Of the 940 patients, 22% were found to have depression, which was associated with medication noncompliance. Those with more severe depression had a higher incidence of medication nonadherence. In addition, women were disproportionately depressed (27% depressed vs 13% not depressed, $P<.001$), and therefore more likely to be noncompliant with their medications; however, breakdown based on gender was not reported.[37]

Despite a significant number of cardiac patients having depression, it is often underrecognized or not treated. Recently, a scientific advisory group of the American Heart Association recognized the high incidence of depression in patients with CVD and published recommendations for screening, referral, and treatment of depression in patients with CHD.[38] It is suggested that, at a minimum, the Patient Health Questionnaire (PHQ-2)[39] should be administered to ascertain whether a patient is depressed, both in the inpatient and outpatient setting. If the patient answers yes to either question, then the PHQ-9 should be administered. If a patient is found to have depression (mild to severe) then he or she should be referred to a health care professional for further diagnosis and treatment. This is easy and quick to administer in patients. Despite the lack of positive beneficial outcomes data, depression should not be ignored or not treated. Many patients may have had unrecognized depression before the cardiac event; this is a key opportunity to catch these patients and make a difference in their lives.

Improved diagnosis and treatment of depression is important as well from a financial standpoint. Data from the WISE study demonstrated that depression in women suspected of myocardial ischemia is expensive and has been shown to substantially increase 5-year cardiovascular costs by 15% to 53%, depending on the diagnostic criteria for depression.[40] These data reiterate the importance of screening for depression and the potential impact on medical costs if depression is treated.

TREATMENT OF DEPRESSION

Depression has a stigma that needs to be disregarded and it needs to be recognized and accepted. There is an increased prevalence of depression in women, especially post-MI, and so screening efforts should be promoted. Theoretically, if depression worsens cardiovascular outcomes, then treatment should result in reduction of its negative impacts. Interestingly, in the late 1960s Dr Thomas Hackett and Dr N.H. Cassem, psychiatrists at Massachusetts General Hospital, found that patients who had experienced an MI recovered much faster from a physical standpoint compared with an emotional standpoint. The "ego infarction" was coined from them, to indicate the devastating changes in body image that the young men experienced but could not verbalize. These two advocated for early post-MI cardiac rehabilitation for both the MI as well as the ego infarction.

Cardiac rehabilitation has been recommended for secondary prevention of CVD[41,42] and has been shown to reduce mortality.[43] Recently, Milani and Lavie[44] assessed the impact of cardiac rehabilitation on depression in 522 patients with CHD enrolled in a rehabilitation program and compared them with a group of 179 patients with CHD who did not complete the rehabilitation program. This study demonstrated a nearly 63% reduction in prevalence of depressive symptoms (17% to 6%, $P<.0001$) in those patients completing cardiac rehabilitation. There was a 73% reduction in mortality (8% vs 30%, $P<.0005$) in depressed patients who completed cardiac rehabilitation compared with depressed patients who did not complete cardiac rehabilitation. These benefits of reduction in depressive symptoms and mortality were seen even with only mild improvements in exercise capacity. Despite the benefits, women are less often referred to cardiac rehabilitation and less likely to participate after referral compared with men.[45] Unfortunately, only 15% of eligible women actually enroll in cardiac rehabilitation programs despite proven cardiovascular benefits.[46] The low enrollment numbers are frequently attributed to underreferral of women by physicians, low social support, and transportation issues. In Toronto, the Women's College Hospital designed a cardiac rehabilitation program for women, and is exploring ways to facilitate more women to participate, including providing social support with fellow participants and professional staff as well as flexible program schedules. Investigation into addressing physician referral patterns and transportation issues are some of the barriers for women that still need to be addressed[47]; one of the most powerful predictors of participation is physician recommendation.[45] Cardiac rehabilitation programs that are specifically tailored to women have also shown reduced depressive symptoms compared with women participating in traditional programs.

In the past, it was known that depression was associated with worse morbidity and mortality as well as slow recovery after an acute MI; however, only a minority of patients were treated for depression. Preliminary treatment of depression was with antidepressants that had cardiotoxic effects. It was not until recent years that selective serotonin reuptake inhibitors (SSRIs) made the market and were less likely to have cardiotoxic effects. The Sertraline Antidepressant Heart Attack Trial (SADHART) was a multicenter, placebo-controlled trial that demonstrated sertraline to be safe and effective in the treatment of depression in hospitalized patients with major depression who had an acute MI or unstable angina.[48]

The Enhancing Recovery in Coronary Heart Disease (ENRICHD) study included 2481 patients post-MI (44% women) with depression or low social support who were randomized to 16 weeks of cognitive behavioral therapy versus usual care. Those patients who had severe depression or did not respond to psychotherapy were also treated with pharmacotherapy, typically with SSRIs. In this study, cognitive behavioral therapy decreased depression and low perceived social support but did not aid in reducing the primary end point of death or MI after 3.5 years. Subgroup analysis of the effect on death and nonfatal MI demonstrated usual care is favored in women and cognitive behavioral therapy in men.[49] Subsequent data from the ENRICHD trial showed patients with an acute MI who are severely depressed and treated with SSRIs have a lower mortality and nonfatal MI rate.[50] This was a retrospective analysis that was not powered to assess SSRIs effectively; randomized trials are warranted. Physicians were notified if their patient had depression, so many of the patients in the usual care group were on an SSRI by the end of the trial. Therefore, it is unclear if treatment of depression truly does not affect cardiac outcomes or if another intervention needs to be selected. Previous studies in cardiac patients have demonstrated poor outcomes in patients with low social support; however, outcomes were measured by rates of rehospitalization and death, as opposed to health status (angina, functional status, and quality of life). One recently published study by Leifheit-Limson and colleagues[51] demonstrated that in the first year post-MI, lower social support is associated with more depressive symptoms and poorer health status compared with those with high social support systems. This was most apparent in women.

SUMMARY

Heart disease and depression are very common, frequently concomitant, conditions that were previously speculated by the World Health Organization to be the first and second leading causes of disability (respectively) by the year 2020.[52] There have been no secondary prevention of CVD trials that have shown treatment of depression reduces cardiovascular events. Women patients are different, all with diverse types of cardiovascular disease and depression, which likely respond to different treatments. More clinical trials are needed to further assess the association of cardiovascular disease and depression, investigate biomarkers and ways to treat depression, as well as evaluating if treatment of depression makes a positive impact on cardiovascular outcomes.

REFERENCES

1. Ferketich AK, Schwartzbaum JA, Frid DJ, et al. Depression as an antecedent to heart disease among women and men in the NHANES I study. National Health and Nutrition Examination Survey. Arch Intern Med 2000;160:1261–8.
2. Wassertheil-Smoller S, Shumaker S, Ockene J, et al. Depression and cardiovascular sequelae in postmenopausal women. The Women's Health Initiative (WHI). Arch Intern Med 2004;164:289–98.
3. Mendes de Leon CF, Krumholz HM, Seeman TS, et al. Depression and risk of coronary heart disease in elderly men and women: New Haven EPESE, 1982–1991. Established Populations for the Epidemiologic Studies of the Elderly. Arch Intern Med 1998;158:2341–8.
4. Thombs BD. Prevalence of depression in survivors of acute myocardial infarction. J Gen Intern Med 2006;21:30–8.
5. Nicholson A, Kuper H, Hemingway H. Depression as an aetiologic and prognostic factor in coronary heart disease: a meta-analysis of 6362 events among 146 538 participants in 54 observational studies. Eur Heart J 2006;27:2763–74.
6. Rutledge T, Reis SE, Olson MB, et al. Depression symptom severity and reported treatment history in the prediction of cardiac risk in women with suspected myocardial ischemia: the NHLBI-sponsored WISE study. Arch Gen Psychiatry 2006;63:874–80.
7. Kessler RC, McGonagle KA, Swartz M, et al. Sex and depression in the National Comorbidity Survey. I: lifetime prevalence, chronicity and recurrence. J Affect Disord 1993;29:85–96.
8. Kornstein SG. Gender differences in depression: implications for treatment. J Clin Psychiatry 1997; 58:12–8.

9. van't Spijker A, Trijsburg RW, Duivenvoorden HJ. Psychological sequelae of cancer diagnosis: a meta-analytical review of 58 studies after 1980. Psychosom Med 1997;59:280–93.
10. Ferketich AK, Binkley PF. Psychological distress and cardiovascular disease: results from the 2002 National Health Interview Study. Eur Heart J 2005; 26:1923–9.
11. Taylor CB, Conrad A, Wilhelm FH, et al. Psychophysiological and cortisol response to psychological stress in depressed and nondepressed older men and women with elevated cardiovascular disease risk. Psychosom Med 2006;68:538–46.
12. Carney RM, Blumenthal JA, Stein PK, Watkins, et al. Depression, heart rate variability, and acute myocardial infarction. Circulation 2001;104:2024–8.
13. Lespérance F, Frasure-Smith N, Théroux P, et al. The association between major depression and levels of soluble intercellular adhesion molecule 1, interleukin-6, and C-reactive protein in patients with recent acute coronary syndromes. Am J Psychiatry 2004;161: 271–7.
14. Empana JP, Sykes DH, Luc G, et al. for the PRIME Study Group. Contributions of depressive mood and circulating inflammatory markers to coronary heart disease in healthy European men: the Prospective Epidemiological Study of Myocardial Infarction (PRIME). Circulation 2005;111:2299–305.
15. Sherwood A, Hinderliter AL, Watkins LL, et al. Impaired endothelial function in coronary heart disease patients with depressive symptomatology. J Am Coll Cardiol 2005;46:656–9.
16. Bruce EC, Musselman DL. Depression, alterations in platelet function, and ischemic heart disease. Psychosom Med 2005;67:S34–6.
17. Vaccarino V, Johnson BD, Sheps DS, et al. Depression, inflammation, and incident cardiovascular disease in women with suspected coronary ischemia, The National Heart, Lung and Blood Institute-sponsored coronary ischemia. J Am Coll Cardiol 2007;50:2044–50.
18. Carney M, Freedland KE, Stein PK, et al. Effects of depression on QT interval variability after myocardial infarction. Psychosom Med 2003;65(2):177–80.
19. Carney RM, Freedland KE, Veith RC. Depression, the autonomic nervous system, and coronary heart disease. Psychosom Med 2005;67(Suppl 1): S29–33.
20. Empana JP, Jouven X, Lemaitre RN, et al. Clinical depression and risk of out-of-hospital cardiac arrest. Arch Intern Med 2006;166:195–200.
21. Whang W, Albert CM, Sears SF Jr, et al. for the TOVA Study Investigators. Depression as a predictor for appropriate shocks among patients with implantable cardioverter-defibrillators: results from the Triggers of Ventricular Arrhythmias (TOVA) study. J Am Coll Cardiol 2005;45:1090–5.
22. Whang W, Kubzansky LD, Kawachi I, et al. Depression and risk of sudden cardiac death and coronary heart disease in women: results from the Nurses' Health Study. J Am Coll Cardiol 2009;53:950–8.
23. Ford DE, Mead LA, Chang PP, et al. Depression is a risk factor for coronary artery disease in men: the precursors study. Arch Intern Med 1998;158:1422–6.
24. Anda R, Williamson D, Jones D, et al. Depressed affect, hopelessness, and the risk of ischemic heart disease in a cohort of US adults. Epidemiology 1993;4:285–94.
25. Barefoot JC, Schroll M. Symptoms of depression, acute myocardial infarction, and total mortality in a community sample. Circulation 1996;93:1976–80.
26. Agatisa PK, Matthews KA, Bromberger JT, et al. Coronary and aortic calcification in women with a history of major depression. Arch Intern Med 2005;165:1229–36.
27. Stewart JC, Janicki DL, Muldoon MF, et al. Negative emotions and 3-year progression of subclinical atherosclerosis. Arch Gen Psychiatry 2007;64: 225–33.
28. Elovainio M, Keltikangas-Jarvinen L, Kivimaki M, et al. Depressive symptoms and carotid artery intima-media thickness in young adults: the Cardiovascular Risk in Young Finns Study. Psychosom Med 2005;67:561–7.
29. Frasure-Smith N, Lesperance F. Depression and cardiac risk: present status and future directions. Postgrad Med J 2010;86:193–6.
30. Frasure-Smith N, Lespérance F, Talajic M. Depression following myocardial infarction. Impact on 6-month survival. JAMA 1993;270:1819–25.
31. Frasure-Smith N, Lesperance F, Juneau M, et al. Gender, depression, and one-year prognosis after myocardial infarction. Psychosom Med 1999;61: 26–37.
32. Lespérance F, Frasure-Smith N, Talajic M, et al. Five-year risk of cardiac mortality in relation to initial severity and one-year changes in depression symptoms after myocardial infarction. Circulation 2002; 105:1049–53.
33. Mallik S, Spertus JA, Reid KJ, et al. Depressive symptoms after acute myocardial infarction: evidence for highest rates in younger women. Arch Intern Med 2006;166:876–83 for the PREMIER Registry Investigators.
34. Parashar S, Rumsfeld JS, Reid KJ, et al. Impact of depression on sex differences in outcome after myocardial infarction. Circ Cardiovasc Qual Outcomes 2009;2:33–40.
35. Gottlieb SS, Khatta M, Friedman E, et al. The influence of age, gender, and race on the prevalence of depression in heart failure patients. J Am Coll Cardiol 2004;43:1542–9.
36. Rieckmann N, Gerin W, Kronish IM, et al. Course of depressive symptoms and medication adherence

after acute coronary syndromes: an electronic medication monitoring study. J Am Coll Cardiol 2006;48: 2218–22.

37. Gehi A, Haas D, Pipkin S, et al. Depression and medication adherence in outpatients with coronary heart disease: findings from the Heart and Soul Study. Arch Intern Med 2005;165:2508–13.
38. Lichtman JH, Bigger JT, Blumenthal JA, et al. Depression and coronary heart disease: recommendations for screening, referral, and treatment. Circulation 2008;118:1768–75.
39. Whooley MA, Simon GE. Managing depression in medical outpatients. N Engl J Med 2000;343: 1942–50.
40. Rutledge T, Vaccarino V, Johnson BD, et al. Depression and cardiovascular health care costs among women with suspected myocardial ischemia: prospective results from the WISE (Women's Ischemia Syndrome Evaluation) study. J Am Coll Cardiol 2009;53:176–83.
41. Balady GJ, Williams MA, Ades PA, et al. Core components of cardiac rehabilitation/secondary prevention programs: 2007 update: a scientific statement from the American Heart Association Exercise, Cardiac Rehabilitation, and Prevention Committee, the Council on Clinical Cardiology; the Councils on Cardiovascular Nursing, Epidemiology and Prevention, and Nutrition, Physical Activity, and Metabolism; and the American Association of Cardiovascular and Pulmonary Rehabilitation. Circulation 2007;115:2675–82.
42. Mosca L, Banka CL, Benjamin EJ, et al. Expert Panel/Writing Group. American Heart Association. American Academy of Family Physicians. American College of Obstetricians and Gynecologists. American College of Cardiology Foundation. Society of Thoracic Surgeons. American Medical Women's Association. Centers for Disease Control and Prevention. Office of Research on Women's Health. Association of Black Cardiologists. American College of Physicians. World Heart Federation. National Heart, Lung, and Blood Institute. American College of Nurse Practitioners. Evidence-based guidelines for cardiovascular disease prevention in women: 2007 update. Circulation 2007;115: 1481–501.
43. Taylor RS, Brown A, Ebrahim S, et al. Exercise-based rehabilitation for patients with coronary heart disease: systematic review and meta-analysis of randomized controlled trials. Am J Med 2004;116: 682–92.
44. Milani RV, Lavie CJ. Impact of cardiac rehabilitation on depression and its associated mortality. Am J Med 2007;120:799–806.
45. Jackson L, Leclerc J, Erskine Y, et al. Getting the most out of cardiac rehabilitation: a review of referral and adherence predictors. Heart 2005;91:10–4.
46. Allen JK, Scott LB, Stewart KJ, et al. Disparities in women's referral to and enrollment in outpatient cardiac rehabilitation. J Gen Intern Med 2004;19: 747–53.
47. Rolfe DE, Sutton EJ, Landry M, et al. Women's experiences accessing a women-centered cardiac rehabilitation program: a qualitative study. J Cardiovasc Nurs 2010;25:332–41.
48. Glassman AH, O'Connor CM, Califf RM, et al. Sertraline Antidepressant Heart Attack Randomized Trial (SADHEART) Group. Sertraline treatment of major depression in patients with acute MI or unstable angina. JAMA 2002;288:701–9.
49. Berkman LF, Blumenthal J, Burg M, et al. Effects of treating depression and low perceived social support on clinical events after myocardial infarction: the Enhancing Recovery in Coronary Heart Disease Patients (ENRICHD) randomized trial. JAMA 2003;289:3106–16.
50. Taylor CB, Youngblood ME, Catellier D, et al. Effects of antidepressant medication on morbidity and mortality in depressed patients after myocardial infarction. Arch Gen Psychiatry 2005;62:792–8.
51. Leifheit-Limson EC, Reid KJ, Kasl SV, et al. The role of social support in health status and depressive symptoms after acute myocardial infarction: evidence for a stronger relationship among women. Circ Cardiovasc Qual Outcomes 2010;3:143–50.
52. Murray CJ, Lopez AD. Global mortality, disability, and the contribution of risk factors: Global Burden of Disease Study. Lancet 1997;349:1436–42.

Later-Life Depression and Heart Failure

Susan M. Maixner, MD[a,*], Laura Struble, PhD, GNP, BC[a,b], Mary Blazek, MD[a], Helen C. Kales, MD[a,c,d]

KEYWORDS

• Mood disorders • Aged • Comorbidity

Mrs B, a 76-year-old married woman with New York Heart Association class II, American College of Cardiology stage C heart failure (HF), hypertension, hyperlipidemia, hypothyroidism, and osteoarthritis, was referred to a geriatric psychiatrist for anxiety. She was a caregiver for her 81-year-old husband, who had Alzheimer disease. The onset of her anxiety was approximately 4 months previously, when she had required more aggressive therapy for her HF. An echocardiogram showed a left ventricular ejection fraction of greater than 55%. She reported anxiety attacks and extreme worry that her prognosis was fatal, and that her husband would be placed in a nursing home. She feared leaving her husband alone, and had missed several doctor appointments. She did not tolerate fluoxetine started by her cardiologist, and had been requiring escalating doses of benzodiazepines (alprazolam), without improvement. She had developed initial insomnia, and had recently been prescribed a sleeping medication, zolpidem, by her primary care physician.

She had been independent in both basic (eg, dressing, bathing) and instrumental (eg, cooking, driving) activities of daily living; however, in the past 2 months, her daughter had begun to oversee bill paying and setting up medicines after Mrs B received a shut-off notice for nonpayment of 2 utility bills, and medication errors occurred for both the patient and her husband.

Mrs B denied feeling sad or having crying spells. However, she admitted to anhedonia; she no longer enjoyed her grandchildren's visits and had stopped attending her weekly card club. She had trouble falling and staying asleep, and described ruminative worries. Her energy level was low. Mrs B had not kept to a low-sodium diet and did not weigh herself daily. She had lost 20 pounds in the previous year, but had gained 5 pounds since she last weighed herself 2 weeks previously. She had difficulty making decisions (eg, what to wear or what to cook), and trouble with concentration, but she denied memory problems. She felt "frantic" from the time she got up until after dinner, but denied classic panic attack symptoms. She had a "short fuse," often losing her temper with her husband. She felt guilty, hopeless, helpless, and worthless. She felt ambivalent about being alive, and even prayed to die in her sleep. However, religious beliefs and duty to her family precluded any active suicidal ideation.

Past psychiatric history was significant for postpartum depression after the birth of her third child, which was treated with electroconvulsive therapy. Her family history included 3 siblings with cardiovascular disease, a daughter with depression, a son with generalized anxiety disorder, and a grandson with bipolar disorder. Her husband required supervision because of his dementia. Her daughter lived 24 km (15 miles) away, whereas

[a] Section of Geriatric Psychiatry, Department of Psychiatry, University of Michigan, 4250 Plymouth Road, Ann Arbor, MI 48109-2700, USA
[b] Division of Acute, Critical, and Long-term Care, School of Nursing, 400 North Ingalls Building , Ann Arbor, MI 48109-5482, USA
[c] Department of Veterans Affairs, Ann Arbor Center of Excellence (COE), 4250 Plymouth Road, Ann Arbor, MI 48109-2700, USA
[d] Department of Veterans Affairs, Serious Mental Illness Treatment, Research, and Evaluation Center (SMITREC), 4250 Plymouth Road, Ann Arbor, MI 48109-2700, USA
* Corresponding author.
E-mail address: smaixner@umich.edu

Heart Failure Clin 7 (2011) 47–58
doi:10.1016/j.hfc.2010.08.009
1551-7136/11/$ – see front matter

her 2 sons lived an hour away. At least one child visited weekly. She was a lifelong nonsmoker and nondrinker.

Results of workup and physical examination including checks of complete blood count, thyroid-stimulating hormone, vitamin B_{12}, folic acid, electrolytes, and renal and hepatic functions were within normal limits. A Folstein Mini-Mental State Examination (MMSE) was administered and Mrs B scored 25 (out of a possible 30 points, missing 2 of the short-term memory items at 3-minute recall, one of the attention items, and orientation to exact date and day).

Cognitive-behavioral therapy focusing on her anxiety and depressive rumination was recommended, but the patient refused. Citalopram was started at 10 mg, and after 1 week increased to 20 mg. Six weeks after antidepressant initiation, she felt slightly less anxious, was more tolerant of her husband, made decisions more easily, and her appetite had begun to improve. Alprazolam was tapered by 0.25 mg/wk to 0.25 mg twice daily, but she did not tolerate a further reduction because of residual anxiety symptoms. Her citalopram was then titrated to 40 mg over 2 weeks. Cognitive-behavioral therapy was again discussed with the patient, and she agreed to this in a group setting. Six weeks later, she was able to discontinue alprazolam after a gradual taper. Initial insomnia returned with discontinuation of zolpidem, so trazodone was initiated at 50 to 100 mg as needed at bedtime. She reported improvement in her anxiety and depressive symptoms. She enlisted more assistance from her children, and was also referred to her county's Area Agency on Aging to locate additional resources for her husband's care. Her guilty feelings remitted and she returned to her previous activities.

Using the case of Mrs B, this article: (1) highlights depression criteria, prevalence, and later-life depression (LLD) presentations; (2) discusses factors contributing to LLD; (3) reviews the interplay between HF and LLD; and (4) suggests screening and treatment recommendations for depression in patients with HF.

LLD: PREVALENCE AND SCOPE OF THE PROBLEM

Depression is the most common psychiatric disorder in the geriatric population, with prevalence estimates of up to 3% in the general population and 12% in medical settings.[1] By 2030, depressive disorders, followed by ischemic heart disease, are projected to be the top 2 causes of disability and disease burden among developed countries worldwide.[2] LLD is associated with increased morbidity and mortality as well as with medical burden, health-service use, longer hospital stays, and disability. With the interplay of medical, psychiatric, and psychosocial factors, detection can be difficult. However, treatments for depression among elderly people do exist, and approximately 60% of depressed older adults recover within 6 months, which is comparable with younger patients.[3]

RELATIONSHIP OF LLD TO MEDICAL ILLNESS

The hallmark of LLD is medical comorbidity.[4] Medical illness is common in elderly patients who have LLD, with 88% of such patients diagnosed with at least one significant medical disorder, and 48% having 3 or more.[5] The prevalence of major depression increases in clinical settings that are marked by high levels of medical illness and physical disability, with rates of major depression less than 3% among elderly people in the community, 10% to 12% in inpatient medical settings,[1] and 20% to 25% among cognitively intact patients in nursing homes.[6] Whereas some illness-specific cohorts, such as patients with coronary heart disease (CHD), seem to have higher than expected rates of depression,[7] in other elderly patients specific medical illnesses are less important than overall medical burden and degree of functional disability. Medical illness has been documented as the most powerful predictor of poor outcomes in patients with LLD. However, depression itself may delay recovery by decreasing motivation and compliance and interfering with rehabilitation, thus prolonging hospitalizations.

LLD AND HF

Over the past 25 years, the importance of screening for depression in patients with heart disease, specifically following acute myocardial infarction and in CHD, has been established. In 2008, the American Heart Association, with the endorsement of the American Psychiatric Association, published recommendations for screening, referral, and treatment of depressive symptoms in patients with CHD.[8] The link between depression and CHD has prompted investigators to explore the relationship between depression and other forms of cardiac disease.

There is an epidemic of HF in the United States that carries serious clinical, psychological, and societal consequences.[9] Studies show high rates of depression in HF compared with the general population.[10–13] The prevalence of depressive symptoms in patients with HF encompasses a wide but high range across studies. A meta-analysis found the prevalence of depression in patients with HF was 21.5%, 4 times the prevalence in the general population.[14] Other research found depressive-symptom prevalence ranging from 13% to 48% in outpatients with HF[15–17] and 35% to 70% in hospitalized patients.[18] The wide range in prevalence estimates likely reflects studies using different diagnostic criteria for HF and depression, in addition to different subject inclusion criteria such as age, gender, and disease severity.[18] Differences in study measurements and design may also explain some of the variance. Depressive symptoms were associated with a worse prognosis, a 2-fold risk of mortality, and increased readmissions compared with patients without depressive symptoms.[11,19] Increased depression has also been directly related to increased health care use, which is more evident with longer follow-up.[20]

The relationship between HF and depression reflects the complex nature of both disease processes. Patients with HF may score higher on depression ratings because self-reported estimates reflect somatic symptoms possibly unrelated to mood.[21] It may be difficult to know whether a particular symptom, such as fatigue, is related to depression, a coexisting medical illness, or both.[22,23] However, evidence suggests a shared pathophysiology between depressive symptoms and HF, including neuroendocrine abnormalities, arrhythmias, elaboration of inflammatory cytokines, and platelet aggregation.[24,25]

Depression often creates significant functional limitations in people without chronic medical conditions.[26] Depression in HF has been associated with reduced functional ability and physical inactivity, which in turn are associated with higher mortality.[27] Therefore, functional limitations from HF and depression may have an additive effect, and successful treatment of depression may improve the patients' level of functioning.[13]

DEPRESSION SYMPTOMS: REVIEW, PRESENTATIONS OF LLD, OVERLAP WITH HF

Major depressive disorder is an illness characterized by at least 2 weeks with 5 or more of the following symptoms (including at least one cardinal symptom): either depressed mood or anhedonia (cardinal symptoms) as well as sleep disturbance, appetite change, reduced energy, decreased interest, guilt feelings (which may include hopelessness, helplessness, worthlessness, or feeling like a burden), psychomotor agitation or retardation, impairment in concentration or decision making, and thoughts of death or suicide.[28] Psychosis may be present. In older adults, cognitive impairment is often seen, although not a criterion. Minor depression/subsyndromal depressive symptoms are also often clinically significant.[29,30] A noteworthy number of older adults present with their first depressive episode in later life, and late-onset depression is more often associated with medical comorbidities.[31]

Depression detection can be more challenging in elderly people. As shown by Mrs B, a significant number of patients with LLD may deny a depressed mood. However, anhedonia (inability to feel pleasure) and most other depressive symptoms are endorsed. The denial of sadness in older adults has been coined masked depression and may be a cohort effect in the current elderly population.[32] Often, anxiety, cognitive issues, and pain/somatic symptoms are a proxy for a depressed mood. This situation shows the necessity of further questioning about depression symptoms, even if sadness is denied.

The 2 depressive symptoms most frequently reported in patients with HF are fatigue and sleep problems.[33] Thus, the overlap of fatigue as a symptom is important to consider in assessment. Sleep disturbances are less likely to evoke stigma/denial, increasing accuracy of patient symptom reports.[34] Other common symptoms of chronic HF that overlap with depressive/anxiety symptoms include shortness of breath, drowsiness, cognitive problems, nocturia (worsening insomnia), weight loss, palpitations, and exercise intolerance.

ADDITIONAL FEATURES UNIQUE TO LLD

Vascular Depression

The linkage of late-onset depression with brain changes on magnetic resonance imaging (white-matter hyperintensities [WMHs]) was noted beginning in the late 1980s.[35] Fujikawa and colleagues[36] described finding silent stroke in most patients with late-onset major depression, notably in the absence of family history of depressive illness or psychosocial stressors. Mounting evidence led to the proposal of the vascular depression hypothesis (VDH) in 1997 by Alexopoulos and colleagues.[37] The VDH describes depression with the following characteristics: (1) late age of onset (after age 65 years) or change in course after early onset; (2) persistent symptoms; and (3) the association of depression with vascular disease or vascular risk factors and diffuse or multifocal cerebrovascular lesions. Indirect support for the VDH includes: high rates of depression in patients with hypertension, hyperlipidemia, and coronary artery disease; the high rate of poststroke depression; the frequency of silent stroke and WMHs in late-onset depression[36,37]; and the infrequent family history of depression found in those with depression and silent stroke.[37]

Cognitive Impairment and Executive Dysfunction

Executive dysfunction is prominent in LLD, involving compromised integrity of frontal structures and subcortical connections (striatofrontal dysfunction[38]) and manifests as impairments in planning, organization, problem solving, and abstraction. Although it is not the only cause of executive dysfunction, ischemic brain damage is believed to be a major potential contributor to such conditions.[39] Other disorders causing executive dysfunction include those affecting subcortical structures, such as Parkinson disease, and other causes involving degeneration of the basal ganglia. Studies of patients with executive dysfunction[39] or vascular depression[40] indicate that these patients have a poorer and delayed response to antidepressants, decreased long-term recovery, increased relapse risk, and more adverse events and disability.

Cognitive impairment is a key feature of HF.[41] The cognitive issues with executive dysfunction in HF may share similar conditions with vascular depression and, as in Mrs B, may manifest as medication noncompliance and difficulty managing finances.

Anxiety

Somatic symptoms are a core feature of anxiety disorders in older patients. Depression associated with clinically significant anxiety, primarily generalized anxiety disorder, or subsyndromal anxiety characterized by generalized anxiety or panic symptoms is found in approximately half of older outpatients with depression.[42] Anxious individuals may be hypervigilant regarding their bodily sensations, and may overestimate the dangerousness of medications or the severity of side effects.[42] Older patients with anxious depression frequently misattribute somatic symptoms of anxiety to adverse medication effects, contributing to both dropout and poor response in antidepressant treatment trials.[43] In addition, older adults with anxiety and a somatic focus may tend to discount psychological explanations for psychiatric symptoms and refuse treatment.[42] Anxious depression is associated with higher rates of suicidality in older patients.[43] However, comorbid anxiety is also modifiable; one study[44] found that psychic and somatic symptoms of anxiety were among the symptoms showing greatest change during adequate antidepressant treatment of LLD. Mrs B described nearly constant generalized anxiety symptoms. These symptoms created an increased reliance on the use of benzodiazepines "to get through the day." In addition, it was believed that the benzodiazepines were contributing to cognitive difficulties, as well as to a potential risk of falling.

Nonadherence

Although rates of antidepressant treatment among elderly patients have increased with the availability of newer antidepressants, among those who begin treatment, nonadherence ranges from 40% to 75%.[45] Although providers are increasingly diagnosing depression and recommending treatment of older patients, there needs to be greater effort to ensure that patients initiate and continue appropriate care throughout the course of their depressive illness.[45] Preliminary data from the Primary Care Research in Substance Abuse and Mental Health for Elderly study suggest that most older adults surveyed from a random primary care sample believe that depression is a medical illness.[46] However, only 50% were willing to take an antidepressant. One study showed that stigma affected treatment discontinuation in older patients, not in younger patients.[47] Complexity of the medication regimen as a result of medical comorbidity may also be associated with decreased medication adherence in elderly patients. Other illness factors that may affect adherence to LLD medication include depression severity, comorbid substance abuse, and cognitive impairment.[45] Adherence is predicated on taking the correct amount of medication at the correct times; intact memory and executive function are needed for these tasks. Nonadherence because of cognitive issues can be improved by the use of pillboxes, caregiver support, and newer technologies such as medication alarm reminder systems; such technologies may have been helpful for Mrs B.

Psychosocial Components

Psychosocial changes occurring in later life include: losses (the death of loved ones or increasing disability); role transitions (retirement, dependency, or caregiving); and changes in social contacts and support networks (as a result of moves and deaths). Although most of these stressors are met with resilience, some increase the risk of depression in later life.[48–50] There is limited research on the effect of many of these psychosocial changes. However, there is ample clinical evidence that these factors may be contributors to poor depression outcomes, including treatment resistance. Widowhood carries a significant risk of bereavement. In the first month after being widowed, about 33% of people are depressed by DSM (Diagnostic and Statistical Manual of Mental Disorders) criteria.[48] Six months following the death of a spouse, about 25% of the survivors still meet depression criteria, with about 15% still being depressed at 13 months.[48] As shown by Mrs B's case, caregivers carry an increased risk for depression, often neglecting their own medical, dental, and mental-health needs. In addition, the caregiving responsibilities may lead to inadequate sleep and nutrition. Social contacts can be reduced as well because of the intensity of the workload. In one meta-analysis, caregivers' rates of major depressive disorder were approximately 22%.[49] Spousal caregivers are believed to be at higher risk of depression because of their older age and medical comorbidities. Caregivers also pay the ultimate price for providing care because of the increased risk of heart disease and higher mortality.[51–54]

Financial issues may also affect the course and treatment of depression. A patient may choose not to fill a medication because of cost. They may not be able to afford a higher copay for mental-health treatment. Although the latter issue may eventually be addressed by parity legislation, it remains a reality for many patients.

Specific to patients with HF, it has been reported that sociodemographic factors increase the likelihood of depression.[55] Depression is associated with higher rates of nonadherence and lower levels of social support, both of which worsen prognosis in HF. However, in an examination of sociodemographic variables relating depression to HF, marital status and living arrangement variables did not show significant differences.[33] Given the lack of effect of these environmental and social factors, these investigators concluded that their results suggested a stronger biologic connection between HF and depression.

TREATMENT OF LLD

Screening and Detection

The American Heart Association has published recommendations for screening for depressive symptoms in patients with CHD (**Fig. 1**).[9] Until specific recommendations can be made for HF, we suggest extrapolating these to the population of patients with HF. The PHQ-2 is the minimum suggested screening instrument for depression, which consists of the first two questions of the PHQ-9, inquiring about anhedonia and depressed mood. If either question is affirmed, then the PHQ-9 should be administered.[56] The PHQ-9, a 9-item depression scale subset of the longer, well-validated Patient Health Questionnaire, is a reliable and valid measure of depression severity (**Fig. 2**).[57] Cognitive status should also be evaluated via screening. The MMSE[58] is a well-studied instrument, but the Montreal Cognitive Assessment[59] detects more frontal and executive dysfunction.

Depression seems to increase the risk of cardiovascular morbidity and mortality, although no evidence exists that depression treatment can alter the cardiovascular morbidity and mortality associated with depression in CHD or HF. Treatment can relieve the suffering of depression in its own right, and improve quality of life.[60] Four time points in HF management have been recommended to identify and treat depression: (1) at the initial diagnosis of HF; (2) if the patient manifests persistent nonadherence; (3) in the case of persistent patient reports of cardiac symptoms unexplained by objective testing; and (4) if the patient reports chronic sleep problems or fatigue.[34] During hospitalization, the initial goals for older adults with acute HF and depression are accurate assessment and pharmacologic treatment of depression. Classic symptoms of depression are often overlooked because patients ascribe somatic symptoms to their heart disease and overlook the emotional associations. Cardiac patients' complaints that suggest an underlying depression include: unusual and chronic tiredness or lack of energy; recent onset of irritability or anger; feeling under stress; weight loss without dieting; and insomnia.[61,62]

General Treatment Considerations

Investigations of pharmacologic and nonpharmacologic treatments of LLD in HF are still in the early stages and thus there are limited data on the use of specific treatment modalities. Treatment must be guided by experience when depression is present in patients with CHD, taking into consideration the cardiovascular effects of specific antidepressant drugs. The axiom of treatment of LLD is "start low, go slow, but don't stop." The last phrase is added because many older patients may receive suboptimal doses over a long period, but older patients with depression may require doses similar to those prescribed to younger patients but titrated more slowly.[63]

In later life, considering other causes of mood disturbance besides depression assists with the differential of LLD. A careful examination, review of medications, and symptom chronology guide the clinician to the correct diagnosis. Remembering the 4 Ds (delirium, depression, dementia, and drugs [medication effect]) is useful. Delirium

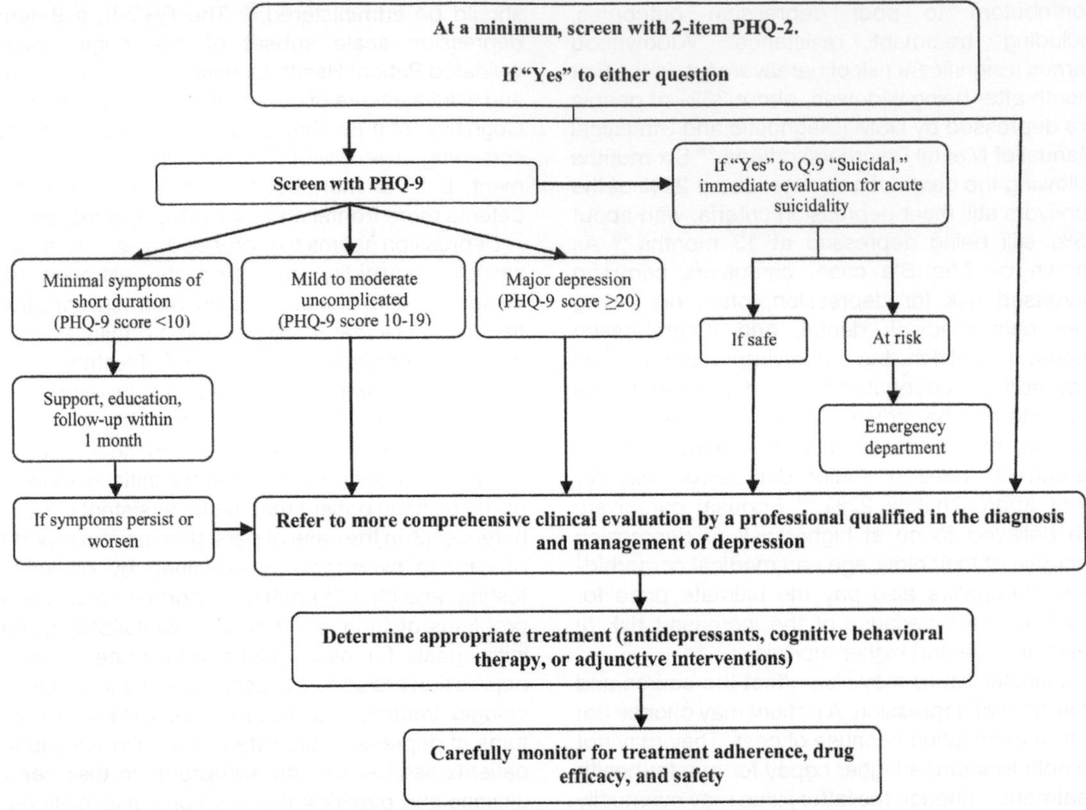

Fig. 1. American Heart Association/American Psychiatric Association recommendations for screening for depression in patients with coronary heart disease.[10] (*From* Lichtman J, Bigger JT, Blumenthal J, et al. Depression and coronary heart disease: recommendations for screening, referral, and treatment: a science advisory from the American Heart Association Prevention Committee of the Council on Cardiovascular Nursing, Council on Clinical Cardiology, Council on Epidemiology and Prevention, and Interdisciplinary Council on Quality of Care and Outcomes Research: endorsed by the American Psychiatric Association. Circulation 2008;118(17):1770; with permission.)

onset is usually within days and is associated with a fluctuating level of consciousness. The onset of depression is usually weeks to months. For a (nonvascular) dementia, onset is typically months to years.

Often treatment goals are not met during an inpatient stay because of shortened hospital stays, changes in physician reimbursement, and lack of continuity.[64] Although judged clinically stable, patients newly discharged from the hospital recovering from an HF exacerbation may show many psychosocial and behavioral risk factors for rehospitalization. Education and psychological support should always accompany an antidepressant prescription. Patient understanding of the side-effect profile and the importance of continuing the medication at home may increase adherence to treatment.[61,62] Use of a comprehensive transitional-care model approach acknowledges the chronicity of HF and the need for continuity of care.[65,66] In a randomized, controlled trial, a 3-month protocol was developed for advanced practice nurse involvement in discharge-planning and home follow-up.[65] The results showed an increased length of time between hospital discharge and readmission or death, reduced total number of rehospitalizations, and decreased health care costs.

Nonpharmacologic Treatments

Psychotherapy

Evidenced-based psychological treatments for depression with the most empiric support are cognitive-behavioral therapy (CBT), interpersonal therapy, and problem-solving therapy (PST).[67–69] Only CBT and PST have been evaluated as stand-alone treatments in LLD. The theoretic assumption behind CBT and PST is that human behaviors are learned, and interventions use strategies related to changing how people process information from their psychosocial environment

PHQ9P

PATIENT HEALTH QUESTIONNAIRE-9				
Over the <u>last 2 weeks</u>, how often have you been bothered by any of the following problems?	**Not at all**	**Several days**	**More than half the days**	**Nearly every day**
1. Little interest or pleasure in doing things	0	1	2	3
2. Feeling down, depressed, or hopeless	0	1	2	3
3. Trouble falling or staying asleep, or sleeping too much	0	1	2	3
4. Feeling tired or having little energy	0	1	2	3
5. Poor appetite or overeating	0	1	2	3
6. Feeling bad about yourself — or that you are a failure or have let yourself or your family down	0	1	2	3
7. Trouble concentrating on things, such as reading the newspaper or watching television	0	1	2	3
8. Moving or speaking so slowly that other people could have noticed? Or the opposite — being so fidgety or restless that you have been moving around a lot more than usual	0	1	2	3
9. Thoughts that you would be better off dead or of hurting yourself in some way	0	1	2	3
	FOR OFFICE CODING			
	0 + ____	+ ____	+ ____	
	=Total Score: ____			

If you checked off <u>any</u> problems, how <u>difficult</u> have these problems made it for you to do your work, take care of things at home, or get along with other people?

Not difficult at all	Somewhat difficult	Very difficult	Extremely difficult
☐	☐	☐	☐

Fig. 2. PHQ-9.[56] (*From* Kroenke K, Spitzer RL, Williams JB. The PHQ-9: validity of a brief depression severity measure. J Gen Intern Med 2001;16(9):606–13. PRIME-MD is a trademark of Pfizer Inc. Copyright 1999 Pfizer Inc. All rights reserved. Reproduced with permission.)

(cognitive restructuring), problem solving and communication-skill building, and mood reregulation (behavioral activation). The processes of behavioral and affective change are different in CBT (affect and cognitive regulation skills) and PST (improving problem-resolution skills).[67] PST may hold particular promise in patients with LLD and executive dysfunction.[69] Clinically, psychological treatments are often combined with pharmacologic treatments but research on combined treatments lags behind practice.

Enhancing social support

Encouraging natural support systems such as family, church, and social or interest groups (eg, bridge and book clubs) builds a stronger social-support system necessary for improved clinical outcomes in HF and depression. In addition, formal support groups, such as HF support groups, provide opportunities for patients to connect with others who have similar concerns, which relieves stress. Community services can be located through each county's Area Agency on Aging, and include visiting nurses, elder care workers, social workers, physical and occupation therapists, rehabilitation specialists, Meals on Wheels, and legal services.

Exercise

Exercise is increasingly recognized as an important part of enhancing mood[70] and memory in later life.[71] Exercise training in patients with stable HF, under the supervision of a trained cardiac rehabilitation team, has been shown to be safe and effective in decreasing anxiety and depression.[72]

Palliative care

HF is the result of cardiovascular disease. It is chronic, and eventually terminal. Honest discussions regarding the progressive nature of HF, including the patient's preferences and expectations, help patients plan for future needs, including advance directives. In a prospective study of individual preference for HF treatment, patients preferred improved symptom control over longer survival time.[73] Palliative care expands the medical-disease model of care to include goals for enhancing quality of life of patients and their families, optimizing function, helping with decision making, and providing opportunities for personal growth.[74] Life-prolonging medical care and palliative care can be delivered concurrently. A multidisciplinary team approach for end-stage HF that includes physician, advanced practice nurse, social work, and spiritual and/or psychological support in either inpatient or outpatient settings provides patients with their last wishes in the environment that they choose.[75]

Pharmacologic Treatment

Initial pharmacologic treatment

First-line pharmacologic treatment continues to be the class of selective serotonin reuptake inhibitors (SSRIs). These drugs have little effect on cardiac functioning other than mild slowing of the heart rate, which is clinically insignificant. Caution should be exercised in patients taking medications that decrease heart rate, especially β-blockers. Interest has been shown in the ability of SSRIs to reduce platelet activation, which may add benefit to patients with coronary disease.[76,77]

In the case of Mrs B, the first choice of antidepressant may have been problematic. As noted in the section on comorbid anxiety, such patients are often prone to attribution of somatic symptoms of anxiety to adverse medication effects, contributing to both dropout and poor response.[42] Thus, the choice of fluoxetine was not optimal in an elderly patient with anxiety. Given that all SSRIs have similar mechanisms of action, the choice should be made based on side-effect and pharmacokinetic profiles. Citalopram or sertraline are the top antidepressant choices for LLD in expert consensus guidelines. Among SSRIs, they have more benign side effect profiles and lower risk of drug interactions compared to fluoxetine or paroxetine.[78] SSRIs are also first-line in dementia with depression,[79] and depression with anxiety.

Other important considerations are to ensure that the patient has a trial of adequate dose and duration (eg, 6 weeks or longer); many antidepressants trials lack this and result in poorer response.[63] With anxiety symptoms, the time to treatment response may be longer, up to 12 weeks, and may require a higher SSRI dose.

Advanced pharmacologic management

After initial treatment of adequate dose and duration and limited response, one could switch to another antidepressant. Choices include a different SSRI, a serotonin-norepinephrine reuptake inhibitor (eg, venlafaxine or duloxetine), bupropion, or mirtazapine.[78] Switching may be preferable to augmentation because the patient only has to take one antidepressant, resulting in better compliance and fewer drug interactions and side effects.[80] A switch to bupropion would not likely be helpful in a case of anxious depression. Mirtazapine may be helpful in patients with reduced sleep and appetite.

Tricyclic antidepressants (TCAs) should not be used as first-line treatment in patients with ischemic heart disease, but are sometimes used only in patients with severe depression who have not responded to other treatments.[81] They can increase the risk of arrhythmias, particularly in patients with HF. Cardiovascular side effects of TCAs include orthostatic hypotension, delayed cardiac conduction through the A-V node-His bundle with potential for heart block, and increased heart rate. TCAs have quinidinelike antiarrhythmic effects that have been shown to increase cardiac mortality in patients with ischemic heart disease. Nortriptyline and desipramine are the preferred TCAs in this population, because they have fewer anticholinergic effects.

In the case of partial antidepressant response, an augmentation or combination therapy strategy could be used.[78] Advantages of this strategy include: (1) maintaining improvements gained by the current antidepressant; (2) preventing a treatment delay when one antidepressant is stopped and another started; and (3) allowing for a longer overall antidepressant trial. Such an augmentation trial would best be undertaken in conjunction with a psychiatrist with ample experience in treating older patients with medical comorbidities. Augmentation strategies[82] include: (1) the addition of bupropion to an SSRI (response rates of > 50%; possible side effects include delirium and seizure); (2) lithium augmentation less than 0.5 mEq/L (use with extreme caution in patients with HF because of increased lithium levels with thiazide diuretics, angiotensin-converting enzyme inhibitors, and nonsteroidals); (3) the use of antipsychotic medication (cautions because of metabolic syndrome, black-box warning in elderly demented patients, but necessary for psychotic depression); and (4) liothyronine T_3.

Vascular Depression

The VDH points to primary prevention of vascular disease, advising the discontinuation of smoking and excessive drinking, and modification of treatable vascular risk factors (eg, blood pressure, cholesterol level).[37] PST has shown improvements in vascular depression (see earlier discussion).

Depression and Comorbid Anxiety

SSRIs are the first-line treatment of anxious depression. If appropriately identified, anxious depression may be effectively managed via: (1) pretreatment accounting of physical symptoms of anxiety for comparison with later adverse effects, which may allow the patient to compare more objectively those physical symptoms that are new and may be drug-related with those that predated the medication and may be caused by the underlying illness; (2) altered antidepressant titration schedules (start low, go slow, aim high, treat long); (3) psychoeducation; (4) early supportive contact[42]; and (5) cognitive-behavioral treatment strategies. Such structured support of older patients with anxious depression may achieve outcomes similar to those achieved in patients without anxiety.[43]

Electroconvulsive Therapy

Electroconvulsive therapy (ECT) remains the most highly effective treatment of LLD and psychotic depression. Although ECT can cause retrograde and anterograde amnesia, it is often effective in the cognitively impaired patient.[83] Recovery rates from amnesia have been shown to be high in elderly patients. ECT can be used safely in patients with HF.[84]

Sedative/Hypnotic Use

Benzodiazepines are efficacious for anxiety but do not treat underlying depression. Older adults can become dependent on this class of medications, and are more sensitive to the adverse effects of cognitive impairment, falls, and hip fractures.[85] Once a response to antidepressant treatment occurs, the goal should be to taper off the benzodiazepines gradually and discontinue. Because this may not be possible in someone who has taken them for years, reduction to lowest effective dose may be an appropriate target for some patients. Interdose rebound anxiety is seen with short-acting agents such as alprazolam. If benzodiazepines must be used, lorazepam is preferred, because it has no active metabolites, it does not undergo phase 1 hepatic metabolism, and its short to medium half-life does not increase with age. Nonbenzodiazepine hypnotics, like Mrs B's zolpidem, are frequently prescribed for sleep in older adults. However, caution must be exercised because these agents have a risk for dependency, and have been associated with doubling the risk of hip fractures[86] and impaired driving in elderly patients.[87] Behavioral sleep therapy interventions, sleep hygiene measures, trazodone, or mirtazapine may be alternative strategies.

SUMMARY

Depression is common and problematic in older patients with HF. Future research is needed to examine the best ways to manage the challenge of older adults with HF and depression to improve quality of life and well-being among this growing population subgroup.

REFERENCES

1. Shanmugham B, Karp J, Drayer R, et al. Evidence-based pharmacologic interventions for geriatric depression. Psychiatr Clin North Am 2005;28(4): 821–35, viii.
2. Mathers CD, Loncar D. Projections of global mortality and burden of disease from 2002 to 2030. PLoS Med 2006;3(11):2011–30.
3. Alexopoulos GS, Meyers BS, Young RC, et al. Recovery in geriatric depression. Arch Gen Psychiatry 1996;53(4):305–12.
4. Friedhoff AJ, et al. Consensus development conference statement: diagnosis and treatment of depression in late life. In: Schneider LS, Reynolds CF III, Lebowitz BD, editors. Diagnosis and treatment of depression in late life. Results of the NIH consensus development conference. Washington, DC: American Psychiatric Press; 1992.

5. Lacro JP, Jeste DV. Physical comorbidity and polypharmacy in older psychiatric patients. Biol Psychiatry 1994;36(3):146–52.
6. Katz IR, Beaston-Wimmer P, Parmelee P, et al. Failure to thrive in the elderly: exploration of the concept and delineation of psychiatric components. J Geriatr Psychiatry Neurol 1993;6(3):161–9.
7. Alexopoulos GS. Interventions for depressed elderly primary care patients. Int J Geriatr Psychiatry 2001; 16(6):553–9.
8. Lichtman J, Bigger JT, Blumenthal J, et al. Depression and coronary heart disease: recommendations for screening, referral, and treatment: a science advisory from the American Heart Association Prevention Committee of the Council on Cardiovascular Nursing, Council on Clinical Cardiology, Council on Epidemiology and Prevention, and Interdisciplinary Council on Quality of Care and Outcomes Research: endorsed by the American Psychiatric Association. Circulation 2008;118(17): 1768–75.
9. Lloyd-Jones D, Adams RJ, Brown TM, et al. Heart disease and stroke statistics–2010 update: a report from the American Heart Association. Circulation 2010;121(7):e46–215.
10. Galbreath AD, Krasuski RA, Smith B, et al. Long-term healthcare and cost outcomes of disease management in a large, randomized, community-based population with heart failure. Circulation 2004;110(23):3518–26.
11. Jiang W, Alexander J, Christopher E, et al. Relationship of depression to increased risk of mortality and rehospitalization in patients with congestive heart failure. Arch Intern Med 2001;161(15):1849–56.
12. Vaccarino V, Kasl SV, Abramson J, et al. Depressive symptoms and risk of functional decline and death in patients with heart failure. J Am Coll Cardiol 2001;38(1):199–205.
13. Havranek EP, Ware MG, Lowes BD. Prevalence of depression in congestive heart failure. Am J Cardiol 1999;84(3):348–50, A349.
14. Rutledge T, Reis V, Linke S, et al. Depression in heart failure: a meta-analytic review of prevalence, intervention effects, and associations with clinical outcomes. J Am Coll Cardiol 2006;48(8):1527–37.
15. Rumsfeld J, Havranek E, Masoudi F, et al. Depressive symptoms are the strongest predictors of short-term declines in health status in patients with heart failure. J Am Coll Cardiol 2003;42(10):1811–7.
16. Gottlieb SS, Khatta M, Friedmann E, et al. The influence of age, gender, and race on the prevalence of depression in heart failure patients. J Am Coll Cardiol 2004;43(9):1542–9.
17. Gottlieb S, Kop W, Thomas S, et al. A double-blind placebo-controlled pilot study of controlled-release paroxetine on depression and quality of life in chronic heart failure. Am Heart J 2007;153(5):868–73.
18. O'Connor C, Joynt K. Depression: are we ignoring an important comorbidity in heart failure? J Am Coll Cardiol 2004;43(9):1550–2.
19. Jiang W, Kuchibhatla M, Clary G, et al. Relationship between depressive symptoms and long-term mortality in patients with heart failure. Am Heart J 2007;154(1):102–8.
20. Fulop G, Strain JJ, Stettin G. Congestive heart failure and depression in older adults: clinical course and health services use 6 months after hospitalization. Psychosomatics 2003;44(5):367–73.
21. Haworth JE, Moniz-Cook E, Clark AL, et al. Prevalence and predictors of anxiety and depression in a sample of chronic heart failure patients with left ventricular systolic dysfunction. Eur J Heart Fail 2005;7(5):803–8.
22. Noel PH, Williams JW Jr, Unutzer J, et al. Depression and comorbid illness in elderly primary care patients: impact on multiple domains of health status and well-being. Ann Fam Med 2004;2(6):555–62.
23. Katon WJ. Clinical and health services relationships between major depression, depressive symptoms, and general medical illness. Biol Psychiatry 2003; 54(3):216–26.
24. Joynt KE, Whellan DJ, O'Connor CM. Depression and cardiovascular disease: mechanisms of interaction. Biol Psychiatry 2003;54(3):248–61.
25. Kjaer A, Hesse B. Heart failure and neuroendocrine activation: diagnostic, prognostic and therapeutic perspectives. Clin Physiol 2001;21(6):661–72.
26. Wells KB, Stewart A, Hays RD, et al. The functioning and well-being of depressed patients. Results from the medical outcomes study. JAMA 1989;262(7):914–9.
27. Zuluaga MC, Guallar-Castillon P, Rodriguez-Pascual C, et al. Mechanisms of the association between depressive symptoms and long-term mortality in heart failure. Am Heart J 2010;159(2):231–7.
28. American Psychiatric Association. Diagnostic and statistical manual of mental disorders, Fourth edition, text revision. Washington, DC: American Psychiatric Association; 2000.
29. Lyness JM, Kim J, Tang W, et al. The clinical significance of subsyndromal depression in older primary care patients. Am J Geriatr Psychiatry 2007;15(3): 214–23.
30. Grabovich A, Lu N, Tang W, et al. Outcomes of subsyndromal depression in older primary care patients. Am J Geriatr Psychiatry 2010;18(3):227–35.
31. Blazer DG. Depression in late life: review and commentary. J Gerontol A Biol Sci Med Sci 2003; 58:249–65.
32. Blazer DG, editor. Diagnosis and treatment of depression in late life. St. Louis (MO): Mosby-Year Book; 1993.
33. Rohyans L, Pressler S. Depressive symptoms and heart failure: examining the sociodemographic variables. Clin Nurse Spec 2009;23(3):138–44.

34. Ketterer MW, Knysz W. Screening, diagnosis & monitoring of depression/distress in CHF patients. Heart Fail Rev 2009;14(1):1–5.
35. Krishnan KR, Goli V, Ellinwood EH, et al. Leukoencephalopathy in patients diagnosed as major depressive. Biol Psychiatry 1988;23(5):519–22.
36. Fujikawa T, Yamawaki S, Touhouda Y. Background factors and clinical symptoms of major depression with silent cerebral infarction. Stroke 1994;25(4):798–801.
37. Alexopoulos GS, Meyers BS, Young RC, et al. 'Vascular depression' hypothesis. Arch Gen Psychiatry 1997;54(10):915–22.
38. Tranel D, Andersen SW, Benton A. Development of the concept of "executive function" and its relationship to frontal lobes. In: Boller F, Spinnerler J, Hendler JA, editors. Handbook of neuropsychology. Amsterdam: Elsevier; 1994. p. 125–48.
39. Alexopoulos GS. New concepts for prevention and treatment of late-life depression. Am J Psychiatry 2001;158(6):835–8.
40. Simpson SW, Jackson A, Baldwin RC, et al. 1997 IPA/Bayer Research Awards in Psychogeriatrics. Subcortical hyperintensities in late-life depression: acute response to treatment and neuropsychological impairment. Int Psychogeriatr 1997;9(3):257–75.
41. Trojano L, Antonelli Incalzi R, Acanfora D, et al. Cognitive impairment: a key feature of congestive heart failure in the elderly. J Neurol 2003;250(12):1456–63.
42. Lenze EJ, Karp JF, Mulsant BH, et al. Somatic symptoms in late-life anxiety: treatment issues. J Geriatr Psychiatry Neurol 2005;18(2):89–96.
43. Lenze EJ, Mulsant BH, Dew MA, et al. Good treatment outcomes in late-life depression with comorbid anxiety. J Affect Disord 2003;77(3):247–54.
44. Nelson JC, Clary CM, Leon AC, et al. Symptoms of late-life depression: frequency and change during treatment. Am J Geriatr Psychiatry 2005;13(6):520–6.
45. Zivin K, Kales HC. Adherence to depression treatment in older adults: a narrative review. Drugs Aging 2008;25(7):559–71.
46. Oslin D, Zubritsky C, Katz I, et al. The impact of beliefs about depression among elderly primary care patients. American Association for Geriatric Psychiatry 16th Annual Meeting. Honolulu (HI), March 1–4, 2003.
47. Sirey JA, Bruce ML, Alexopoulos GS, et al. Perceived stigma as a predictor of treatment discontinuation in young and older outpatients with depression. Am J Psychiatry 2001;158(3):479–81.
48. Zisook S, Shuchter SR. Depression through the 1st year after the death of a spouse. Am J Psychiatry 1991;148(10):1346–52.
49. Cuijpers P. Depressive disorders in caregivers of dementia patients: a systematic review. Aging Ment Health 2005;9(4):325–30.
50. Oxman TE, Hull JG. Social support and treatment response in older depressed primary care patients. J Gerontol B Psychol Sci Soc Sci 2001;56(1):P35–45.
51. Shaw WS, Patterson TL, Ziegler MG, et al. Accelerated risk of hypertensive blood pressure recordings among Alzheimer caregivers. J Psychosom Res 1999;46(3):215–27.
52. Lee S, Colditz GA, Berkman LF, et al. Caregiving and risk of coronary heart disease in U.S. women: a prospective study. Am J Prev Med 2003;24(2):113–9.
53. Schulz R, Beach SR. Caregiving as a risk factor for mortality: the caregiver health effects study. JAMA 1999;282(23):2215–9.
54. Christakis NA, Allison PD. Mortality after the hospitalization of a spouse. N Engl J Med 2006;354(7):719–30.
55. Havranek EP, Spertus JA, Masoudi FA, et al. Predictors of the onset of depressive symptoms in patients with heart failure. J Am Coll Cardiol 2004;44(12):2333–8.
56. Whooley MA, Avins AL, Miranda J, et al. Case-finding instruments for depression: two questions are as good as many. J Gen Intern Med 1997;12:439–45.
57. Kroenke K, Spitzer RL, Williams JB. The PHQ-9: validity of a brief depression severity measure. J Gen Intern Med 2001;16(9):606–13.
58. Folstein MF, Robins LN, Helzer JE. The mini-mental state examination. Arch Gen Psychiatry 1983;40(7):812.
59. Nasreddine ZS, Phillips NA, Bedirian V, et al. The Montreal Cognitive Assessment, MoCA: a brief screening tool for mild cognitive impairment. J Am Geriatr Soc 2005;53(4):695–9.
60. Shapiro PA. Treatment of depression in patients with congestive heart failure. Heart Fail Rev 2009;14(1):7–12.
61. Lesperance F, Frasure-Smith N. Depression in patients with cardiac disease: a practical review. J Psychosom Res 2000;48(4–5):379–91.
62. Lesperance F, Frasure-Smith N, Juneau M, et al. Depression and 1-year prognosis in unstable angina. Arch Intern Med 2000;160(9):1354–60.
63. Mulsant BH, Alexopoulos GS, Reynolds CF, et al. Pharmacological treatment of depression in older primary care patients: the PROSPECT algorithm. Int J Geriatr Psychiatry 2001;16(6):585–92.
64. Fonarow GC. The Acute Decompensated Heart Failure National Registry (ADHERE): opportunities to improve care of patients hospitalized with acute decompensated heart failure. Rev Cardiovasc Med 2003;4(Suppl 7):S21–30.
65. Naylor MD, Brooten DA, Campbell RL, et al. Transitional care of older adults hospitalized with heart failure: a randomized, controlled trial. J Am Geriatr Soc 2004;52(5):675–84.

66. Moser DK, Rich MW. Heart failure in the critically ill older patient. In: Foreman MD, Milisen K, Fulmer TT, editors. Critical care nursing of older adults. 3rd edition. New York: Springer; 2010. p. 503–29.
67. Arean PA, Cook BL. Psychotherapy and combined psychotherapy/pharmacotherapy for late life depression. Biol Psychiatry 2002;52(3):293–303.
68. Lett HS, Davidson J, Blumenthal JA. Nonpharmacologic treatments for depression in patients with coronary heart disease. Psychosom Med 2005; 67(Suppl 1):S58–62.
69. Alexopoulos GS, Raue P, Arean P. Problem-solving therapy versus supportive therapy in geriatric major depression with executive dysfunction. Am J Geriatr Psychiatry 2003;11(1):46–52.
70. Warburton DE, Nicol CW, Bredin SS. Health benefits of physical activity: the evidence. CMAJ 2006; 174(6):801–9.
71. Colcombe SJ, Kramer AF, Erickson KI, et al. Cardiovascular fitness, cortical plasticity, and aging. Proc Natl Acad Sci U S A 2004;101(9):3316–21.
72. Kulcu DG, Kurtais Y, Tur BS, et al. The effect of cardiac rehabilitation on quality of life, anxiety and depression in patients with congestive heart failure. A randomized controlled trial, short-term results. Eura Medicophys 2007;43(4):489–97.
73. Stanek EJ, Oates MB, McGhan WF, et al. Preferences for treatment outcomes in patients with heart failure: symptoms versus survival. J Card Fail 2000;6(3):225–32.
74. National Consensus Project for Quality Pallative Care: clinical Practice Guidelines for quality palliative care, executive summary. American Academy of Hospice and Palliative Medicine; Center to Advance Palliative Care; Hospice and Palliative Nurses Association; Last Acts Partnership; National Hospice and Palliative Care Organization. J Palliat Med 2004;7(5):611–27.
75. Coviello JS, Hricz-Borges L, Masulli PS. Accomplishing quality of life in end-stage heart failure: a hospice multidisciplinary approach. Home Healthc Nurse 2002;20(3):195–8.
76. Serebruany VL, Glassman AH, Malinin AI, et al. Platelet/endothelial biomarkers in depressed patients treated with the selective serotonin reuptake inhibitor sertraline after acute coronary events: the Sertraline AntiDepressant Heart Attack Randomized Trial (SADHART) Platelet Substudy. Circulation 2003;108(8):939–44.
77. Parissis J, Fountoulaki K, Paraskevaidis I, et al. Sertraline for the treatment of depression in coronary artery disease and heart failure. Expert Opin Pharmacother 2007;8(10):1529–37.
78. Alexopoulos GS, Katz IR, Reynolds CF III, et al. Pharmacotherapy of depression in older patients: a summary of the expert consensus guidelines. J Psychiatr Pract 2001;7(6):361–76.
79. Katz IR. Diagnosis and treatment of depression in patients with Alzheimer's disease and other dementias. J Clin Psychiatry 1998;59(Suppl 9):38–44.
80. Papakostas GI, Fava M, Thase ME. Treatment of SSRI-resistant depression: a meta-analysis comparing within- versus across-class switches. Biol Psychiatry 2008;63(7):699–704.
81. Glassman AH, Roose SP, Bigger JT Jr. The safety of tricyclic antidepressants in cardiac patients. Risk-benefit reconsidered. JAMA 1993;269(20):2673–5.
82. Dodd S, Horgan D, Malhi GS, et al. To combine or not to combine? A literature review of antidepressant combination therapy. J Affect Disord 2005;89(1–3): 1–11.
83. Kamholz BA, Mellow AM. Management of treatment resistance in the depressed geriatric patient. Psychiatr Clin North Am 1996;19(2):269–86.
84. Rayburn BK. Electroconvulsive therapy in patients with heart failure or valvular heart disease. Convuls Ther 1997;13(3):145–56.
85. Sorock GS, Shimkin EE. Benzodiazepine sedatives and the risk of falling in a community-dwelling elderly cohort. Arch Intern Med 1988;148(11): 2441–4.
86. Wang PS, Bohn RL, Glynn RJ, et al. Zolpidem use and hip fractures in older people. J Am Geriatr Soc 2001;49(12):1685–90.
87. Leufkens TR, Vermeeren A. Highway driving in the elderly the morning after bedtime use of hypnotics: a comparison between temazepam 20 mg, zopiclone 7.5 mg, and placebo. J Clin Psychopharmacol 2009;29(5):432–8.

Anxiety and Depression in Implanted Cardioverter-Defibrillator Recipients and Heart Failure: A Review

Vicki Freedenberg, RN, MSN[a], Sue A. Thomas, RN, PhD[b,*], Erika Friedmann, PhD[b]

KEYWORDS

- Psychological distress
- Implantable cardioverter-defibrillator
- Gender • Age • Shocks • ICD

Implanted cardioverter-defibrillators (ICDs) are surgically implanted automatic electrical devices designed to terminate ventricular arrhythmias and prevent sudden cardiac death (SCD). They provide antitachycardic pacing and/or deliver a low-energy shock to the heart.[1] In the last decade the use of ICDs has expanded from secondary prevention in patients who have experienced significant ventricular arrhythmias to primary prevention in patients who are at risk for significant ventricular arrhythmias. The clinical use of ICDs for primary prevention in patients with heart failure (HF) escalated rapidly after the Multicenter Automatic Defibrillator Implantation Trial II (MADIT-II)[2] and Sudden Cardiac Death in Heart Failure trial (SCD-HeFT)[3] demonstrated their benefits for reducing mortality in patients with HF or reduced ejection fraction and without significant ventricular arrhythmias. The positive results of these clinical trials, improved ICD technology, and ease of insertion are leading to a rapid expansion in use of these devices. Guidelines specifically recommend ICDs for primary prevention to reduce SCD in patients with ischemic and nonischemic HF who have left ventricular ejection fractions of less than 35% with New York Heart Association (NYHA) functional class II or III, optimal medical management, and a reasonable life expectancy of 1 year or more.[4,5]

Although ICDs clearly reduce mortality, their effects on patients' psychological status are equivocal, with a substantial number of patients becoming depressed or anxious after ICD implantation. Depressive symptoms occur in 24% to 33% of patients who received ICDs for secondary prevention.[6] From 24% to 87% of recipients of ICDs for secondary prevention report increased symptoms of anxiety, and 13% to 35% are clinically anxious.[7]

Although the ICD provides patients with potential protection from SCD, the ICD may increase anxiety and depression in vulnerable patients with HF. Extensive evidence supports depression in patients with HF as an independent predictor of worsening HF, increased hospitalizations, and increased mortality[8–17] Anxiety in outpatients with HF ranges from 18% to 45%.[18,19] Depression occurs in 13%[20] to 48%[21] of outpatients with HF. The combination of anxiety or depression in

[a] Department of Cardiology, Children's National Medical Center, 111 Michigan Avenue, NW, Washington, DC 20010, USA
[b] University of Maryland School of Nursing, 655 West Lombard Street, Baltimore, MD 21201, USA
* Corresponding author.
E-mail address: thomas@son.umaryland.edu

Heart Failure Clin 7 (2011) 59–68
doi:10.1016/j.hfc.2010.08.008
1551-7136/11/$ – see front matter

heartfailure.theclinics.com

patients with HF who receive ICDs may prove deleterious to the patients' health.

Our prior review in 2006 concluded that anxiety and depression are common in patients who received ICDs for secondary prevention.[22] Younger age, female gender, and shocks were the predictors of worse anxiety and depression in ICD recipients. The current review was undertaken to examine the effects of ICD on anxiety and depression in studies published since that review, and expands to include studies of ICDs in patients with HF. Using the search terms "depression," "anxiety," or "psychological" and "implantable cardioverter-defibrillator" or "implant" and "defibrillator," we searched PubMed and PsychInfo for articles in English on adults (April 2005–February 2010) and any articles in pediatric populations that had been excluded from our previous review. We also scrutinized all references in the articles we obtained for additional articles missed in the electronic database searches.

Twenty-one additional studies were identified that assessed anxiety and/or depression in ICD recipients (**Table 1**). Two studies[23,24] were in pediatric populations and found contrasting results. DeMaso and colleagues[23] found only 12.5% of the patients to be depressed and Eicken and colleagues[24] found 30% anxious and 70% depressed. Nine studies included substantial numbers of patients with HF. Prevalence of anxiety was similar in studies including patients with (19%–48%) and without (13%–46%) HF; prevalence of depression was also similar among studies including patients with (13%–35%) and without (7%–41%) HF.

One study of patients with HF who received ICDs as primary prevention examined longitudinal changes in anxiety and depression in 2 years of follow-up.[25] In linear mixed models analysis, anxiety decreased in patients with NYHA class III HF but remained stable in those with NYHA class II HF. Patients with more severe HF were more anxious at the time of ICD implantation and decreased to levels of anxiety similar to those patients with less severe HF by the end of the 2-year follow-up. Overall depression decreased in time, but increased in patients who received shocks. Age and gender did not predict longitudinal changes in anxiety or depression. A longitudinal study of anxiety among ICD recipients, 42% of whom had received ICDs for HF, found that more than half of the ICD recipients who were anxious at insertion remained anxious 1 year later.[26]

AGE

Earlier reviews[22,27,28] found younger age of the ICD recipient to be associated with increased psychological distress. In reviewing the literature since 2005, the authors found 9 studies of adults[11,29–36] and 2 of children[23,24] in which the relationship of age to depression and/or anxiety was examined (**Table 2**). Six studies[29–33,35] found no relationship of anxiety and/or depression to age and 3 studies[11,34,36] found that younger adult patients were more distressed. The 2 studies of the pediatric population[23,24] found conflicting results when examining the relationship of anxiety and depression to age.

In the 3 studies that found a relationship of psychological distress to age, anxiety, depression, or both, anxiety and depression were related to younger age. In a small cross-sectional study of patients with ICDs,[11] age was negatively correlated with state anxiety, trait anxiety, and depression. In a multicenter clinical trial examining predictors of ICD shocks, depression was more common among younger than older patients.[36] Among ICD recipients, initial anxiety was negatively related to age after controlling for gender.[34]

HF status of the ICD recipients was described in 4[31,32,34,36] of the studies that examined the relationship of psychological distress to age. Three of these studies[32,34,36] included more than 100 participants with HF. In 2 of these studies,[34,36] psychological distress was related to younger age. One study[32] found no relationship with age and anxiety and/or depression among 610 ICD recipients with a mean age of 62.4 years, 25% of whom had HF. Smith and colleagues[34] examined both depression and anxiety among 240 ICD recipients, 78% of whom had HF, with a mean age of 58.4 years; anxiety was associated with lower age. Whang and colleagues[36] examined depression but not anxiety among 645 ICD recipients, 49% of whom had HF, with a mean age of 64.1 years. Depression was associated with lower age of ICD recipients. These studies suggest that ICD recipients with HF who are younger may be more depressed or anxious.

GENDER

In the general population, women are 1.9 times as likely to experience significant depression (95% confidence interval [CI] 1.8, 2.0) and 1.7 times as likely to experience anxiety (95% CI 1.6, 1.8) in their lifetimes compared with men.[37] Findings regarding the relationship of gender to depression and/or anxiety in the ICD literature are limited because most ICD recipients in the studies are male. Although women in the general population have increased prevalence of anxiety and depression, this relationship is not consistent in the ICD population. In the review of the literature since

Table 1
Psychological status, depression and anxiety in ICD recipients

Author	Year Published	Sample Size	Tool	% Anxiety	% Depression	% HF, NYHA Class II–IV
Pediatric Population						
DeMaso et al[23]	2004	20	RCMA, RADS	0	12.5	NA
Eicken et al[24]	2005	10	DISYPS-KJ	30	70	NA
No Indication of Patient HF Status						
Pedersen et al[40]	2005	182	HADS	32	28	NS
Bilge et al[29]	2006	91	HADS	46	41	NS
Friedmann et al[11]	2006	48	STAI, BDI	32 state 41 trait	21 mild 6 moderate	NS
Leosdottir et al[33]	2006	44	BAI, BDI	15 mod–severe	10 mod–severe	NS
Luyster et al[38]	2006	100	STAI, BDI	21	22	NS
Crossmann et al[30]	2007	35	STAI, BAI	Not calculated	Not assessed	NS
Lemon and Edelman[62]	2007	49	DASS	33	10	NS
Newall et al[63]	2007	46	HADS	13	7	NS
Pedersen et al[42]	2008	211	HADS	25	25	NS
Spindler et al[35]	2009	535	HADS	37	19	NS
Include Patients with HF						
Whang et al[36]	2005	645	CES-D	Not assessed	18	49
Smith et al[34]	2006	240	STAI, BDI–II	Not calculated	Not calculated	78
Johansen et al[32]	2008	610	HADS	19	13	25
Dougherty and Hunziker[39]	2009	168	STAI, CES-D	33	23	55
Dunbar et al[44]	2009	246	STAI, BDI-II	37	23	32-Class III–IV; 67- Class I–II
Jacq et al[31]	2009	65	MINI, HADS	27	28	77
Luyster et al[57]	2009	88	STAI, BDI	36	24	61
Thomas et al[25]	2009	153	STAI, BDI	25	35	100
ven den Broek et al[41]	2009	391	STAI, BDI	48	35	82

Abbreviations: BAI, Beck Anxiety Inventory; BDI, Beck Depression Inventory; BDI-II, Beck Depression Inventory-II; CES-D, Center for Epidemiologic Studies Depression Scale; DASS, Depression, Anxiety, and Stress Scale; DISYPS-KJ, Diagnostik System für psychische Störungen im Kindes-und Jugendalther nach ICD-10 und DSM-IV; HADS, Hospital Anxiety and Depression Scale; MINI, Mini International Neuropsychiatric Interview; NA, not applicable; NS, not specified; NYHA, New York Heart Association; RADS, Revised Children's Manifest Anxiety Scale; RCMA, Reynold Adolescent/Child Depression Scales.

Table 2
Summary of studies relating age to anxiety and/or depression

Author	Year	N	Age Range	Mean Age (y)	Findings
Pediatric Population					
DeMaso et al[23]	2004	20	9–19	14.8	No increase in anxiety or depression
Eicken et al[24]	2006	16	4–15.9	Median 12.2	7/10 subjects had generalized depression and/or anxiety
No Indication of Patient HF Status					
Bilge et al[29]	2006	91	18–86	53 ± 14	No significant relationship between age and anxiety/depression
Crossmann et al[30]	2007	35	35–65	57 ± 6.3	Age does not predict anxiety (depression not measured)
Friedmann et al[11]	2006	48	34–90	66 ± 12.1	Younger age, increased anxiety and depression
Leosdottir et al[33]	2006	41	23–85	61.8 ± 14.2	Younger patients had better scores but not statistically significant, except on GHQ
Spindler[35]	2009	535		61.5 ± 14.4	Age not related to anxiety/depression
Includes Patients with HF					
Whang et al[36]	2005	645		64.1±	Age inversely related to depression (anxiety not measured)
Smith et al[34]	2006	240		58.4±	Age negatively related to anxiety controlling for gender
Johansen et al[32]	2008	610	8–85	62.4 ± NA	Age not related to anxiety/depression
Jacq et al[31]	2009	65		59.8 ± 14.8	No relationship between age and anxiety/depression

2005, the authors found 8 studies[29–32,34–36,38] addressing gender differences in depression and anxiety among patients (**Table 3**); 3 studies[32,34,36] included a significant number of patients with HF. Women comprised from 5.5% to 25% of the participants in the 8 studies. Two of the studies included fewer than 10 women.[30,31] Of the remaining 6 studies, 1 found greater anxiety and depression among women,[29] 2 of the 5 that assessed anxiety found greater anxiety among women,[32,35] and 2 found greater depression among women.[36,38] Reflecting the population in general, women had more psychological distress than men. Of the 5 studies[29,32,35,36,38] that found increased psychological distress, 2[32,36] included ICD recipients with HF.

Most of the studies used simple chi squares for frequencies or *t*-tests to compare the average scores between men and women. Smith and colleagues[34] used multivariate analysis to compare average anxiety with depression scores between men and women after controlling for age (for anxiety) and HF (for depression) in a group of 240 ICD recipients, 78% of whom had HF. After controlling for these variables, there were no significant differences in anxiety or depression. In this study, HF contributed significantly to depression, but not anxiety. These findings suggest that both female gender and HF are associated with higher depression among ICD recipients independent of age. Female gender also seems to be associated with higher anxiety among ICD recipients independent of HF status and age.

SHOCKS

The shocks generated by ICDs are both life saving and frightening and have the potential to cause

Table 3
Summary of studies relating gender to anxiety and/or depression

Author	Year	N	Women (%)	Women (N)	Anxiety	Depression
No Indication of Patients' HF Status						
Bilge et al[29]	2006	91	15	12	W>M	W>M
Luyster et al[38]	2006	100	19	19	NS	W>M
Crossmann et al[30]	2007	35	14.3	5	NS	NS
Spindler et al[35]	2009	535	5.5	97	W>M	NS
Includes Patients with HF						
Whang et al[36]	2005	645	18.3	118	NA	W>M
Smith et al[34]	2006	240	25	60	NS	NS
Johansen et al[32]	2008	610	17.7	108	W>M	NS
Jacq et al[31]	2009	65	13.8	9	NS	NS

Abbreviations: M, men; NA, not assessed; NS, $P>.05$; S, $P<.05$; W, women.

anxiety and depression in patients. In previous reviews,[22,27,28] the number and frequency of shocks were related to negative psychosocial status and increased anger, depression, and anxiety. The authors found 13 studies not included in our previous review that address the effect of shocks on ICD recipient's psychological status (**Table 4**).[23,24,29,31,32,36,38–41] Four of these studies included significant numbers of ICD recipients with HF,[32,36,39,41] and 2[23,24] were pediatric studies.

Table 4
Summary of studies relating shocks to anxiety and/or depression

Author	Year Published	Sample Size	Anxiety	Depression	% Shocked
Pediatric Population					
DeMaso et al[23]	2004	20	NS	NS	40
Eicken et al[24]	2005	10	Anxiety > shocks	NS	30
No Indication of Patients' HF Status					
Pedersen et al[40]	2005	182	Anxiety > shocks	NS	30
Bilge et al[29]	2006	91	Anxiety > shocks	NS	62
Leosdottir et al[33]	2006	44	NS	NS	15
Luyster et al[38]	2006	100	NS	Depr > shocks	26
Crossmann et al[30]	2007	35	NS	NA	64
Pedersen et al[42]	2008	211	Anxiety > shocks	Depr > shocks	13
Includes Patients with HF					
Whang et al[36]	2005	645	NA	Depr > shocks	9
Johansen et al[32]	2008	610	Anxiety > shocks	Depr > shocks	43
Dougherty and Hunziker[39]	2009	168	Anxiety tends > shocks	NS	33
Jacq et al[31]	2009	65	Anxiety > shocks (MINI)	Depr > shock (HADS)	62
ven den Broek et al[41]	2009	391	Anxiety + type D > shocks	NS	19

Abbreviations: Depr, depression; HADS, Hospital Anxiety and Depression Scale; MINI, Mini International Neuropsychiatric Interview; NA, not assessed; NS, $P>.05$.

Nine of the studies of adult ICD recipients found higher anxiety and depression related to ICD shocks[29,31,32,36,38–42]; 2 did not.[30,33] In 7 of 10 adult studies that included assessment of anxiety, anxiety was higher among those who received shocks than among those who did not.[29,31,32,39–42] In all studies that included patients with HF, anxiety was higher among those who were shocked.[31,32,36,39,41] In 5 of the 10 adult studies that examined the relationship of depression to ICD shock, depression was higher among those who were shocked.[31,32,36,38,42] In 3 of the 5 studies that included patients with HF, depression was higher among those who were shocked than among those who were not.[31,32,36]

Several studies that included patients with HF used multivariate analyses to examine the relationship of shocks and psychological status. In multivariate time-to-event analysis, greater depression severity was associated with ICD shocks after controlling for age and gender.[36] In multivariate logistic regression, both female gender and ICD shocks were significant predictors of anxiety, but not depression.[36] In a similar multivariate logistic regression analysis, female gender (odds ratio [OR] 2.38), symptomatic HF (OR 5.15), and ICD shocks (OR 2.21) independently predicted anxiety after controlling for psychotropic medication, and multiple covariates. Symptomatic HF (OR 6.82), ICD shocks (OR 2.0), and psychotropic medication (OR 2.75) independently predicted depression after controlling for age and numerous covariates.[32] In a study with a different perspective, the odds of receiving ICD shocks within the first 12 months after implantation were higher in patients with chronic obstructive pulmonary disease (OR 3.1), HF (OR 3.1), and implantation for unmonitored syncope or ventricular tachycardia lasting longer than 10 seconds (OR 4.45). High anxiety at the time of ICD implantation approached statistical significance (OR 2.82, $P = .09$).[39]

Two studies examined the effects of shocks on mood in pediatric populations.[23,24] Among pediatric ICD recipients (N = 10), the 3 who were shocked in the past 6 months exhibited severe signs of anxiety.[24] Among 20 pediatric ICD recipients, including 40% who experienced shocks, neither anxiety nor depression differed according to shock experience.[23] The ability to generalize from the findings of these studies is severely hampered by the small number of participants.

Two studies[29,31] examined the relationship of number of ICD shocks to psychological distress. The greater number of ICD shocks was associated with both anxiety and depression in 1 study[29] and depression in another.[31]

Most studies examining the relationship of shocks to depression and/or anxiety used psychological scales to rate the severity of psychological distress. The 2 studies, 1 of pediatric patients[24] and 1 of adults,[31] that included interviews found that anxiety was more common among patients who received ICD shocks than among those who did not, but found no differences in frequency of depression. The later study[31] also included the Hospital Anxiety and Depression Scale (HADS). Depression scores were significantly higher among patients who received ICD shocks than among those who did not, but anxiety scores did not differ. Both HF and shocks predict psychosocial distress. Interventions to reduce distress may be particularly important for ICD recipients with HF and those who receive ICD shocks.

CLINICAL IMPLICATIONS

Prevention of the development of anxiety and depression is essential for the effective use of ICDs in patients with HF. Medical management of patients with HF with ICDs must be optimized to slow the progression of HF and decrease the number of ICD shocks. Screening for anxiety and depression before ICD implantation for all patients with HF can identify those with pre-ICD depression and anxiety. Younger patients and women are particularly vulnerable. Repeated assessment of anxiety and depression every 6 months is warranted in these groups and patients who receive ICD shocks.

TREATMENT OF DEPRESSION AND ANXIETY IN ICD RECIPIENTS WITH HF

No large clinical trials have examined pharmacologic treatment of anxiety or depression in ICD recipients with HF. Pharmacologic treatment of anxiety and depression in patients with HF is addressed in the article by Echols and Jiang elsewhere in this issue.

Five recent randomized controlled trials of nonpharmacologic interventions were identified for ICD patients (**Table 5**). Nonpharmacologic intervention in ICD recipients positively affects depression, anxiety, psychosocial distress, and overall adaptation.[43–46] Cognitive behavioral therapy (CBT) shows promise at improving anxiety and psychological symptoms related to living with an ICD.[45,46] A home-based CBT program for patients with ICDs was associated with decreased anxiety and depression compared with a usual hospital-based program.[45] A 6-week CBT intervention was more effective than a 4-hour psychoeducational workshop at controlling psychological distress including anxiety and depression over

Table 5
Summary of recent randomized clinical trials (evidence level A) of nonpharmacologic interventions in ICD recipients

Author	Year Published	N	Intervention	Reduction in Psychological Distress	% HF
Dougherty et al[43]	2005	168	Telephone intervention information and support	S	Not assessed
Edelman et al[47]	2007	22	Informational session	NS	Not assessed
Sears et al[46]	2007	30	Cognitive behavioral	S	Not assessed
Dunbar et al[44]	2009	246	Psychoeducational telephone or in-hospital group counseling	S	32% NYHA class III–IV; 67% NYHA class I–II
Lewin et al[45]	2009	192	Cognitive behavioral	S	77

4 months.[46] There was no difference in device acceptance, which improved with time, between the groups. One of these studies, in which a nonpharmacologic intervention was effective, included a significant proportion of ICD recipients with HF.[45] Psychoeducational interventions have also proved effective. A structured 8-week posthospital telephone intervention led to 6- and 12-month improvements in anxiety and distress compared with usual care.[43] A combined in-hospital/out-of-hospital psychoeducational intervention was more effective than usual care for reducing anxiety and depression at 12 months. A telephone intervention in the same timeframe was equally effective.[44] One of these studies included a significant number of patients with HF with ICDs.[44] One trial found that a single session lasting 60 to 90 minutes that provided information and reassurance was not effective at reducing ICD-related distress[47]; the small sample size precludes sufficient power to conclude that this intervention is ineffective.

Nonpharmacologic interventions positively affect depression, anxiety, psychosocial distress, and overall adaptation in patients with HF who have not received ICDs.[48,49] CBT may be superior to pharmacotherapy in preventing relapsing depression in patients with HF.[48] In the Support, Education, and Research in Chronic Heart Failure (SEARCH) study, a nonrandomized clinical trial of depression, anxiety, and HF symptoms, depressed patients with HF (n = 208) improved more at 1 year following an 8-week mindfulness-based psychoeducational intervention compared with usual care.[49]

Computer-based CBT intervention may be a viable application in the population of patients with ICDs, based on its successful use in other clinical populations.[50] As cited in our previous review, patients with ICDs benefit from group support and forums to discuss their shared experiences, whether in person or via online chat rooms.[46,50,51] Nurses have successfully implemented patient programs such as telephone intervention, verbal and written patient education materials, coping skill training, and patient support groups.[43,44,51–53]

Overall, there remains a paucity of randomized controlled trials examining interventions to improve anxiety, depression, and psychological distress in the population of patients with ICDs, especially among those with HF. In addition, the authors found no studies addressing interventions among pediatric patients, whereas the number of ICD implants in this truly young population is increasing as ICDs become small enough to implant in younger children. The use of cognitive behavior therapy and other nonpharmacologic interventions is appropriate for the treatment of psychological distress in ICD recipients with HF. This area of research is ripe for investigation.

DISCUSSION

Anxiety and depression are common in patients with HF with ICDs and occur at rates similar to those of other patients with HF. In view of the high prevalence of anxiety and depression among ICD recipients with HF, psychosocial issues must be addressed at implantation and for at least the first 2 years.

ICD recipients with HF who are younger may be more depressed or anxious. Both female gender and HF are associated with higher anxiety and depression among ICD recipients. The strongest predictor of psychological distress is receiving ICD shocks. Screening and interventions to reduce psychological distress among ICD recipients are particularly important for those who are younger than 60 years old, female, and those who receive ICD shocks.

Additional examination of factors associated with increased anxiety and depression in patients with HF with ICDs is warranted. Two longitudinal studies[25,26] suggest that patients with more severe HF and those who are psychologically distressed require close monitoring of psychological status and may benefit from intervention at time of implantation.

Shared pathophysiologic pathways and behavioral risk factors emphasize the importance of a holistic approach to screening, diagnosis, and treatment of anxiety and depression in ICD recipients with HF. Depression, anxiety, and HF share elements of common neuroendocrine pathways. These pathways include increased activation of the hypothalamic-pituitary-adrenal axis, autonomic dysregulation, immune system alterations, and increased platelet activation.[54] Health behaviors common in patients who are anxious and depressed may contribute to poorer health outcomes. Poor medication and diet adherence and decreased exercise are frequently associated with anxiety and depression.[55–60] Limited evidence on the effects of pharmacologic and nonpharmacologic therapy for depression and anxiety in patients with HF precludes the development of treatment guidelines for this population at this time.[61] CBT[45,46] and psychoeducational programs[43,44] show promise for reducing psychological distress in ICD recipients with HF.[45]

REFERENCES

1. Glikson M, Friedman PA. The implantable cardioverter defibrillator. Lancet 2001;357(9262):1107–17.
2. Moss AJ, Brown M, Cannon DS, et al. Multicenter automatic defibrillator implantation trial-cardiac resynchronization therapy (MADIT-CRT): design and clinical protocol. Ann Noninvasive Electrocardiol 2005;10(Suppl 4):34–43.
3. Bardy GH, Lee KL, Mark DB, et al. Amiodarone or an implantable cardioverter-defibrillator for congestive heart failure. N Engl J Med 2005;352(3):225–37.
4. Hunt SA, Abraham WT, Chin MH, et al. ACC/AHA 2005 guideline update for the diagnosis and management of chronic heart failure in the adult: a report of the American College of Cardiology/American Heart Association Task Force on Practice Guidelines (Writing Committee to Update the 2001 guidelines for the evaluation and management of heart failure): developed in collaboration with the American College of Chest Physicians and the International Society for Heart and Lung Transplantation: endorsed by the Heart Rhythm Society. Circulation 2005;112(12):154–235.
5. Zipes DP, Camm AJ, Borggrefe M, et al. ACC/AHA/ESC 2006 guidelines for management of patients with ventricular arrhythmias and the prevention of sudden cardiac death: a report of the American College of Cardiology/American Heart Association Task Force and the European Society of Cardiology Committee for Practice Guidelines (Writing Committee to Develop Guidelines for Management of Patients With Ventricular Arrhythmias and the Prevention of Sudden Cardiac Death). J Am Coll Cardiol 2006;48(5):e247–346.
6. Sears SF Jr, Stutts LA, Aranda JM Jr, et al. Managing congestive heart failure patient factors in the device era. Congest Heart Fail 2006;12(6):335–40.
7. Sears SF Jr, Todaro JF, Lewis TS, et al. Examining the psychosocial impact of implantable cardioverter defibrillators: a literature review. Clin Cardiol 1999;22(7):481–9.
8. DeJong JM, Moser DK, Chung ML. Predictors of health status for heart failure patients. Prog Cardiovasc Nurs 2005;20(4):155–62.
9. Faller H, Stork S, Schowalter M, et al. Depression and survival in chronic heart failure: does gender play a role? Eur J Heart Fail 2007;9(10):1018–23.
10. Faris R, Purcell H, Henein MY, et al. Clinical depression is common and significantly associated with reduced survival in patients with non-ischaemic heart failure. Eur J Heart Fail 2002;4:541–51.
11. Friedmann E, Thomas SA, Inguito P, et al. Quality of life and psychological status of patients with implantable cardioverter defibrillators. J Interv Card Electrophysiol 2006;17:65–72.
12. Jiang W, Alexander J, Christopher E, et al. Relationship of depression to increased risk of mortality and rehospitalization in patients with congestive heart failure. Arch Intern Med 2001;161(15):1849–56.
13. Jiang W, Kuchibhatla M, Cuffe MS, et al. Prognostic value of anxiety and depression in patients with chronic heart failure. Circulation 2004;110(22):3452–6.
14. Murberg TA. Long-term effect of social relationships on mortality in patients with congestive heart failure. Int J Psychiatry Med 2004;34(3):207–17.
15. Rumsfeld JS, Haveranek EP, Masoudi F, et al. Depressive symptoms and the strongest predictors of short-term declines in health status in patients with heart failure. J Am Coll Cardiol 2003;42:1811–7.
16. Sherwood A, Blumenthal JA, Trivedi R, et al. Relationship of depression to death or hospitalization in patients with heart failure. Arch Intern Med 2007;167(4):367–73.

17. Westlake C, Dracup K, Fonarow G, et al. Depression in patients with heart failure. J Card Fail 2005;11(1): 30–5.
18. Friedmann E, Thomas SA, Liu F, et al. Relationship of depression, anxiety, and social isolation to chronic heart failure outpatient mortality. Am Heart J 2006; 152(5):940–8.
19. Haworth JE, Moniz-Cook E, Clark AL, et al. Prevalence and predictors of anxiety and depression in a sample of chronic heart failure patients with left ventricular systolic dysfunction. Eur J Heart Fail 2005;7(5):803–8.
20. Murberg TA, Bru E, Aarsland T, et al. Functional status and depression among men and women with congestive heart failure. Int J Psychiatry Med 1998;28(3):273–91.
21. Gottlieb SS, Khatta M, Friedmann E, et al. The influence of age, gender, and race on the prevalence of depression in heart failure patients. J Am Coll Cardiol 2004;43(9):1542–9.
22. Thomas SA, Friedmann E, Kao CW, et al. Quality of life and psychological status of patients with implantable cardioverter defibrillators. Am J Crit Care 2006;15(4):389–98.
23. DeMaso DR, Lauretti A, Spieth L, et al. Psychosocial factors and quality of life in children and adolescents with implantable cardioverter-defibrillators. Am J Cardiol 2004;93(5):582–7.
24. Eicken A, Kolb C, Lange S, et al. Implantable cardioverter defibrillator (ICD) in children. Int J Cardiol 2006;107(1):30–5.
25. Thomas SA, Friedmann E, Gottlieb SS, et al. Changes in psychosocial distress in heart failure (HF) outpatients with implantable cardioverter defibrillators. Heart Lung 2009;38:109–20.
26. Pedersen SS, van den Broek KC, Theuns DA, et al. Risk of chronic anxiety in implantable defibrillator patients: a multi-center study. Int J Cardiol 2009. [Epub ahead of print].
27. Bostwick JM, Sola CL. An updated review of implantable cardioverter/defibrillators, induced anxiety, and quality of life. Psychiatr Clin North Am 2007;30(4):677–88.
28. Sears SF Jr, Conti JB. Quality of life and psychological functioning of ICD patients. Heart 2002;87(5): 488–93.
29. Bilge AK, Ozben B, Demircan S, et al. Depression and anxiety status of patients with implantable cardioverter defibrillator and precipitating factors. Pacing Clin Electrophysiol 2006;29(6):619–26.
30. Crossmann A, Pauli P, Dengler W, et al. Stability and cause of anxiety in patients with an implantable cardioverter-defibrillator: a longitudinal two-year follow-up. Heart Lung 2007;36(2):87–95.
31. Jacq F, Foulldrin G, Savoure A, et al. A comparison of anxiety, depression and quality of life between device shock and nonshock groups in implantable cardioverter defibrillator recipients. Gen Hosp Psychiatry 2009;31(3):266–73.
32. Johansen JB, Pedersen SS, Spindler H, et al. Symptomatic heart failure is the most important clinical correlate of impaired quality of life, anxiety, and depression in implantable cardioverter-defibrillator patients: a single-centre, cross-sectional study in 610 patients. Europace 2008;10(5):545–51.
33. Leosdottir M, Sigurdsson E, Reimarsdottir G, et al. Health-related quality of life of patients with implantable cardioverter defibrillators compared with that of pacemaker recipients. Europace 2006;8(3):168–74.
34. Smith G, Dunbar SB, Valderrama AL, et al. Gender differences in implantable cardioverter-defibrillator patients at the time of insertion. Prog Cardiovasc Nurs 2006;21(2):76–82.
35. Spindler H, Johansen JB, Andersen K, et al. Gender differences in anxiety and concerns about the cardioverter defibrillator. Pacing Clin Electrophysiol 2009; 32(5):614–21.
36. Whang W, Albert CM, Sears SF Jr, et al. Depression as a predictor for appropriate shocks among patients with implantable cardioverter-defibrillators: results from the Triggers of Ventricular Arrhythmias (TOVA) study. J Am Coll Cardiol 2005;45(7):1090–5.
37. Seedat S, Scott KM, Angermeyer MC, et al. Cross-national associations between gender and mental disorders in the World Health Organization World Mental Health Surveys. Arch Gen Psychiatry 2009; 66(7):785–95.
38. Luyster FS, Hughes JW, Waechter D, et al. Resource loss predicts depression and anxiety among patients treated with an implantable cardioverter defibrillator. Psychosom Med 2006;68(5):794–800.
39. Dougherty CM, Hunziker J. Predictors of implantable cardioverter defibrillator shocks during the first year. J Cardiovasc Nurs 2009;24(1):21–8.
40. Pedersen SS, van Domburg RT, Theuns DA, et al. Concerns about the implantable cardioverter defibrillator: a determinant of anxiety and depressive symptoms independent of experienced shocks. Am Heart J 2005;149(4):664–9.
41. van den Broek KC, Nyklicek I, van der Voort PH, et al. Risk of ventricular arrhythmia after implantable defibrillator treatment in anxious type D patients. J Am Coll Cardiol 2009;54(6):531–7.
42. Pedersen SS, Theuns DA, Erdman RA, et al. Clustering of device-related concerns and type D personality predicts increased distress in ICD patients independent of shocks. Pacing Clin Electrophysiol 2008;31(1):20–7.
43. Dougherty CM, Thompson EA, Lewis FM. Long-term outcomes of a telephone intervention after an ICD. Pacing Clin Electrophysiol 2005;28(11):1157–67.
44. Dunbar SB, Langberg JJ, Reilly CM, et al. Effect of a psychoeducational intervention on depression, anxiety, and health resource use in implantable

cardioverter defibrillator patients. Pacing Clin Electrophysiol 2009;32(10):1259–71.
45. Lewin RJ, Coulton S, Frizelle DJ, et al. A brief cognitive behavioural preimplantation and rehabilitation programme for patients receiving an implantable cardioverter-defibrillator improves physical health and reduces psychological morbidity and unplanned readmissions. Heart 2009;95(1):63–9.
46. Sears SF, Sowell LD, Kuhl EA, et al. The ICD shock and stress management program: a randomized trial of psychosocial treatment to optimize quality of life in ICD patients. Pacing Clin Electrophysiol 2007;30(7):858–64.
47. Edelman S, Lemon J, Kirkness A. Educational intervention for patients with automatic implantable cardioverter defibrillators. Aust J Adv Nurs 2007;24(3):26–32.
48. O'Hea E, Houseman J, Bedek K, et al. The use of cognitive behavioral therapy in the treatment of depression for individuals with CHF. Heart Fail Rev 2009;14(1):13–20.
49. Sullivan MJ, Wood L, Terry J, et al. The Support, Education, and Research in Chronic Heart Failure Study (SEARCH): a mindfulness-based psychoeducational intervention improves depression and clinical symptoms in patients with chronic heart failure. Am Heart J 2009;157(1):84–90.
50. Kuhl EA, Sears SF, Conti JB. Using computers to improve the psychosocial care of implantable cardioverter defibrillator recipients. Pacing Clin Electrophysiol 2006;29(12):1426–33.
51. Vogt A. Establishing an ICD support group. A framework. Adv Nurse Pract 2006;14(9):59–60.
52. Dougherty CM, Lewis FM, Thompson EA, et al. Short-term efficacy of a telephone intervention by expert nurses after an implantable cardioverter defibrillator. Pacing Clin Electrophysiol 2004;27(12):1594–602.
53. Dunbar SB, Funk M, Wood K, et al. Ventricular dysrhythmias: nursing approaches to health outcomes. J Cardiovasc Nurs 2004;19(5):316–28.
54. Thomas SA, Chapa DW, Friedmann E, et al. Depression in patients with heart failure: prevalence, pathophysiological mechanisms, and treatment. Crit Care Nurse 2008;28(2):40–55.
55. DiMatteo MR, Lepper HS, Croghan TW. Depression is a risk factor for noncompliance with medical treatment: meta-analysis of the effects of anxiety and depression on patient adherence. Arch Intern Med 2000;160(14):2101–7.
56. Gary R, Lee SY. Physical function and quality of life in older women with diastolic heart failure: effects of a progressive walking program on sleep patterns. Prog Cardiovasc Nurs 2007;22(2):72–80.
57. Luyster FS, Hughes JW, Gunstad J. Depression and anxiety symptoms are associated with reduced dietary adherence in heart failure patients treated with an implantable cardioverter defibrillator. J Cardiovasc Nurs 2009;24(1):10–7.
58. Redeker NS. Sleep disturbance in people with heart failure: implications for self-care. J Cardiovasc Nurs 2008;23(3):231–8.
59. Riegel B, Moser DK, Anker SD, et al. State of the science: promoting self-care in persons with heart failure: a scientific statement from the American Heart Association. Circulation 2009;120(12):1141–63.
60. van der Wal MH, Jaarsma T, Moser DK, et al. Compliance in heart failure patients: the importance of knowledge and beliefs. Eur Heart J 2006;27(4):434–40.
61. Watson K, Summers KM. Depression in patients with heart failure: clinical implications and management. Pharmacotherapy 2009;29(1):49–63.
62. Lemon J, Edelman S. Psychological adaptation to ICDs and the influence of anxiety sensitivity. Psychol Health Med 2007;12(2):163–71.
63. Newall EG, Lever NA, Prasad S, et al. Psychological implications of ICD implantation in a New Zealand population. Europace 2007;9(1):20–4.

Screening and Identification of Depression Among Patients with Coronary Heart Disease and Congestive Heart Failure

Kenneth R. Yeager, PhD[a,*], Philip F. Binkley, MD, MPH[a], Radu V. Saveanu, MD[a], Deanna M. Golden-Kreutz, PhD[b], Allard E. Dembe, ScD[c], Laxmi S. Mehta, MD[b], Subhdeep Virk, MD[a]

KEYWORDS

• AHA • Depression • Cardiovascular • CHD

In September 2008, the American Heart Association (AHA) released a multispecialty AHA Science Advisory that endorsed depression screening, referral, and treatment of individuals with coronary heart disease (CHD). In support to this endorsement, the AHA Science Advisory Group noted that more than 60 prospective studies over the past 40 years have examined the link between established indices of depression and prognosis in individuals with known CHD. Initial review articles examining this connection were published in the late 1990s. Since then, more than 100 reviews, including several meta-analyses, have been published, examining the role of depression on cardiovascular morbidity and mortality. Despite differences in samples, duration of follow-up, and assessment techniques, these studies have demonstrated relatively consistent results and suggest an important connection between cardiovascular morbidity and mortality in patients with depressive symptoms or major depression.[1,2]

Depression is also a relatively common condition among persons with congestive heart failure (CHF). It is estimated that comorbid depression ranges between 24% and 40% of patients diagnosed with stable ambulatory heart failure.[3–5] This article discusses the current best practices for the screening, identification, and treatment of depression in patients with CHD and CHF, as well as the financial aspects associated with care management.

THE IMPORTANCE OF DEPRESSION SCREENING IN CARDIOVASCULAR MORBIDITY AND MORTALITY

Depression occurring concurrently with cardiovascular diseases is associated with poor outcomes that range from low functional status or poor

[a] Department of Psychiatry, The Ohio State University, 1670 Upham Drive, Columbus, OH 43210, USA
[b] Department of Internal Medicine, The Ohio State University, Columbus, OH, USA
[c] Division of Health Services Management & Policy, College of Public Health, The Ohio State University, Columbus, OH, USA
* Corresponding author.
E-mail address: kenneth.yeager@osumc.edu

Heart Failure Clin 7 (2011) 69–74
doi:10.1016/j.hfc.2010.08.007
1551-7136/11/$ – see front matter. Published by Elsevier Inc.

quality-of-life ratings to recurrent cardiac events to, in the most severe cases, higher mortality rates.[6] Vaccarino and colleagues[7] documented that an increasing number of depressive symptoms is a negative prognostic factor for patients with heart failure, just as it is for patients with CHD. Nicholson and colleagues[8] suggest that nearly half of the variance identified between depression and heart disease is explained away when left ventricular ejection fraction is added to prediction models.

Barth and colleagues[9] sought to quantify the effect of depressive symptoms (eg, Beck Depression Inventory, hospital anxiety and depression scale) or depressive disorders (major depression) on cardiac or all-cause mortality. Results of a meta-analysis of 29 publications reporting on 20 studies indicate that depressive symptoms increase the risk of mortality in patients with CHD. Within the first 6 months, depressive disorders are found to have no significant effect on mortality. However, after 2 years, the risk is more than 2 times higher for patients with CHD with clinical depression.

Ferketich and Binkley[10] published, perhaps, the largest population analysis of measures of distress in patients with heart disease, relying on the National Health Interview Survey. This analysis showed that patients with CHF had the highest prevalence of distress of all patients with cardiovascular illness. In addition, the prevalence of distress in patients with other cardiovascular diseases exceeded that in those without such a history. Whooley[11] suggests that primary care providers should routinely screen patients with cardiovascular disease for depression, because depression requires treatment regardless of its cardiovascular effects, and screening plus collaborative care is cost-effective in primary care settings.

However, these findings are not without controversy. According to Ziegelstein and colleagues,[12] although a large number of patients with CHD may screen positive for depression, few actually meets the diagnostic criteria. Further, it is indicated that depression treatment in patients with CHF results in a little variance in depression symptom change scores, and there is no evidence that screening for depression improves CHD outcomes.

Despite these various schools of thought, the negative effect of depression on the patient with cardiac illness is generally accepted among both cardiologists and psychiatrists. The AHA Science Advisory Group notes that depression is commonly present in patients with CHD and is independently associated with increased cardiovascular morbidity and mortality. Screening tests for depressive symptoms should be performed to identify patients who may require further assessment and treatment.[1] Physicians and staff at The Ohio State University (OSU) Ross Heart Hospital and the OSU Harding Hospital recognized the critical need for expert diagnosis and management in this patient population. The remainder of this article discusses how a collaborative cardiovascular disease and depression-screening program was formed at The Ohio State University Medical Center (OSUMC) to meet the needs of this patient population and how an electronic screening process was established.

OSUMC DEPRESSION AND CARDIAC DISEASE COLLABORATIVE

The OSUMC depression and cardiac disease collaborative was initially created in 2006 by 2 of the authors (P.B. and R.S.) in response to the growing amount of data that showed a significant association between depression and CHD. The collaborative consisted of faculty from the Department of Psychiatry, Division of Cardiology, and College of Public Health. The group met on a monthly basis and the initial goals were

- To study the incidence and prevalence of depression in the patient population admitted to the OSU Ross Heart Hospital and compare it with the national data.
- To establish a better mechanism of detection of depressive symptoms in this inpatient population.
- To establish an outpatient psychiatric program that would provide ongoing clinical care to patients with depression and CHD after discharge from the heart hospital.
- To establish research protocols that would provide further understanding of the incidence/prevalence of depression in CHD across various patient populations, its genetic and neurobiological markers, and the efficacy of various psychiatric treatments.

The OSUMC depression and cardiac disease collaborative was enthusiastically endorsed by the Medical Center Leadership and various hospital boards and is moving toward accomplishing these goals.

DEVELOPMENT ISSUES

The screening development process revealed important issues that needed to be addressed early in the stages of this project. Staff from both the departments had questions concerning who would be screening the patient for depression, which screening tool was most appropriate for the patient population, and at what point screening should occur. In addition, issues associated with stigma in depression were presented. Initial trials of various paper-and-pencil depression screening tools were met with differing levels of receptivity by patients completing the questionnaire and the staff who were asked to administer them.

Time constraints also quickly became apparent. Hospitalizations are normally short in the acute care environment, and patient care staff must work quickly to accomplish all the work that needs to be done before the patient is discharged. Feedback from both patients and staff revealed that a depression-screening tool should

- Use portable technology
- Be easily accessed, read, and understood by the patient
- Remain in a secure password-protected environment behind the hospital information systems fire wall
- Have the ability to interface with the medical record and other electronic data-collection tools
- Provide instant feedback to both the patient and health care professionals
- Contain recommendations stratified to reflect risk factors associated with patient presentation.

Patient safety was also a topic of discussion on several levels. Although development of a portable screening tool seemed to be the most desirable option, feedback and input were required from epidemiology and information technology staff to recommend cleaning and disinfecting processes that met hospital standards and that could be used with electronic components. In addition, staff had concerns that asking a patient to sit on the edge of a bed to use a computer on wheels might present an increased fall risk.

FINDING AND USING THE RIGHT TOOL: THE 9-ITEM PATIENT HEALTH QUESTIONNAIRE

After beta tests of several different types of instruments, and with feedback from patients and staff, the best screening tool for the patients with cardiac illness was determined to be a computer-based version of the 9-item Patient Health Questionnaire (PHQ-9). PHQ-9 is a brief depression-screening instrument that most patients are able to complete within 5 minutes without assistance. In addition, a considerable amount of literature supports the use of the PHQ-9 in cardiologic depression screening.[13–15]

PHQ-9 begins with the question, "Over the last 2 weeks, how often have you been bothered by any of the following problems?" Options for response for each item of the scale progress from "not at all" to "several days," "more than half the days," and "nearly everyday." Items are scored as 0, 1, 2, and 3, respectively. Questions in PHQ-9 correlate nicely with the *Diagnostic and Statistical Manual of Mental Disorders (Fourth Edition, Text Revision)* diagnostic categories, and PHQ-9 presents with an impressive sensitivity of 83% and specificity of 90% when using the structured clinical interview for *Diagnostic and Statistical Manual of Mental Disorders (Fourth Edition)* as the criterion standard.[16]

Timing of the screening process is an important factor that must be considered when determining accuracy of any tool. The screening should be given neither too soon after the cardiac event to allow enough time for patients to adjust to their situation nor too close to the discharge to become a barrier to further assessment and follow-up. In the authors' case, a 6-month trial using nursing staff to initiate the screening process met with only fair results. The authors believe that this result occurred because of several reasons:

- The cardiology nursing staff is responsible for a large number of tasks on a day-to-day basis and does not always have time to administer questionnaires
- Processes vary within different areas of the heart hospital
- Variances in patients' level of care and severity create different levels of workload and patient turnover.

Following careful consideration and process analysis, it was determined that the optimal area for depression screening in the authors' program was cardiac rehabilitation. All patients are seen in cardiac rehabilitation before discharge. At this point, the patient is well enough to complete the physical assessment, and depression screening can be done parallel with other tasks, such as linking the patient to community resources. In the authors' program, a referral to cardiac rehabilitation autotriggers depression screening, unless circumstances have dictated the patients be screened earlier in their hospital stay.

When referred to cardiac rehabilitation, PHQ-9 is one of several questionnaires that the patient completes. During the initial "rehab" appointment, the patient is provided with a computer, and the initial window to the PHQ-9 screening tool opens.

The computer welcomes the patient to the screening process, and an informational letter explains the importance of depression screening in all patients. The patient clicks "next" to navigate through the pages of screening questions. The patient is instructed to answer each question by clicking on the radio dial next to the most appropriate statement. Once the screening tool is completed the patient sees a thank you note for completing the process. For the patient, the screening process is complete.

Cardiac rehabilitation staff connects to the secure server, enters the patient identification number, and prints the results screen. A summary of the answers and depression score is related to the treatment team who determine the most appropriate next steps. The electronic screening tool has both a calculated score and specific recommendations for depression management, depending on the severity of depression detected. In cases of severe depression, or potential suicidal ideation, immediate notification is sent to the physician of record. All screening results appear in the medical record under questionnaires and are flagged for immediate attention should the level of depression be recognized as severe or if suicide risk is noted. The screening process at a glance is shown in **Fig. 1**, and proposed recommendations included in the "view results page" are shown in **Fig. 2**.

Depression screening can generate several false-positive results; therefore, it is important to meet with the patient to discuss the outcome of screening results and the meanings behind questions answered in the affirmative indicating severe depression or suicidal ideation. For example, one patient indicated, "I would rather die…"; however, the patient did not finish the statement by stating "than deal with the pain following the surgery procedure." Collaborative efforts between cardiology and psychiatry have been established to systematically screen patients with moderately severe and severe depression ratings that address such situations.

DATA RECORDING, MANAGEMENT, AND RETRIEVAL

Screening is completed on a secure Web page housed on the medical center's network behind the fire wall. Secure Internet access enables staff from multiple locations to connect to the screening tools through the use of portable devices, such as room computers and laptop computers on wheels. Once connected to the screening tool, the staff member enters a username and secure password to access the database. All professional clinical staff, including physicians, nurses, social workers, have access to the depression-screening tool.

Once the patient completes the screening process, answers are saved to the server. Information gathered in the screening process are electronically transferred and integrated into the medical center's information warehouse (IW). The IW is an Oracle-based data repository that gathers information including patient demographics, diagnosis, orders, and health history as well as a large variety of other important information, such as pharmacy and laboratory data. During development of the screening tool, data access provisions were made for a limited number of research and professional staff working on this CHF and Depression project. Staff with IW access are able

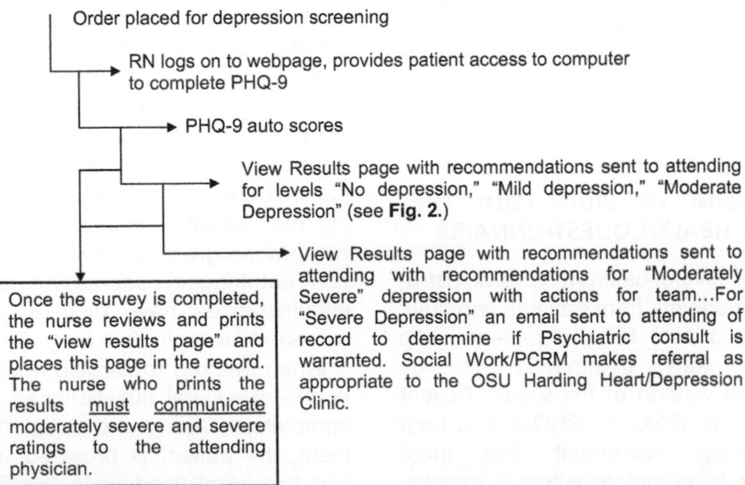

Fig. 1. The screening process at a glance. PCRM, patient care resource manager.

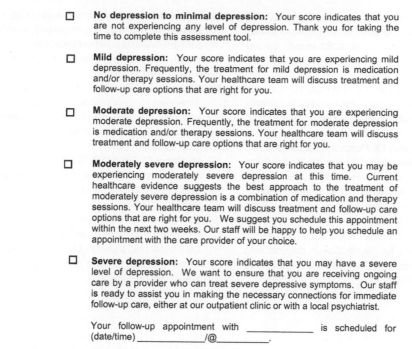

☐ **No depression to minimal depression:** Your score indicates that you are not experiencing any level of depression. Thank you for taking the time to complete this assessment tool.

☐ **Mild depression:** Your score indicates that you are experiencing mild depression. Frequently, the treatment for mild depression is medication and/or therapy sessions. Your healthcare team will discuss treatment and follow-up care options that are right for you.

☐ **Moderate depression:** Your score indicates that you are experiencing moderate depression. Frequently, the treatment for moderate depression is medication and/or therapy sessions. Your healthcare team will discuss treatment and follow-up care options that are right for you.

☐ **Moderately severe depression:** Your score indicates that you may be experiencing moderately severe depression at this time. Current healthcare evidence suggests the best approach to the treatment of moderately severe depression is a combination of medication and therapy sessions. Your healthcare team will discuss treatment and follow-up care options that are right for you. We suggest you schedule this appointment within the next two weeks. Our staff will be happy to help you schedule an appointment with the care provider of your choice.

☐ **Severe depression:** Your score indicates that you may have a severe level of depression. We want to ensure that you are receiving ongoing care by a provider who can treat severe depressive symptoms. Our staff is ready to assist you in making the necessary connections for immediate follow-up care, either at our outpatient clinic or with a local psychiatrist.

Your follow-up appointment with ____________ is scheduled for (date/time) ____________/@__________.

Fig. 2. Proposed recommendations included in the "view results page."

to monitor a variety of process measures, including patient history for treatment of depression, medication management, relative laboratory data, length of stay, and readmission rates.

SUMMARY

In the light of perspectives reported in this article combined with the ease of screening using an Internet-based, standardized, and effective measure, it is difficult to observe a negative effect on cardiologists performing depression screening. Our preliminary experience using the PHQ-9 screening questionnaire has been positive. An expanded version of the PHQ-9 questionnaire with four additional items related to past depression history and stressful life events among cardiac patients is being developed and will be incorporated into the screening program. Although there is some evidence that treating depression alters the course of heart disease, it is clearly known that recognizing and treating depression is essential for the overall health and well-being of patients and that this comorbid condition must be addressed in a collaborative manner by all health care professionals.

REFERENCES

1. Lichtman JH, Bigger JT Jr, Blumenthal JA, et al. Depression and coronary heart disease: recommendations for screening, referral, and treatment. A Science Advisory from the American Heart Association Prevention Committee of the Council on Cardiovascular Nursing, Council on Clinical Cardiology, Council on Epidemiology and Prevention, and Interdisciplinary Council on Quality of Care and Outcomes Research. Circulation 2008; 118:1768–75.
2. Musselman DL, Evans DL, Nemeroff CB. The relationship of depression to cardiovascular disease: epidemiology, biology, and treatment. Arch Gen Psychiatry 1998;55:580–92.
3. Havranek EP, Ware MG, Lowes BD. Prevalence of depression in congestive heart failure. Am J Cardiol 1999;84:348–50.
4. Koening HG. Depression in hospitalized older patients with congestive heart failure. Gen Hosp Psychiatry 1998;20:29–43.
5. Skotzko CE, Krichten C, Zietowski G, et al. Depression is common and precludes accurate assessment of functional status in elderly patients with congestive heart failure. J Card Fail 2000;6: 300–5.
6. Van Melle JP, de Jonge P, Spijkerman TA, et al. Prognostic association of depression following cardiovascular events: a meta-analysis. Psychosom Med 2004;66:814–22.
7. Vaccarino V, Kasl SV, Abramson J, et al. Depressive symptoms and risk of functional decline and death in patient with heart failure. J Am Coll Cardiol 2001;38:199–205.

8. Nicholson A, Kuper H, Hemingway H. Depression as an aetiologic and prognostic factor in coronary heart disease: a meta-analysis of 6362 events among 146538 participants in 54 observational studies. Eur Heart J 2006;27:2763–74.
9. Barth J, Schumacher M, Herrmann-Lingen C. Depression as a risk factor for mortality in patients with coronary heart disease: a meta-analysis. Psychosom Med 2004;66:802–13.
10. Ferketich AK, Binkley PF. Psychological distress and cardiovascular disease: results from the 2002 national health interview survey. Eur Heart J 2005;26:1923–9.
11. Whooley MA. To screen or not to screen? Depression in patients with cardiovascular disease. J Am Coll Cardiol 2009;54:891–4.
12. Ziegelstein RC, Thombs BD, Coyne JC, et al. Routine screening for depression in patients with coronary heart disease: never mind. J Am Coll Cardiol 2009;54:886–90.
13. Bigger JT Jr. Screening for depression in cardiac patients. Available at: http://www.physweeklyarchives.com/article.asp?issueid=669&articleid=5572. PhysWeeklyArchives.com, March 2009;26(10). Accessed June 5, 2010.
14. Gilbody S, Richards D, Brealey S, et al. Screening for depression in medical settings with the patient health questionnaire (PHQ): a diagnostic meta-analysis. J Gen Intern Med 2007;22:1596–602.
15. McManus D, Pipkin SS, Whooley MA. Screening for depression in patients with coronary heart disease (data from the Heart and Soul study). Am J Cardiol 2005;96:1076–81.
16. Davidson KW, Kupfer DJ, Bigger J, et al. Assessment and treatment of depression in patients with cardiovascular disease: National Heart, Lung and Blood Institute working group report. Psychosom Med 2006;68:645–50.

Diagnosing Depression in Congestive Heart Failure

Radu V. Saveanu, MD[a,*], Tara Mayes, MD[a,b]

KEYWORDS

• Depression • Congestive heart failure • Diagnosis
• Assessment

How often do practitioners utter the phrase "This patient is depressed, but he has good reason to be depressed"?

If someone suffers from a major medical condition, patients and doctors alike assume that depression becomes the natural state of being. Sadness is expected. Dysphoric mood, poor sleep, and lack of interest are the natural consequences of physical illness. Correct?

Studies show otherwise. In truth, fewer than half of medically compromised patients meet the diagnostic criteria for major depression.[1] This includes terminal cancer patients, individuals with acquired immunodeficiency syndrome (AIDS), and those with compromised cardiac function.[2–6] The remainder frequently demonstrate symptoms of a depressive illness that are waved off by physicians, because mood disturbances are expected.

"If I were him I would be depressed too." Licensed professionals frequently make statements like this to alleviate the stress of caring for a patient that exhibits symptoms of depression. Having a reason for a patient's dysphoria makes it easier to disregard a potential psychiatric condition.

Researchers have shown that it is possible to tease apart depression from major nonpsychiatric comorbidities. Studies have demonstrated that major depression is an independent illness and not merely the result of diabetes, fibromyalgia, or acute coronary syndrome.[7–10]

"Patients with diabetes are twice as likely to experience depression as those without diabetes."[7] Many physicians assume that loss of vision and sexual capacity, fear of amputations and dialysis, and strict diet control with constant blood sugar monitoring adequately explain the increase in mood disorders seen in this patient population. However, studies show that this line of thinking is insufficient.

Although coping with diabetes is challenging, depressive episodes frequently preceded the diagnosis of diabetes. Also, a family history of depression indicates a far greater risk of depression in patients with diabetes regardless of their medical state.[7] Patients with fibromyalgia and concurrent depression are "significantly more likely to live alone, report elevated functional limitations, and display more maladaptive thoughts than nondepressed patients."[9]

Nondepressed patients with fibromyalgia are significantly more likely to have pursued treatment recommendations such as participating in physical therapy.[9] Hallmark symptoms of fibromyalgia like pain, positive tender points, and hypersensitivity to pressure are evident in both depressed and nondepressed patients. Thus, physicians should look at lifestyle and thought processes in separating out depression, and not simply treat fibromyalgia as a masked form of depression.

DIAGNOSING DEPRESSION IN HEART DISEASE

For decades physicians have struggled with diagnosing depression in people with heart disease. Commonly, the symptoms of depression and the

The authors have nothing to disclose.
[a] Department of Psychiatry, The Ohio State University Medical Center, 1670 Upham Drive, Suite 130, Columbus, OH 43210, USA
[b] Twin Valley Behavioral Health, 2200 West Broad Street, Columbus, OH 43223, USA
* Corresponding author.
E-mail address: Radu.Saveanu@osumc.edu

Heart Failure Clin 7 (2011) 75–79
doi:10.1016/j.hfc.2010.08.010
1551-7136/11/$ – see front matter. Published by Elsevier Inc.

symptoms of weak cardiac function overlap and are difficult to tease apart. In addition, heart failure often begets depression, which can in turn worsen cardiac function. Sometimes depression leads to a myocardial event that results in an even worse depressive episode. No matter how one approaches the issue, major depression and heart failure are inextricably linked, and the difficulty in separating the two illnesses often leads to compromised patient care.

New data from the Sertraline Antidepressant Heart Attack Randomized Trials (SADHART) suggest that half of the episodes of major depression began long before the cardiac event and were not caused by acute coronary syndrome (ACS).[10] "Contrary to expectation, half of the episodes of MDD associated with ACS began before rather than after the onset of ACS."[10] The original assumption that in-hospital depression is reactive is now being revised. Although depression and ACS can influence the course of one another, they are two distinct syndromes.

Currently, prior episodes of major depression are not a diagnostic criterion for major depressive disorder, and previous episodes are not considered when determining whether to treat depression in heart failure patients. However, SADHART found a 23% reduction in life-threatening events for patients treated with the selective serotonin reuptake inhibitor (SSRI) sertraline.[10] Therefore, accurately diagnosing depression and treating it appropriately clearly impact health, mood, and longevity in this population.

The first step in differentiating the syndromes of depression and heart failure is understanding the definition of major depression. While sad feelings can be a natural part of experiencing a physical illness, these alone do not constitute a major depressive episode. Neither do overlapping symptoms of decreased energy, anorexia, and insomnia comprise a major depressive episode.

In fact, patients are not even required to feel sad to meet criteria for major depression. According to the *Diagnostic and Statistical Manual of Mental Disorders,* Fourth Edition (DSM-IV), a patient must have either a depressed mood or suffer from anhedonia (markedly diminished interest or pleasure in all or almost all activities) for a period of 2 weeks to be considered for the diagnosis. In addition, patients must demonstrate at least four additional symptoms during the same 2-week period. These symptoms may include

- Insomnia or hypersomnia
- Significant weight or appetite change (increase or decrease)
- Psychomotor agitation or retardation
- Fatigue or loss of energy
- Feelings of worthlessness or excessive or inappropriate guilt
- Diminished ability to think or concentrate
- Recurrent thoughts of death or suicidal ideation.[11]

Thus, even patients who do not complain of a depressed mood can still meet criteria for major depression and respond to treatment.

The SADHART-Congestive Heart Failure (CHF) study reports that "the adverse effect of depression on the prognosis of heart failure is comparable to the impact of aging or ischemic etiology on heart failure prognosis and is independent of those factors."[12] SSRIs are generally benign when used in cardiac patients and are efficacious in treating major depression, particularly in persons with a history of depression that preceded their coronary events.

Who should be treated with antidepressants? How does one distinguish patients who are psychiatrically depressed from those who are demonstrating signs of physical illness only? There are several approaches that one can use.

- The first is the inclusive approach, which includes all signs and symptoms described by the patient regardless of whether his or her complaints can be attributed to his or her heart condition.[1]
- Second is the etiologic approach, which includes symptoms of depression only if they cannot be accounted for by the physical illness.[1]
- Next is the substitutive approach, which recommends exchanging cognitive symptoms of depression for neurovegetative ones. For example, one could substitute pessimism for decreased energy, since the cardiac condition could potentially be responsible for the lack of energy.[1]
- The final approach is the exclusive approach, which completely ignores any symptom that could be the result of the medical condition.[1]

Each approach has its drawbacks. The inclusive approach may potentially overdiagnose depression and lead to false positives. The etiologic approach is often unreliable and requires a clear understanding of causality that is not always apparent. The substitutive approach recommends changing the DSM-IV criteria for depression. Although the changes serve a purpose, they ignore important diagnostic symptoms that have existed for decades and that have been adopted by practicing physicians the world over. Lastly, the exclusive approach eliminates symptoms, undoubtedly resulting in missed diagnoses and false negatives.

So, which approach is best? How does one determine who gets treated with an SSRI for depression and who gets treated for heart failure in isolation?

Trying to decide which symptoms qualify as part of the diagnostic criteria for depression is controversial at best. The potential for disagreement is especially high for symptoms such as fatigue, decreased appetite, psychomotor retardation, and poor concentration. These complaints are manifestations of both heart failure and mood disturbance, and separating the mental contributions from the physical components may be an insurmountable task.

The standard inclusive approach counts all symptoms toward the diagnosis of depression, making it the most reliable approach to take. Patients are rarely overlooked with the inclusive strategy, as all complaints are considered valid signs of mental illness. The withdrawn, anhedonic heart failure patient is given the same diagnosis as the sobbing, agitated heart failure patient. Unfortunately, this approach may lead to inflated rates of depression, and diagnostic validity is compromised in favor of reliability. In addition, the overdiagnosis of depression may lead to an excess of treatment expenditures. Because resources may at times be allocated to patients not truly in need, inclusiveness has the potential to become an expensive approach to health care.

The DSM uses the etiologic approach to diagnosing mental illness, stating that major depression can only be diagnosed if the mood abnormalities are not "due to the direct physiologic effects of a substance,"[11] or "due to the direct physiologic effects of a general medical condition."[11] The individual clinician is responsible for judging how to interpret a patient's presentation. Thus, some physicians may attribute a patient's anorexia to heart failure, while others may attribute it to depression. Without further guidelines as to how a symptom should be interpreted, the etiologic method often fails to be a reliable approach. In the end the etiologic approach becomes a judgment call.

The substitutive approach attempts to eliminate confusion by discarding those symptoms of depression that are most likely to be confused with symptoms of a medical illness. New symptoms are substituted for the original criteria to help avoid ambiguity. Possible substitutions are irritability for loss of energy, tearfulness for weight loss, social withdrawal for psychomotor impairments. Physicians theorize that symptoms of cognitive or affective nature are less likely to be misunderstood as complications of a physical condition like heart failure. Although many find this approach intellectually appealing, to date there has been no agreement on which symptoms are appropriate for either disposal or substitution. Until consensus is reached, there will be difficulties with this method, because it requires each provider to adopt his or her own diagnostic criteria.

Finally, the exclusive approach removes diagnostic criteria that are ambiguous in nature. Symptoms that have the potential to arise from either physical or mental illness are discounted (eg, changes in sleep, appetite, energy). Physicians using exclusion end up working with a shorter list of symptoms. Fewer patients will be identified using this approach, since several of their mood symptoms will no longer be attributed to their emotional well being but instead attributed strictly to their physical health. Although reducing false positives, exclusion will miss patients who might benefit from treatment.

Each of the described approaches has benefits and drawbacks. Without a diagnostic scheme that demonstrates a clear advantage, physicians are left to choose which approach works best with their treatment style.

CASE HISTORY

A 59-year-old white man with known cardiomyopathy starts to experience shortness of breath and fatigue a week before presenting to his neighborhood emergency room. Medical work-up demonstrates a congestive heart failure (CHF) exacerbation, and he is admitted to the cardiology service for diuresis and symptom management. When hospitalized, the patient experiences several episodes of tearfulness, stating he is sick of all the medical procedures and just wants to go home, where "whatever happens, happens." He endorses difficulty sleeping due to the noise in the critical care unit and complains he has no appetite for hospital food. He refuses to get up for the physical therapist, stating he is too tired and repeatedly asks the team to stop wasting its time on him. He denies suicidal ideations but wonders if his "time is up." The cardiology team consults psychiatry to rule out major depression and provide treatment recommendations.

If the consulting psychiatrist uses the inclusive approach, then the patient will undoubtedly be treated for depression. He appears to be experiencing mood fluctuations, poor sleep, poor appetite, decreased energy and motivation, and passive thoughts of death. If the psychiatrist employs the etiologic approach, however, then the patient may or may not be treated for a mood disorder. The tearfulness and ruminating thoughts could be attributed to frustration with his physical health and being trapped in the hospital. Like most cardiac patients, he has difficulty sleeping. In the intensive care units, this is undoubtedly due to nighttime interruptions from staff, alarming monitors, overhead pages, and frequent medical emergencies. Hospital food appeals to very few, and fatigue is a natural consequence of a CHF exacerbation. Therefore, depending on whether the psychiatrist elects to attribute the patient's experience to a mood disorder or his cardiac condition will determine if an antidepressant is used. Equally ambiguous is the substitutive approach. If the psychiatrist feels the patient's neurovegetative symptoms cannot be separated from his heart failure and the patient denies alternative symptoms like indecisiveness and self-pity, then once again the patient may not receive treatment for depression. Finally, all the complaints listed in the case study are possible sequelae of heart failure. Therefore, the patient's insomnia, decreased appetite, and poor energy are likely to disqualify him from receiving a diagnosis of major depression if the exclusive approach is used. This case example illustrates that depending on the exact symptoms endorsed by the patient and the approach used by the psychiatrist, treatment initiation may only occur 25% of the time. In this case, only one of the four approaches identified the patient as needing treatment. How many depressed patients are missed then if the inclusive approach is not used by everyone?

Scientists have long wondered why depression and heart failure seem to go together like donuts and high cholesterol. Clearly patients do not need one to have the other, but the two illnesses seem to fuel one another in a way researchers are just beginning to understand. Currently "heart failure is the fastest growing cardiovascular disorder in the United States," and it is expected to be the leading cause of death by 2020.[13] Depression is the second most frequent reason people call off sick from work according to a recent study funded by the National Institute of Mental Health.[14] Current figures estimate that one in three outpatients with CHF present with a co-occurring depression.[15]

Despite the documented overlap, however, there are no proven theories explaining the comorbidity of heart failure and depression. Proposed mechanisms for the contribution of depression to heart disease include increased activation of the hypothalamic-pituitary-adrenal axis, hyperactivity of the sympathoadrenal system, changes in the activity level of the autonomic nervous system via decreased heart rate variability, and problems with the platelet activation cascade.[16] Newer models suggest a link between cytokines, depression, and heart failure. However, more studies need to be done before a causal link can be established.

Major functions of cytokines include regulating the immune system and priming the body to respond to infection. In heart failure patients, abundant proinflammatory cytokines are released following myocardial injury. Interleukin (IL)-6 and tumor necrosis factor (TNF)-α are the most commonly observed, but IL-1β and IL-2 are also thought to play a role in heart failure.[13] Higher levels of circulating cytokines correspond with an increasing severity of heart failure symptoms.

From a psychiatric standpoint, researchers like Michael Maes have shown that activation of the inflammatory response system also occurs in major depression. Additionally, monoamine deficits associated with major depression are associated with abnormalities in the immune system. Overproduction of IL-6 and IL-1β, two of the proinflammatory cytokines connected with heart failure, have been linked with a severe form of depression known as melancholic depression.[17,18]

Other reinforcing evidence comes from case studies of individuals treated with the cytokine interferon (INF)α for hepatitis C. Patients receiving INFα frequently become depressed, and the depression responds positively to traditional antidepressants.[19]

These findings and others are consistent with the idea that depression is tied to heart failure patients through an elevation in blood level cytokines and that depression in CHF patients may equally respond to conventional antidepressant treatment.

SUMMARY

Deciding whom to treat for depression is a daunting task. Each of the approaches described (inclusive, exclusive, etiologic, and substitutive) has risks and benefits. However, the real risk appears to be in neglecting treatment of mood disordered patients. SADHART shows that people with acute coronary syndrome benefit from treatment with an SSRI, and studies are underway to demonstrate success in CHF patients as well.

Although major depression is difficult to separate from the physical ailments of heart failure, attention to the strict criteria set forth by the DSM-IV can provide guidance in distinguishing between the two diseases. Despite their unique properties, both depression and heart failure are associated with significant morbidity and mortality. Together, they present a significant health risk.

Given the high level of association between the two maladies, the authors recommend using an inclusive approach to treatment. The low level of risk using SSRIs in acute coronary syndrome has already been demonstrated by the SADHART study. An extrapolation of those results would suggest similar success for other cardiac patients. Although by using the inclusive approach one might anticipate a potential excess of false-positive diagnoses of depression in CHF patients, the relatively benign nature of SSRI treatment may justify this overinclusiveness as worthwhile. Until future studies provide better guidance, providers should err on the side of their patients and actively diagnose and treat depression. As stated in a recent issue of *Circulation*, "The opportunity to screen for and treat depression in cardiac patients should not be missed, as effective depression treatment may improve health outcomes."[20]

REFERENCES

1. McDaniel JS, Brown FW, Cole SA. Assessment of depression and grief reactions in the medically ill. In: Stoudemire A, Fogel BS, Greenberg DB, editors. Psychiatric care of the medical patient. Oxford (United Kingdom): Oxford University Press; 2000. p. 149–64.
2. Bukberg J, Penman D, Holland JC. Depression in hospitalized cancer patients. Psychosom Med 1984;46:199–212.
3. Rodin G, Voshart K. Depression in the medically ill: an overview. Am J Psychiatry 1986;143:696–705.
4. Stoudemire A. Depression in the medically ill. In: Michaels R, Cavenar J, Brodie HS, editors. Psychiatry. Philadelphia: J.B. Lippincott; 1985. p. 1–8.
5. Wells KB, Hays RD, Burnam A, et al. Detection of depressive disorders for patients receiving prepaid or fee-for-service care. JAMA 1989;262:3298–302.
6. Stober DR, Schwartz JA, McDaniel JS, et al. Depression and HIV disease: prevalence, correlates, and treatment. Psychiatr Ann 1997;27:372–7.
7. Lustman PJ, Anderson R. Depression in adults with diabetes. Psychiatr Times 2002;19:1069–78.
8. Kirmayer LJ, Robbins JM, Kapusta MA. Somatization and depression in fibromyalgia syndrome. Am J Psychiatry 1988;145:950–4.
9. Okifuji A, Turk DC, Sherman JJ. Evaluation of the relationship between depression and fibromyalgia syndrome: why aren't all patients depressed? J Rheumatol 2000;1:212–9.
10. Glassman AH, Bigger JT, Gaffney M, et al. Onset of major depression associated with acute coronary syndrome. Arch Gen Psychiatry 2006;63:283–8.
11. Task Force on DSM-IV. Mood disorders. In: First MB, editor. Diagnostic and statistical manual of mental disorders. 4th edition. Arlington (VA): American Psychiatric Association; 2000. p. 345–428.
12. Jiang W, O'Connor C, Silva SG, et al. Safety and efficacy of sertraline for depression in patients with CHF (SADHART-CHF): a randomized, double-blind, placebo-controlled trial of sertraline for major depression with congestive heart failure. Am Heart J 2008;156:437–44.
13. Pasic J, Levy WC, Sullivan MD. Cytokines in depression and heart failure. Psychosom Med 2003;65:181–93.
14. Merikangas KR, Ames M, Cui L, et al. The impact of comorbidity of mental and physical conditions on role disability in the US adult population. Arch Gen Psychiatry 2007;64:1180–8.
15. Konstam V, Moser DK, De Jong MJ. Depression and anxiety in heart failure. J Card Fail 2005;11:455–63.
16. Jiang W, Kuchibhatla M, Clary GL, et al. Relationship between depressive symptoms and long-term mortality in patients with heart failure. Am Heart J 2007;154:102–8.
17. Maes M, Scharpe S, Meltzer HY, et al. Relationship between interleukin-6 activity, acute phase proteins, and function of the hypothalamic–pituitary axis in severe depression. Psychiatry Res 1993;49:11–27.
18. Maes M. Evidence for an immune response in major depression: a review and hypothesis. Prog Neuropsychopharmacol Biol Psychiatry 1995;19:11–38.
19. Gleason OC, Yates WR. Five cases of interferon-alpha-induced depression treated with antidepressant therapy. Psychosomatics 1999;40:510–2.
20. Lichtman JH, Bigger JT Jr, Blumenthal JA, et al. Depression and coronary heart disease: recommendations for screening, referral, and treatment. Circulation 2008;118:1768–75.

Clinical Trial Evidence for Treatment of Depression in Heart Failure

Melvin R. Echols, MD[a], Wei Jiang, MD[b,*]

KEYWORDS

• Depression • Heart failure • Depression treatment

Depression is continuously recognized to have high prevalence and negative impact on the prognosis of many comorbid diseases, particularly chronic heart failure (CHF) and other populations of cardiovascular disease (CVD).[1] As more is understood about the chronicity of depression and the underappreciated obstacles presented in disease-specific treatment for patients with comorbid depression and heart failure, more research efforts are now requiring a multidisciplinary collaboration to provide optimal management.[2,3] The management of depression in patients with CHF is increasingly challenging as the field continues to advance in evidence-based research and care, requiring more patient initiative to comply with complex treatment strategies.

Although depression and heart failure appear to have negative synergism in terms of morbidity and mortality as comorbid diseases,[4,5] there have been limited and finite amounts of data provided supporting optimal treatment of depression in heart failure patients. Optimal treatment of depression in heart failure patients also has been hindered due to the rapid development of various classes of antidepressant medications over the past several decades.[6–8] There are very few studies that have attempted to prospectively evaluate the role of antidepressants on the outcome of depression in heart failure patients. Therefore, this article will encompass the data available pertaining to clinical trial efforts of depression management in heart failure patients.

Approximately 20% of patients with CHF are estimated to have depression, representing about 1 million people in the United States who are currently dealing with the comorbid conditions of depression and heart failure.[7] Realistically, this is most likely a conservative estimation of prevalence in the overall clinical practice environment. Although the motivation to understand the impact of depression in CVD has focused on various specific populations in acute or subacute phases of CVD, the chronic heart failure patient population has become a much more emphasized group for evaluation over the past decade. There are many possible reasons for this direction, such as the substantial cost of care related to depression treatment in CHF, as well as the significant rates of comorbid depression in these patients.[8,9] Even so, there are still many questions left unanswered pertaining to the adequacy and efficacy of the modern-day treatments available for depression in heart failure patients.

Rutledge and colleagues[6] performed a meta-analysis of depression in heart failure to review the reported prevalence, intervention effects, and association of depression to clinical outcome in heart failure patients. These investigators collected information on 27 articles reporting prevalence information, 14 studies presenting prospective associations of depression and heart failure, and 6 studies reporting the degree of change in depression from treatment baseline. After the considerations of study heterogeneity,

[a] Department of Internal Medicine, Duke Clinical Research Institute, Duke University Medical Center, PO Box 31246, Durham, NC 27710, USA
[b] Departments of Psychiatry and Behavioral Sciences, and Internal Medicine, PO Box 3366, Duke University Medical Center, Durham, NC 27710, USA
* Corresponding author.
E-mail address: jiang001@mc.duke.edu

Heart Failure Clin 7 (2011) 81–88
doi:10.1016/j.hfc.2010.08.004
1551-7136/11/$ – see front matter

the investigators reported a combined prevalence of approximately 20% to 38% across all included studies. The prevalence of detected depression within the heart failure patients varied according to questionnaire completion or diagnostic interview (33.6% vs 19.3%, respectively). This is a subtle yet important difference, as much of the diagnosis of depression within clinical trials relies heavily on the use of patient self-administered questionnaires such as the Beck Depression Inventory (BDI). The results of this meta-analysis suggested that use of such questionnaires was probably more helpful in depression detection. The investigators also reported the consistent finding across several studies (ie, higher rates of death and secondary events in depressed patients with heart failure). The results of this analysis further solidified the impact and significance of depression in heart failure patients, as well as the need for more aggressive management.

There are a few pharmacologic and nonpharmacologic interventions that have been pursued within depressed heart failure patients that may have promise for future treatment strategies. However, there remain many questionable issues related to prevalence and associated clinical outcomes of patients with depression and heart failure that have led some investigators to provide a more detailed basic foundation of past efforts to understand the global challenges in managing these two diseases.

ANTIDEPRESSANTS AND CHF

As the number of medical therapies for heart failure management has exploded within the past 20 years, so have antidepressant therapeutic developments for the treatment of depression. Although the research efforts for both diseases have produced somewhat of a parallel productivity in the pharmaceutical industry, there has been very limited understanding of the impact these medical therapies have on interaction with other disease states. For instance, there have been data in the past management of heart failure care to suggest that some of the disease-specific therapies, such as beta-blockers, may affect incidence of depression in patients with heart failure.[10] Although there continue to be conflicting thoughts of the significance of these findings, several investigators have attempted to provide similar information pertaining to antidepressants and safety related to heart failure care.

Tricyclic Antidepressants

Very few data have reported efficacy and safety results of the use of tricyclic antidepressants (TCAs) in heart failure, yet the previous data are noteworthy, since there remains a fair amount of ambiguity for optimal medical treatment of depression in heart failure patients. Roose and colleagues helped to develop the initial work of evaluating TCAs in CVD, primarily with the study of drugs such as imipramine. As with a number of the TCAs, imipramine was known to have a possible modest antiarrhythmic effect, which initially was thought beneficial in the treatment of acute coronary syndrome, but which was later countered by the adverse effects of antiarrhythmic in the Cardiac Arrhythmia Suppression Trial (CAST). These drugs were also noted to have an impact on heart rate, secondary to many of the anticholinergic properties.[11,12] The cardiotoxic effects related to arrhythmia provocation have been noted with TCAs at therapeutic and massive dosages; these effects include QTc prolongation, conduction delays, significant blocking of the AV nodal and bundle branches, and even increased mortality.[13,14]

Imipramine also was shown to have a significant rate of drug discontinuation secondary to the profound incidence of orthostatic hypotension. This phenomenon was best shown in a small cohort of heart failure patients who were treated with imipramine or bupropion in a random, double-blinded crossover study.[15] There were no effects reported on the worsening or improvement of ejection fraction in this study. Roose and colleagues subsequently evaluated nortriptyline among 21 depressed heart failure patients and found no association of worsening ejection fraction or symptoms within this group. The investigators also noted that there was significantly less severe orthostatic hypotension within this group compared with patients treated in previous trials with imipramine (5% vs 50%, respectively). Those data by Roose and colleagues[16] suggest that certain TCAs may be tolerated and possibly beneficial in patients with left ventricular impairment. However, due to the very small number of these cohorts and lack of a control arm, these data did not support clear superiority benefits of nortriptyline over imipramine, or whether both are superior to other antidepressants. As many of the cardiac research efforts began to appreciate the value of sympathetic antagonism by this time, the drug class continued to lose favor among first-line therapies for depression management in CVD.

The data related to TCAs and other antidepressant therapies also were heavily persuaded by the accepted definitions of heart failure at the time. Most of the data for TCAs and heart failure were in patients with ischemic heart failure. The modest 1A antiarrhythmic activity of the TCAs becomes more significant when considering TCA use for the management of depression in patients with ischemic heart disease. The findings of the CAST suggest that agents with type 1A antiarrhythmic activity, including TCAs, should not be used in patients with ischemic heart disease.[17,18] The hypothesis supported by the CAST study suggested that suppression of ventricular premature depolarizations following myocardial infarction (MI) would reduce cardiac mortality. At the end of the follow-up period, however, the data associated increased mortality to the class 1A and 1C antiarrhythmic agents moricizine, encainide, and flecainide when compared with placebo. The underlying mechanism for these finding is not yet understood, but evidence points to an interaction between class 1 antiarrhythmic agents and ischemic myocardium, which results in greater vulnerability to ventricular fibrillation during an ischemic event.[19] There is not a tremendous level of understanding for TCA use in nonischemic cardiomyopathy. Therefore, the role of this drug class as it relates to present day heart failure care is not fully understood. There is little chance that this drug class may receive an unbiased review of efficacy at present due to the progressive advancement of newer drug classes. However, further evaluation of drugs within this class may be beneficial for optimal treatment of depression in heart failure management.

Selective Serotonin Reuptake Inhibitors

As sympathetic antagonism has become a main focus point for heart failure management, the theory for inhibition of neurosynaptic serotonin reuptake has been just as valuable in managing depression. The appearance of fluoxetine in the 1980s was quickly followed by several competing medications within the same class that were all marketed with reasonable cardiac tolerance.[7] The primary mechanism of action of selective serotonin reuptake inhibitors (SSRIs) results in increased serotonin circulation by blocking presynaptic serotonin receptors. This results in a down-regulation of the actual receptors, sustaining the level of circulating of serotonin.[7,8] This effect has been shown to improve the mood in depressed patients, decreasing the prevalence of clinical depression. Although there is an acceptance of cardiac tolerance for this drug class, there are also some varying degrees of anticholinergic effects, sedation, and weight gain for different SSRIs. There are also some minor changes in heart rate, although not clinically significant.[6,20]

The clinical trial data for the use of SSRIs in patients with CVD vary significantly in terms of disease focus. Much of the data have focused on the use of SSRIs in patients with cardiac ischemia or postacute coronary syndrome. However, a few of investigators have produced evidence to support the safety and efficacy of SSRI use in heart failure patients.[16–18]

Roose and colleagues[20] provided valuable information pertaining to the use of SSRIs in depressed patients with CVD. In 1998, these investigators evaluated the cardiovascular effects of fluoxetine in 27 depressed patients with cardiac disease (CHF, conduction disease, or ventricular arrhythmia) in an open-label trial. Patients were treated up to a maximum dose of 60 mg/d of fluoxetine for 7 weeks. The primary outcome was based on measures of heart rate, ejection fraction, electrocardiogram (ECG) findings, and other secondary parameters. Baseline values of these measures were compared at 2 and 7 weeks. At the end of follow-up, fluoxetine was shown to have very modest effects on decreasing heart rate and increasing supine systolic blood pressure and ejection fraction. The data of the patients taking fluoxetine were compared with 60 patients with a similar disease proportion taking TCAs. Patients taking fluoxetine were found to have fewer adverse effects (4% for fluoxetine, 20% for TCAs), although very little could be concluded from these comparisons because of trial design.

Gottlieb and colleagues[21] assessed the efficacy of controlled released paroxetine on depression and quality of life in CHF through a double-blind, randomized, placebo-controlled design. The investigators evaluated the reductions in depression following 12 weeks of treatment with paroxetine compared with patients taking placebo (total cohort n = 27). Patients who had BDI score greater than 10 and had symptomatic heart failure were eligible for the trial. The BDI was assessed at baseline, 4, 8, and 12 weeks of treatment. At the end of follow-up, patients taking controlled-release paroxetine were associated with a higher percentage of recovery from depression when compared with patients taking placebo, based on BDI greater than 10 (69% vs 23%, $P = .018$). Patients treated with paroxetine also had better improvements in quality of life and consistently lower BDI scores. These findings were encouraging and helped to support the more recent findings of larger clinical efforts.

Alves and colleagues[22] evaluated the use of an SSRI in elderly patients with heart failure to assess the potential benefits of cognitive improvement of sertraline. Through the use of a prospective case–control trial design and the Cambridge Mental Disorders of the Elderly Examination battery (CAMCOG), the investigators assessed the cognitive impairment in 20 patients with major depressive disorder and CHF, 23 nondepressed heart failure patients, and 18 healthy controls. After treatment with sertraline, the investigators reported significant improvements of cognitive function in all groups as representated by CAMCOG scoring. These data supported the potential of antidepressant use in elderly heart failure patients to sustain optimal cognitive function.

Although the results of those studies indicate SSRIs may be effective and safe in depression heart failure patients, certain concerns exist about the sample sizes that are very small and whether such intervention may improve the poor prognosis related to depression.

The Safety and Efficacy of Sertraline for Depression in Patients with Chronic Heart Failure (SADHART-CHF) is a prospective, randomized, double-blind, placebo-controlled trial that has sought to evaluate whether sertraline can improve cardiac outcomes in CHF patients with major depressive disorder.[23] The trial design is presented in **Fig. 1**. Although the primary results of the analysis are unpublished, the preliminary data for this trial were presented at the Heart Failure Society of America conference in 2008.[24] The trial design also incorporated a standard level of nurse-facilitated and intervention support for both the sertraline and the placebo groups. Eligible patients for this trial were aged at least 45 years and had a left ventricular ejection fraction of no more than 45%. These patients also had to have a BDI score of at least10 as well as meet the *Diagnostic and Statistical Manual of Mental Disorders* (Fourth Edition) (DSM-IV) criteria for major depressive disorder.

The inclusion criteria developed by the investigators helped to define a much more specific population of patients with heart failure as well as criteria-specific major depressive disorder. Hamilton Depression Rating Scale (HDRS) that has been used broadly in trials assessing antidepressant effect was the primary measure of depression severity in the SADHART-CHF trial. While the detailed results of the study are being published, according the abstract presentation at the Heart Failure Society of America conference in 2008,[24] the study had randomized 469 heart failure patients with major depressive disorder to either sertraline (n = 234) or placebo (n = 235). Patients

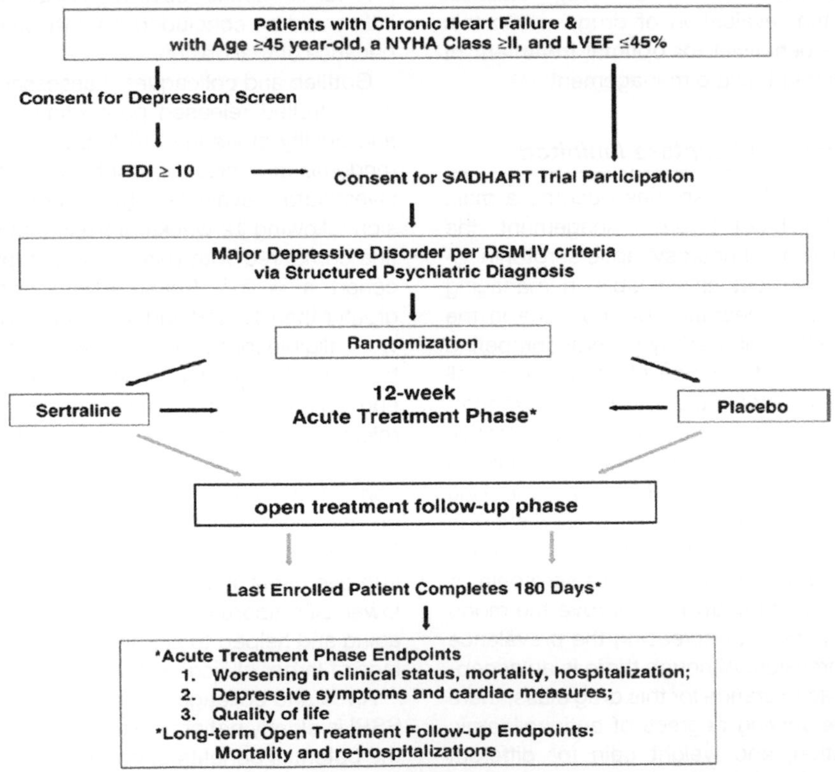

Fig. 1. Flowchart of trial design for SADHART-CHF (Safety and Efficacy of Sertraline for Depression in Patients with Chronic Heart Failure). (*From* Jiang W, O'Connor C, Silva SG, et al. SADHART-CHF Investigators. Safety and efficacy of Sertraline for depression in patients with CHF (SADHART-CHF): a randomized, double-blind, placebo-controlled trial of sertraline for major depression with congestive heart failure. Am Heart J 2008;156:437–44; with permission.)

initially were treated with 50 mg/d of sertraline or placebo with potential titration to a maximum of 200 mg/d for the first 12 weeks of treatment. The primary end points for this trial were change in HDRS at 12 weeks and worsening in clinical status, mortality, or hospitalizations, depressive symptoms, and quality of life. Long-term end point assessments consisted primarily of mortality and rehospitalizations up until the last randomized patient completed the 6-month follow-up, although the study was not powered to adequately evaluate these end points.

At the end of the 12-week treatment, there were no significant differences in depression between either the patients taking sertraline or the patients taking placebo. Even so, both groups had significant improvement in depression independently. There were no differences in the incidence of death, cardiovascular death, or hospitalizations for worsening heart failure between the groups either. The high response rate might have been influenced by the assistance of nurse-facilitated support, which was quite extensive in this trial. The psychiatric-trained nursing staff called the patients at 1, 2, 4, 8, and 10 weeks and coordinated face-to-face home or clinic visits during weeks 6 and 12. The intensity of these nursing efforts is thought to have had a significant influence on the results of this study. Many previous studies did not facilitate nursing support in this manner. The results of this trial helped to emphasize the understated need of more supportive care in patients with depression and heart failure. More study is required to understand if nurse-facilitated interventions or other nonpharmacologic methods may be equivocal or superior to medical therapy in this population.

It is expected that the SADHART-CHF study will provide insights for characteristics of patients who respond to the intervention and who do not and change of quality of life and perceived social stress with intervention and depression responses. Characteristically, approximately 40% of the participants were African American, and 40% were women. Perhaps more will be learned about whether there is any difference with depression intervention in regards to sex and ethnicity.

As the evidence builds for more effective outcome analysis for the impact of depression management in CHF, investigators have continued to design clinical trials to help provide more optimal understanding of treatment for both diseases. The Morbidity, Mortality and Mood in Depressed Heart Failure (MOOD-HF) study is an ongoing prospective, randomized, double-blind, multicenter trial investigating the efforts of the SSRI escitalopram on morbidity and mortality, severity of depression, anxiety, cognitive function, and quality of life in an estimated 700 patients.[25] This trial is the largest clinical trial evaluating the effects of an SSRI on adequately powered hard end points of clinical outcome. The trial design is presented in **Fig. 2**.

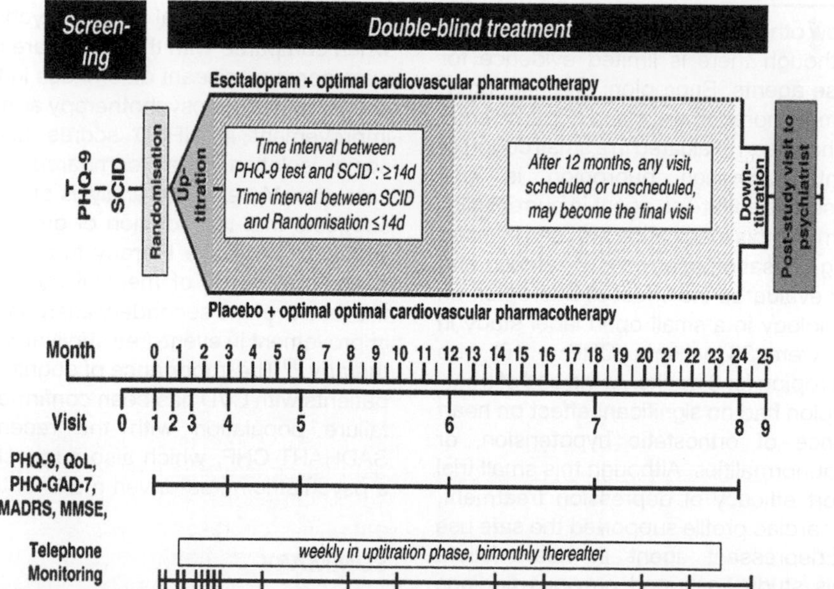

Fig. 2. Flowchart of trial design for MOOD-HF (Morbidity, Mortality and Mood in Depressed Heart Failure). (*From* Angermann CE, Gelbrich G, Störk S, et al. Rationale and design of a randomised, controlled, multicenter trial investigating the effects of selective serotonin reuptake inhibition on morbidity, mortality, and mood in depressed heart failure patients (MOOD-HF). Eur J Heart Failure 2007;9(12):1212–22; with permission.)

Escitalopram was chosen as the SSRI of choice secondary to more selective serotonin receptor inhibition, as well as demonstrated superior efficacy in a meta-analysis of over 4500 patients treated with various antidepressants, including other SSRIs.[26] Eligible patients for MOOD-HF are patients older than 18 years, systolic heart failure of any etiology with New York Heart Association greater than or equal to II and ejection fraction less than 45%. All patients are to have a current episode of depression according to the DSM-IV and the Structured Clinical Interview for Depression (SCID). The primary end point for this analysis is time to first event of either death or unplanned hospitalization. MOOD-HF also has included evaluation of four predefined substudies to

- Evaluate the positive predictive value of the Patient Health Questionnaire (PHQ-9)
- Assess the effect of escitalopram on platelet aggregation
- Assess vasoreactivity in depressed heart failure patients in response to treatment
- Assess various gene polymorphisms that may possibly predispose patients to depression in CHF.[25]

The results of the primary analysis of MOOD-HF and subset studies will hopefully provide valuable insight on the need for more aggressive depression treatment in heart failure patients.

Other Antidepressants

There are a few other medical therapies noteworthy in effect, although there is limited evidence for many of these agents. Bupropion, an antidepressant with primary noradrenergic and dopaminergic effects, also has been evaluated in a small cohort of CVD patients. Although bupropion is less commonly used as a first-line agent in current clinical management, this medication also can be used as a smoking cessation treatment.[7,27] Roose and colleagues[28] evaluated the effect of bupropion on cardiac physiology in a small open label study in 1991. There were 36 patients (CHF = 15) who received bupropion for 3 weeks. At the end of treatment, bupropion had no significant effect on heart rate, incidence of orthostatic hypotension, or conduction abnormalities. Although this small trial did not report efficacy of depression treatment, the low-risk cardiac profile supported the safe use of this antidepressant agent in heart failure patients. This study confirmed previous findings from a small study evaluating the use of bupropion compared with imipramine, suggesting less hemodynamic and cardiac abnormalities with buproprion.[15]

There is much less understanding of other available agents for depression treatment in patients with CVD. Certain agents, such as monoamine oxidase (MAO) inhibitors have much less evidence for use in patients with CVD, and have significant degrees of cardiovascular side effects, including orthostatic hypotension and possible hypertensive crisis.[7,8] This drug class is most likely not beneficial for a CHF population and should be avoided.

Psychotherapy trial evidence

Much of the research effort for depression management in heart failure has focused on pharmacologic management, yet recent data suggest that more emphasis on behavioral or cognitive therapy may help decrease the prevalence of clinical depression in patients with CVD. The Enhancing Recovery in Coronary Heart Disease Patients (ENRICHD) trial was a randomized, controlled trial that evaluated the use of cognitive–behavioral psychotherapy in patients who suffered from myocardial infarction with either low social support or depression.[29] The cognitive therapy was provided in a randomized manner after the indexed myocardial infarction (median time to initiation approximately 11 days), with supplementation of an SSRI when indicated. The primary outcome measure for the cohort of approximately 2500 patients was a composite of death or MI at 6 months, although the secondary outcome measure included change in Hamilton Rating Scale for Depression. At the end of the follow-up period, there were no significant differences in the event-free survival for the psychotherapy arm when compared with the usual care cohort. There were some significant differences in the degree of depression in the psychotherapy arm, including an improvement in HRSD scores and decreased social isolation, when compared with the usual care arm. More recent analysis of these data also suggests that the addition of group therapy with individual cognitive therapy further benefited the patients in terms of medical outcome, although the results of the secondary analysis did not report improvement in event-free survival with this added therapy.[30] The importance of cognitive therapy for patients with CVD has been confirmed in the heart failure population with the recent results of SADHART-CHF, which also suggested benefit in a psychiatric nurse-driven mode of therapy.[24]

SUMMARY

Although there is growing evidence of need for larger clinical trials to assist in the understanding of depression management in heart failure patients, the reported data have initiated more questions as the optimal balance of pharmacologic and nonpharmacologic care is attempted in the management of depression for heart failure patients. The treatment of depression is quite complex in patients without significant cardiovascular disease, requiring significant follow-up and dedication to compliance. The presence of comorbid heart failure in depressed patients has the potential to change the prognosis of not only clinical outcomes of depression, but also the pathway of heart failure treatment compliance and hospitalization. There is significant harmful potential in leaving depression untreated in heart failure patients. Continued efforts to aggressively diagnose and manage depression in heart failure patients ultimately could provide better clinical outcomes as well as improve quality of life for patients. The challenges of depression management in heart failure patients require much attention and ideally will require more specific trial evidence to support the complex management of such patients.

REFERENCES

1. Jiang W, Alexander J, Christopher E, et al. Relationship of depression to increased risk of mortality and rehospitalization in patients with congestive heart failure. Arch Intern Med 2001;161(15): 1849–56.
2. O'Connor CM, Jiang W, Kuchibhatla M, et al. Antidepressant use, depression, and survival in patients with heart failure. Arch Intern Med 2008;168(20): 2232–7.
3. Pozuelo L, Tesar G, Zhang J, et al. Depression and heart disease: what do we know, and where are we headed? Cleve Clin J Med 2009;76(1):59–70.
4. Jiang W, Hasselblad V, Krishnan RR, et al. Patients with CHF and depression have greater risk of mortality and morbidity than patients without depression. J Am Coll Cardiol 2002;39(5):919–21.
5. Jiang W. Impacts of depression and emotional distress on cardiac disease. Cleve Clin J Med 2008;75(Suppl 2):S20–5.
6. Rutledge T, Reis VA, Linke SE, et al. Depression in heart failure a meta-analytic review of prevalence, intervention effects, and associations with clinical outcomes. J Am Coll Cardiol 2006;48(8):1527–37.
7. Shapiro PA. Treatment of depression in patients with congestive heart failure. Heart Fail Rev 2009;14(1): 7–12.
8. Watson K, Summers KM. Depression in patients with heart failure: clinical implications and management. Pharmacotherapy 2009;29(1):49–63.
9. O'Connor CM, Joynt KE. Depression: are we ignoring an important comorbidity in heart failure? J Am Coll Cardiol 2004;43(9):1550–2.
10. Messerli FH, Bangalore S, Yao SS, et al. Cardioprotection with beta-blockers: myths, facts, and Pascal's wager. J Intern Med 2009;266(3):232–41.
11. Glassman AH, Johnson LL, Giardina EG, et al. The use of imipramine in depressed patients with congestive heart failure. JAMA 1983;250(15): 1997–2001.
12. Glassman AH, Roose SP, Bigger JT Jr. The safety of tricyclic antidepressants in cardiac patients. Risk-benefit reconsidered. JAMA 1993;269(20):2673–5.
13. Raisfeld IH. Cardiovascular complications of antidepressant therapy. Interactions at the adrenergic neuron. Am Heart J 1972;83(1):129–33.
14. Jiang W, Krishnan RR, O'Connor CM. Depression and heart disease: evidence of a link, and its therapeutic implications. CNS Drugs 2002;16(2):111–27.
15. Roose SP, Glassman AH, Giardina EG, et al. Cardiovascular effects of imipramine and bupropion in depressed patients with congestive heart failure. J Clin Psychopharmacol 1987;7(4):247–51.
16. Roose SP, Glassman AH, Giardina EG, et al. Nortriptyline in depressed patients with left ventricular impairment. JAMA 1986;256(23):3253–7.
17. The Cardiac Arrhythmia Suppression Trial II Investigators. Effect of the antiarrhythmic agent moricizine on survival after myocardial infarction. N Engl J Med 1992;327(4):227–33.
18. Echt DS, Liebson PR, Mitchell LB, et al. Mortality and morbidity in patients receiving encainide, flecainide, or placebo. The Cardiac Arrhythmia Suppression Trial. N Engl J Med 1991;324(12):781–8.
19. Greenberg HM, Dwyer EM Jr, Hochman JS, et al. Interaction of ischaemia and encainide/flecainide treatment: a proposed mechanism for the increased mortality in CAST I. Br Heart J 1995;74(6):631–5.
20. Roose SP, Glassman AH, Attia E, et al. Cardiovascular effects of fluoxetine in depressed patients with heart disease. Am J Psychiatry 1998;155(5): 660–5.
21. Gottlieb SS, Kop WJ, Thomas SA, et al. A double-blind placebo-controlled pilot study of controlled-release paroxetine on depression and quality of life in chronic heart failure. Am Heart J 2007;153(5): 868–73.
22. Alves TC, Rays J, Telles RM, et al. Effects of antidepressant treatment on cognitive performance in elderly subjects with heart failure and comorbid major depression: an exploratory study. Psychosomatics 2007;48(1):22–30.
23. Jiang W, O'Connor C, Silva SG, et al. Safety and efficacy of sertraline for depression in patients with CHF (SADHART-CHF): a randomized, double-blind, placebo-controlled trial of sertraline for major depression with congestive heart failure. Am Heart J 2008;156(3):437–44.
24. Mehra MR, Rockman HA, Greenberg BH. Highlights of the 2008 Scientific Sessions of the Heart Failure

Society of America. Toronto, Ontario, Canada, September 20–23, 2008. J Am Coll Cardiol 2009; 53(6):514–22.

25. Angermann CE, Gelbrich G, Störk S, et al. Rationale and design of a randomised, controlled, multicenter trial investigating the effects of selective serotonin reuptake inhibition on morbidity, mortality, and mood in depressed heart failure patients (MOOD-HF). Eur J Heart Fail 2007;9(12):1212–22.
26. Kennedy SH, Andersen HF, Thase ME. Escitalopram in the treatment of major depressive disorder: a meta-analysis. Curr Med Res Opin 2009;25(1): 161–75.
27. Swanson NA, Burroughs CC, Long MA, et al. Controlled trial for smoking cessation in a Navy shipboard population using nicotine patch, sustained-release bupropion, or both. Mil Med 2003;168(10):830–4.
28. Roose SP, Dalack GW, Glassman AH, et al. Cardiovascular effects of bupropion in depressed patients with heart disease. Am J Psychiatry 1991;148(4):512–6.
29. Berkman LF, Blumenthal J, Burg M, et al. Effects of treating depression and low perceived social support on clinical events after myocardial infarction: the Enhancing Recovery in Coronary Heart Disease Patients (ENRICHD) Randomized Trial. JAMA 2003;289(23):3106–16.
30. Saab PG, Bang H, Williams RB, et al. The impact of cognitive behavioral group training on event-free survival in patients with myocardial infarction: the ENRICHD experience. J Psychosom Res 2009; 67(1):45–56.

A Review on the Putative Association Between Beta-Blockers and Depression

Daniëlle E.P. Verbeek, MD[a,1,*], Jerry van Riezen, MD[b], Rudolf A. de Boer, MD, PhD[c], Joost P. van Melle, MD, PhD[c], Peter de Jonge, PhD[b,d]

KEYWORDS

• β-Blockers • Depression • Cardiovascular disease • Heart failure • Review

β-Blockers are among the most commonly prescribed drugs in the world. They are registered for a wide range of indications, including angina pectoris, arrhythmias, hypertension, heart failure (HF), and secondary prevention after myocardial infarction (MI). The beneficial effects in reducing anginal complaints and improving prognosis in patients post-MI is undisputed.[1] In patients with HF, β-blockers were initially deemed harmful, but now they have become the cornerstone of the treatment of chronic HF.[2] Small- and large-scale trials[3–7] have undisputedly proved that β-blockers reduce HF-related mortality and morbidity. β-Blocker use is associated with a 35%[4,7] to 65%[3] reduction in total mortality in patients with HF. In the elderly, a 15% reduction in mortality is achieved.[5] Both sudden cardiac death and death caused by worsening HF are significantly reduced. Therefore, current guidelines strongly recommend to prescribe β-blockers for all patients with symptomatic and asymptomatic HF, regardless of the cause, and to titrate to the maximum tolerated dose.[8]

Despite their proven efficacy, β-blocker therapy has its limitations. Particularly, in patients with advanced HF, titration can be troublesome and is not without potential danger (ie, cardiogenic shock). In addition, there are (relative) contraindications to beta-blockade, such as asthma, chronic obstructive pulmonary disease (COPD), conduction system disease or inadequate function of the sinus node with or without bradycardia, diabetes, and peripheral vascular disease. However, recent studies have shown that the use of cardioselective β-blockers in patients with COPD, mild to moderate asthma, diabetes, and mild to moderate peripheral vascular disease is safe.[9–13]

Still, the use of β-blockers is associated with potential adverse effects. Fatigue, sleep disturbances, nightmares, sexual dysfunction, and depression are commonly cited adverse effects, and these effects may be the reasons for the lower-than-desired use of β-blockers.[14] Among these adverse effects, β-blocker–induced depression raised particular attention. For a diagnosis of

[1]From February 1, 2011: Department of Internal Medicine, University Medical Center Groningen, Huispost AA 41, PO Box 30.001, 9700 RB Groningen, The Netherlands.

[a] Department of Internal Medicine, Ziekenhuisgroep Twente, PO Box 7600, 7600 SZ Almelo, The Netherlands

[b] Interdisciplinary Center for Psychiatric Epidemiology, University Medical Centre Groningen, University of Groningen, PO Box 30.001, CC;72, 9700 RB Groningen, The Netherlands

[c] Department of Cardiology, Thorax Center, University Medical Center Groningen, PO Box 30.001, 9700 RB Groningen, The Netherlands

[d] Faculty of Social and Behavioural Sciences, University of Tilburg, Centre of Research on Psychology in Somatic Diseases (CoRPS), Postbus 90153, 5000 LE Tilburg, The Netherlands

* Corresponding author.

E-mail address: verbeek.dep@gmail.com

Heart Failure Clin 7 (2011) 89–99
doi:10.1016/j.hfc.2010.08.006
1551-7136/11/$ – see front matter

depression, according to the Diagnostic and Statistical Manual of Mental Disorders (Fourth Edition) criteria,[15] at least 5 symptoms have to be present, including at least 1 of the 2 main symptoms, that is, depressed mood or loss of interest. In addition, at least 4 of 7 other symptoms of depression should be present: (1) significant change of weight and/or appetite, (2) insomnia or hypersomnia, (3) psychomotoric retardation or agitation, (4) energy loss and fatigue, (5) feelings of worthlessness or increased feelings of guilt, (6) thoughts about death and/or suicidal ideation, and (7) reduced concentration and impaired cognitive capacity. These symptoms have to be present for most part of the day, for at least 2 weeks. The annual prevalence of depression in the general population is estimated at 3% to 5%.[16] Despite the strong clinical suspicion that β-blockers can cause depression, studies on this association often showed conflicting results. The importance of reaching a consensus on the issue may be obvious; depression is a severe condition that greatly affects both cardiovascular prognosis[17,18] and quality of life.[19] In this article the authors review the literature on the alleged association between β-blocker use and depression, describe the putative underlying physiologic working mechanisms, and come to a final conclusion with clinical recommendations for the cardiovascular patient.

INITIAL SIGNS OF POSSIBLE DEPRESSOGENIC PROPERTIES

The discussion on β-blockers and depression started as early as 1967, when Waal[20] reported a conspicuously high incidence of depression among a group of hypertensive patients using propranolol as an antiarrhythmic therapy. Subsequently, several case reports appeared in the literature describing patients with depressive symptoms after the use of the highly lipophilic propranolol.[21–25] Also some other β-blockers were described in case reports to have a depressogenic effect, such as the highly lipophilic timolol,[26–28] which is topically administered to patients with glaucoma. In most patients, depressive symptoms started quickly after the administration of β-blocker therapy; symptoms increased with increasing dosage of the drug but rapidly cleared when the drug was withdrawn or replaced with a more hydrophilic β-blocker. In some cases, there even was a rechallenge, after which depressive symptoms emerged again.[22,24]

Several comments can be made on these reports. The most important problem with these case reports is the lack of controls. Because depression is highly prevalent among the general population and β-blockers are prescribed often, depression is likely to occur by chance in people taking a β-blocker.[29] Besides, many of the described patients had a personal or family history of depression. However, according to the Naranjo criteria (a method for establishing the probability of adverse drug reactions),[30] many patients described in the case reports have a Naranjo score suggesting a likely causal relationship, and most of these case reports involved the lipophilic propranolol or the lipophilic topically (ophthalmic) administered timolol, which also enters the systemic circulation.[31]

Therefore, these case reports raised a strong suspicion that β-blockers, especially the more lipophilic ones that more readily cross the blood-brain barrier, are able to cause depression. **Table 1** provides an overview of the β-blockers and their lipophilicities. Other neuropsychological symptoms, such as drowsiness, fatigue, lethargy, sleep disorders, nightmares, and hallucinations, were also often mentioned.[32]

PRESUMED UNDERLYING MECHANISMS

The exact mechanisms underlying these central nervous system (CNS) adverse effects are still speculated about, but commonly, 4 general mechanisms that were extensively described by Koella[33] are referred to:

1. A centrally mediated specific β-adrenergic mechanism: β-blockers that penetrate the brain in sufficiently high amounts (especially the lipophilic ones) bind to adrenergic receptors. By

Table 1
Lipophilicity of β-blockers

β-Blocker	Lipophilicity
Alprenolol	Lipophilic
Atenolol	Hydrophilic
Bisoprolol	Lipophilic
Bucindolol	Lipophilic
Carvedilol	Lipophilic
Metoprolol	Lipophilic
Nadolol	Hydrophilic
Nebivolol	Lipophilic
Oxprenolol	Lipophilic
Pindolol	Lipophilic
Practolol	Hydrophilic
Propranolol	Lipophilic
Sotalol	Hydrophilic
Timolol	Lipophilic

blocking the adrenergic receptors, they suppress information flow in noradrenergic β-receptor–mediated channels and change activity in a variety of networks that are under beta-adrenergic control. Both β_1- and β_2-adrenergic receptors are found in the human brain.[34]

2. A centrally mediated specific serotonergic mechanism: β-blockers that penetrate through the blood-brain barrier also (1) bind with high affinity to nonadrenergic (eg, serotonergic) receptors, (2) interfere with the signal flow in nonadrenergic pathways, and (3) disturb the activity and reactivity in networks controlled by these pathways, thus disturbing the behavioral/neuropsychological activities organized by these networks. It was demonstrated in rats that certain (lipophilic) β-blockers (propranolol, pindolol, oxprenolol, alprenolol) indeed stereospecifically bind to serotonin receptors and act as serotonin receptor antagonists, whereas other (hydrophilic) β-blockers (atenolol, practolol) fail to enter into such a binding.[35,36]
3. A centrally mediated nonspecific mechanism: β-blockers that penetrate the brain silence some especially sensitive neurons in the CNS because of their membrane stabilizing characteristics (they prevent the neurons to get excited).
4. A peripherally mediated mechanism in which β-blockers induce changes in the autonomic activity in the periphery, which are relayed to the CNS to induce changes in the activity of a variety of central systems.

The relative weight with which any of these 4 mechanisms modifies the functioning of the CNS would depend on the characteristics of the specific β-blocker, for example, the degree of lipophilicity, affinity to nonadrenergic receptors, membrane stabilizing properties, and dose and route of administration. Because β-blockers differ in these characteristics, they may differ in the kind and degree of adverse effects that they exert on the CNS. Illustratively, concentrations of propranolol in the human brain tissue have been found to be 10 to 20 times higher than concentrations of the hydrophilic atenolol. The brain tissue/plasma concentration ratio for propranolol was 26:1 compared with 0.2:1 for atenolol.[37]

SYSTEMATIC STUDIES ON β-BLOCKERS AND DEPRESSION

Following the case reports, many investigators tried to verify the putative association between β-blockers and depression in systematic studies. These studies can be categorized into 4 main categories, depending on their design (**Table 2**).[38] (1) Studies linking β-blocker use to antidepressant prescriptions; (2) randomized controlled trials (RCTs) on the efficacy of β-blockers in various patient categories, in which side effects, including depression, have been recorded; (3) studies on β-blocker use and depression, in which depression has been measured in a protocolized way using standardized questionnaires or structured interviews, for example, the Beck Depression Inventory (BDI) or Diagnostic Interview Schedule (DIS), respectively; and (4) reviews that have been published on this subject. Several studies are discussed in more detail.

One of the first studies to investigate the relationship between β-blockers and depression more systematically was conducted by Avorn and colleagues.[39] In this study, a relatively large random stratified sample of Medicaid recipients using antihypertensive medications were screened for concurrent antidepressant use within a period of 2 years. To control for the possibility that depressive symptoms might have resulted from the presence of chronic medical illness per se (confounding by indication), as well as the possibility that increased physician visits might result in additional diagnoses or therapies even without an increase in prevalence of the condition, patients taking other antihypertensive drugs and patients taking antidiabetics were also studied. Patients using β-blockers were found to have a relative risk (RR) of 1.5 (95% confidence interval [CI], 1.4–1.6) of being prescribed tricyclic antidepressants as compared with patients using hydralazine or antidiabetics. In addition, the magnitude of the association declined with advancing age.

With this study design, however, some problems arise with the interpretation of the results. The study was cross-sectional, raising the problem of an unclear temporal relationship; there was a maximum time window of 2 years between the 2 prescriptions. Besides, the antidepressant use could as well have preceded the β-blocker use in the study patients. In this context, it may be important to know that tricyclic antidepressants have arrhythmogenic properties, which may have triggered clinicians to subsequently prescribe β-blockers. But may be the most important drawback, acknowledged by the investigators themselves, is that the use of antidepressants was used as a marker of depression. On the one hand this would yield an underestimate of the real number of patients with depression because only a part of the population with a depressed mood visits a doctor and is prescribed an

Table 2
Overview of studies on β-blockers and depression

Study Design	Author	Year	β-Blocker	Number of Patients	Measure of Depression	Population	Association
Case reports	McNeill et al[21]	1982	Propranolol	1	Clinical diagnosis	Patient with MI	+
	Petrie et al[24]	1982	Propranolol	3	Clinical diagnosis	Hypertension and arrhythmia	+
	Nolan[26]	1982	Timolol	1	Clinical diagnosis	Glaucoma patient	+
	Russell & Schuckit[75]	1982	Nadolol	1	Clinical diagnosis	Hypertensive patient	+
	Cremona-Barbaro[22]	1983	Propranolol	2	Clinical diagnosis	Hypertensive patients	+
	Pollack et al[25]	1985	Propranolol	3	Clinical diagnosis	Hypertensive patients	+
	Parker[23]	1985	Propranolol	2	Clinical diagnosis	Patients with angina and hypertension	+
	Schweitzer & Maguire[27]	2008	Timolol	1	Clinical diagnosis	Patient with glaucoma	+
Studies linking β-blocker use to antidepressant prescriptions	Avorn et al[39]	1986	Propranolol, metoprolol, nadolol	8235[a]	Tricyclic antidepressants prescriptions	Medicaid recipients	+
	Thiessen et al[40]	1990	Atenolol, nadolol (hydrophilic), labetolol, metoprolol, oxprenolol, pindolol, propranolol, timolol	3218[b]	Antidepressants prescriptions	Registries in a drug registry	±[c]
	Bright & Everitt[43]	1992	Propranolol, metoprolol, nadolol	4302	Antidepressants prescriptions, depression diagnosis, or ECT	Medicaid recipients	–
	Hallas[44]	1996	Propranolol, other β-blockers, not specified	9375[d]	Antidepressants prescriptions	Incident antidepressant users	–
	Johnson & Wallace[41]	1997	Propranolol (2804), atenolol, nadolol, sotalol (1593), acebutolol, labetolol, metoprolol, oxprenolol, pindolol, timolol (2699)	7096[e]	Antidepressants prescriptions	Registries in a drug registry	±[c]
	Kaiserman et al[76]	2006	β-Blockers, not specified	6597	Antidepressants use	Glaucoma patients	–
	Johnell & Fastbom[42]	2008	Propranolol (7731), carvedilol, pindolol, metoprolol, labetolol (135,848), sotalol, atenolol, bisoprolol (115,583)	256,679	Antidepressants prescriptions	Registries in a drug registry	±[c]

RCTs (efficacy of β-blocker)	Hansteen et al[48]	1982	Propranolol	560	Spontaneously admitted adverse effects	Patients with MI	+
	Julian et al[49]	1982	Sotalol	1456	Questioned for suspected adverse effects. At 6 mo, questionnaire about symptoms and adverse effects	Patients with MI	+
	BHAT[50]	1982	Propranolol	3837	Questioned for frequent depression that interfered with work, recreation, or sleep	Patients with MI	–
	Coope et al[45]	1986	Atenolol	884	Self-administered general symptom questionnaire	Hypertensive patients	–
	Dahlöf et al[46]	1991	Atenolol, metoprolol, pindolol	1627	Adverse effects as a group were not specified	Hypertensive patients	–
	Perez-Stable et al[47]	1995	Propranolol	312	Questioned about possible adverse effects and significant clinical events	Hypertensive patients	+
	Packer et al[3]	1996	Carvedilol	1094	Not specified	Patients with HF	–
	BEST[51]	2001	Bucindolol	2708	Not specified	Patients with HF	–
Association between β-blockers and depression (standardized instruments)	Stoudemire et al[52]	1984	Propranolol	35	Zung SDS	Hypertensive nondepressed patients	–
	Griffin & Friedman[53]	1986	Propranolol	34	Ham-D, HGCS	Men with cardiovascular problems requiring propranolol treatment	+
	Blumenthal[54]	1987	Atenolol, propranolol	26	POMS, SCL	Hypertensive patients	–
	Wurzelman et al[60]	1987	Propranolol	488	Zung SDS	Elderly volunteers	–
	Adler[56]	1988	Atenolol, propranolol	31	BDI, Ham-D, POMS, SCL	Hypertensive patients	–
	Goldstein et al[58]	1990	Metoprolol	690	ADL, Zung SDS	Hypertensive patients	–
	Prisant et al[61]	1991	Both high (66) and low (20) lipophilic β-blockers, not specified	466	Zung SDS	Hypertensive patients	–
	Sorgi et al[55]	1992	Nadolol	50	HRDS, BPRS, NOSIE	Psychiatric in-patients with chronic aggressive behavior	–
	Head et al[57]	1996	Propranolol, metoprolol	20	POMS	Healthy student volunteers	+
	Perez-Stable et al[63]	2000	Propranolol	312	BDI, CES-D	Hypertensive patients	–
	Ried et al[62]	2005	Atenolol (558)	1125	CES-D	Hypertensive patients with coronary artery disease	–
	Crane et al[59]	2006	Metoprolol, atenolol, Toprol-XL, sotalol, propranolol, carvedilol	84	GDS	Patients with MI	–

(*continued on next page*)

Table 2
(continued)

Study Design	Author	Year	β-Blocker	Number of Patients	Measure of Depression	Population	Association
Association between β-blockers and depression (structured instruments)	Carney et al[64]	1987	β-Blockers, not specified	77	Semistructured diagnostic interview	CAG patients	–
	Bartels et al[65]	1988	Propranolol	127	DIS	Hypertension, migraine, or angina pectoris patients	–
	Schleifer et al[66]	1991	β-Blockers, not specified	335	SADS-C	Patients with MI	–
	van Melle et al[67]	2006	Metoprolol, sotalol, bisoprolol, atenolol, carvedilol, pindolol, celiprolol	381	CIDI	Patients with MI	–
Reviews	Ried et al[68]	1998	Various β-blockers	26 studies	Various depression measurements used in the included studies	Various indications for β-blocker use	–
	Kohn[29]	2001	Propranolol	26 studies	Various depression measurements used in the included studies	Various indications for β-blocker use	–
	Lama[69]	2002	Various β-blockers	11 studies	Various depression measurements used in the included studies	Various cardiovascular indications for β-blocker use	–
	Ko et al[70]	2002	Various β-blockers	15 studies	Various depression measurements used in the included studies	Various cardiovascular indications for β-blocker use	–
	Patten & Barbui[71]	2004	Various β-blockers	23 studies	Various depression measurements used in the included studies	Various indications for β-blocker use	–
Miscellaneous	Waal[20]	1967	Propranolol	89	Medical chart review	Hypertensive patients with arrhythmia	+
	Yudofsky[77]	1992	Various β-blockers	9 studies	Various depression measurements	β-Blocker users	–
	Gerstman et al[78]	1996	Various β-blockers, also specific propranolol	1290	Record review	Hypertensive patients	–
	Mabuchi et al[79]	2008	β-Blocker eye drops, not specified	230	HADS	Patients with primary open-angle glaucoma	–

Abbreviations: ADL, activities of daily living; BDI, beck depression scale; BPRS, brief psychiatric rating scale; CAG, coronary angiography; CES-D, center for epidemiological studies depression scale; CIDI, composite international diagnostic interview; ECT, electroconvulsive therapy; DIS, diagnostic interview schedule; GDS, geriatric depression scale; HADS, hospital anxiety and depression scale; Ham-D, Hamilton depression scale; HGCS, Hudson generalized contentment scale; HRDS, 24-item Hamilton rating scale for depression; NOSIE, nurses observation scale for inpatient evaluation; POMS, profile of mood states; SADS-C, schedule of affective disorder and schizophrenia; SCL, the symptom checklist-90-R; SDS, self-rating depression scale.

[a] A total of 8235 β-blocker users from a sample of 143,253 patients.
[b] A total of 3218 new β-blocker users, from a total study population of 15,398 patients.
[c] These studies found a positive association for propranolol but not for other β-blockers with increased antidepressant prescriptions.
[d] A total of 11,244 incident users of antidepressants; 9375 β-blocker users (3764 propranolol), of whom 762 used both medicines in the study period.
[e] A total of 7096 β-blocker users.

antidepressant. On the other hand, one can expect an overestimate because antidepressants are also used for indications other than depression, for example, sensory neuropathies and anxiety disorders.

Nevertheless, more studies linking β-blocker use to antidepressant prescriptions have been published since, with inconsistent findings. Thiessen and colleagues,[40] in a retrospective cohort study, accurately recorded the time window between the 2 prescriptions, thereby addressing the problem of unknown temporal relationship and found an increased RR of 2.6 of antidepressant prescriptions subsequent to β-blocker use. Subgroup analyses showed that it was mainly propranolol that accounted for this elevated risk (RR of 4.8); hydrophilic or other lipophilic β-blockers yielded no elevated risk for antidepressant prescriptions. Strikingly, in accordance with the findings of Avorn and colleagues,[39] Thiessen and colleagues[40] found this risk to be highest among the youngest patients; propranolol users aged 20 to 39 years had a RR of 17.2 of being prescribed an antidepressant. Johnson and Wallace,[41] who studied new β-blocker users for concurrent antidepressant use (<34 days), also found higher rates of use of antidepressants in patients using propranolol, but not other β-blockers, especially in the younger age group (20–39 years). However, the authors found that this increased risk could not solely be attributed to propranolol because migraine headache was much more prevalent among propranolol users and probably accounts partly for the increased risk of depression. Recently, even in a population older than 75 years,[42] an increased risk for antidepressants use in propranolol users was found. The investigators also suggested confounding by indication (migraine and tremor) to play a role in this finding.

In contrast to the positive findings in the abovementioned studies, 2 other studies[43,44] did not find the use of β-blockers to be associated with an increase in antidepressant prescriptions. Hallas[44] performed a prescription-sequence symmetry analysis in new β-blocker users and found no increased risk for either propranolol or the group of β-blockers as a whole. Strikingly, the number of patients who started antidepressant therapy after the use of β-blockers was similar to the number of persons following the opposite order, thereby illustrating the importance of registering the temporal relationship between the drugs. Bright and Everitt[43] studied ongoing β-blocker use and included various potential confounders and effect modifiers. After controlling for benzodiazepine use, frequent outpatient visits, and frequent other medications, there was a null effect of β-blockers on antidepressant prescriptions.

The second category of more systematic studies are controlled RCTs on the efficacy of beta-blockade in reducing morbidity and/or mortality for various indications, in which the occurrence of side effects, including depression, is also recorded. Patient categories studied included patients with hypertension,[45–47] post-MI patients,[48–50] and patients with HF.[3,51] These studies have important methodological strengths because of the randomization, resulting in equal distribution of possible confounding variables between the compared groups. However, as measuring the side effects of β-blocker use has not been the main purpose of these studies, the studies mainly used simple checklist responses,[45,49] single questions,[50] or self-report of complaints by patients to evaluate the occurrence of side effects.[49] For measuring depressive disorder, these methods are not reliable and valid. Three of these studies found an increased risk of β-blockers on depression; in 2, the study drug was propranolol,[47,48] and in the third, it was the hydrophilic sotalol.[49] In the Beta-Blocker Heart Attack Trial (BHAT),[50] depression was registered far more often than in the other studies (around 40% compared with <5% in the other studies), but was equal for both β-blocker users and controls. The Beta-Blocker Evaluation of Survival Trial (BEST)[51] on bucindolol versus placebo found 9% versus 12% patients with depression, respectively, indicating a small protective effect of bucindolol on depression. RCTs that studied the efficacy of β-blockers have used measures of depression that had suboptimal validity and reliability. They generally reported low rates of depression, with inconsistent findings concerning increased risks for β-blocker users versus non–β-blocker users to develop depression.

The third category consists of 12 studies, which used standardized measures of depression, for example, the BDI, Hamilton Depression Rating Scale, or Profile of Mood States. However, many of these studies had small sample sizes (≤50 patients),[52–57] with the consequence of an increased risk of type II error and little power. Follow-up period varied from 4 days[57] to 1 year.[47,58,59] Five studies[58,60–63] with a more adequate sample size (>300 patients) found no increased risk for depressive symptoms with the use of a β-blocker. One study had a cross-sectional design,[60] one was a prospective cohort study,[61] and 3 were RCTs with a baseline measurement of depression.[58,62,63]

Only a few studies have used structured diagnostic instruments to diagnose a major depressive disorder. Examples of these instruments are the DIS and Composite International Diagnostic Interview. One study using a semistructured diagnostic psychiatric interview had a small sample size and only 25% power[64]; 1 had a control group largely consisting of volunteers.[65] To the authors' knowledge, only 2 prospective studies used a structured instrument to diagnose a depressive disorder. Both studies were conducted in post-MI populations. The first study found that the use of digitalis but not β-blockers predicted the development of depression.[66] However, depression at baseline was not assessed. The second study[67] did measure baseline depression, and the investigators controlled for many other potential confounders like age, gender, left ventricular ejection fraction, benzodiazepine use, digitalis use, COPD, diabetes mellitus, and previous MI. In addition, they controlled for changes in β-blocker use during the follow-up period of 1 year. The study found no differences between β-blocker users and non–β-blocker users in the prevalence of depressive disorder.[67]

In the last decade, several reviews have been published on this subject.[29,68–71] An often-cited review is that of Ko and colleagues,[70] who included only trials with an RCT design. As already mentioned, these studies generally were not designed for measuring depression. The investigators found that the putative increased risk of depression with β-blocker use was not substantiated. They computed an annual increase in risk of reported depressive symptoms of 6 per 1000 patients (95% CI, −7 to 19). β-Blockers were associated with a small increase in the risk of reported fatigue: 18 per 1000 patients (95% CI, 5–30). In reviews that included not only RCTs but also other studies, the same conclusion as that of Ko and colleagues was reached, namely, there is not enough evidence for a depressogenic effect. Some of these studies did find evidence for other neuropsychological adverse effects of β-blockers, such as fatigue and sedation,[70,72] possibly confounding the issue.

DISCUSSION

Looking back on about 40 years of literature on β-blockers and depression, the discussion started with an impressive amount of case reports strongly suggesting a relationship between the use of a β-blocker and the development of depression in the individual patients described. More systematic studies that have been conducted subsequently did not in general find an increase in the rates of depression. Searching for reasons for the discrepancies between the case reports and the findings in the more systematic studies, the following issues can be considered.

First, as stated before, because depression is quite prevalent in the general population and β-blockers are used widely, cases of beta-blockade and depression are likely to occur at the same time by chance, giving the impression of a medication-induced depression. Nevertheless, Naranjo scores of the case reports did suggest causality in at least some of them.[31]

Second, most of the case reports discussed the effects of the lipophilic β-blockers propranolol and timolol. In contrast, most of the more systematic studies on β-blockers and depression have studied the effect of a group of various β-blockers, including the more frequently used, less-lipophilic, second-generation β-blockers like metoprolol and atenolol. Some studies were able to do subgroup analyses on propranolol solely and found an increase in depression rates for only propranolol,[40–42,53,57] not for other β-blockers. When pooled in a group of other less-lipophilic drugs, this specific effect could be easily missed. At present, propranolol is hardly used for the indications of hypertension, HF, or post-MI. The sole indications for which propranolol is still used are migraine, tremor, hyperthyroidism, and portal hypertension. For hypertension, β-blockers are no longer the first line of treatment.[73] For HF and post-MI, as discussed earlier, there is sound evidence that beta-blockade reduces morbidity and mortality. Besides second-generation β-blockers, third-generation β-blockers such as nebivolol and carvedilol are increasingly prescribed. Both nebivolol and carvedilol are lipophilic, like propranolol, so on theoretical grounds, vigilance regarding potential depressogenic effects can be justified. However, the studies in which a depressogenic effect of propranolol was suggested are of poor methodological quality, because of inadequate measures of depression (ie, antidepressant prescriptions, single questions as a marker) or small study populations, creating a doubt of whether this is a true effect.

Third, in many studies, an increase in fatigue was noticed with β-blocker use. Because fatigue is one of the symptoms of depression, this could have confounded the issue. Indeed, many of the symptoms of depression are also seen in patients with HF, making the diagnosis of depression more complicated.

A question therefore arises if one should not worry at all about a possible depressogenic effect of the commonly prescribed β-blockers. To answer this question, it is worth looking at some general presumptions about drug adverse effects. Referring to the Rothman model of multifactorial etiology,[74] Patten and Barbui[71] expressed that there seems to be an assumption that drugs can act as a sufficient cause of depression. However, "most diseases have a multifactorial etiology, and there are various sets of *contributing* causes, that together may constitute a *sufficient* cause for a disease or disorder. If a drug, in the absence of any other etiological factors, is a sufficient cause of depression, then exposure to that drug should predictably lead to the occurrence of depression in all subjects taking it. No such drug has yet been identified. However, certain drugs may be capable of increasing the risk of depression or triggering depression in some, but not all people. This suggests that the population is characterized by the presence or absence of various other contributing causes, and that exposure to a drug may complete (render sufficient) certain otherwise incomplete *sets* of contributing factors, together amounting to a sufficient cause. The occurrence of depression in a person exposed to a drug may appear unpredictable because at least some of the other contributing causes are unknown or unmeasured."[71] Looking at the case reports, it was noticed that many individuals who developed depression after β-blocker use had a positive personal or family history with depression. Therefore, genetic profile could be one of the important contributing factors, leading to an increased susceptibility for β-blockers in some, but not most, people.

CLINICAL IMPLICATIONS

In patients with cardiovascular problems in general, including HF patients, one should not be reluctant to prescribe β-blockers out of fear of inducing a depression. It is not ruled out that-although based on weak scientific evidence-epecially, the highly lipohilic propranolol has a depressogenic effect. Also, patients with a positive personal or family history of depression might be at an increased risk. One should stay vigilant, and when there is a strong suspicion of β-blocker–induced depression, it seems worthwhile to evaluate the effect of discontinuing the β-blocker, possibly followed by a rechallenge. However, the risk seems small, and considering its clear positive effect on morbidity and mortality, one should not withhold β-blockers in advance because of the fear of inducing depression.

REFERENCES

1. Freemantle N, Cleland J, Young P, et al. Beta blockade after myocardial infarction: systematic review and meta regression analysis. BMJ 1999; 318:1730–7.
2. Waagstein F, Bristow MR, Swedberg K, et al. Beneficial effects of metoprolol in idiopathic dilated cardiomyopathy. Metoprolol in Dilated Cardiomyopathy (MDC) Trial Study Group. Lancet 1993;342: 1441–6.
3. Packer M, Bristow MR, Cohn JN, et al. The effect of carvedilol on morbidity and mortality in patients with chronic heart failure. U.S. Carvedilol Heart Failure Study Group. N Engl J Med 1996;334:1349–55.
4. The Cardiac Insufficiency Bisoprolol Study II (CIBIS II): a randomised trial. Lancet 1999;353(9146):9–13.
5. Flather MD, Shibata MC, Coats AJ, et al. Randomized trial to determine the effect of nebivolol on mortality and cardiovascular hospital admission in elderly patients with heart failure (SENIORS). Eur Heart J 2005;26:215–25.
6. Bristow M, Port JD. Beta-adrenergic blockade in chronic heart failure. Scand Cardiovasc J Suppl 1998;47:45–55.
7. Effect of metoprolol CR/XL in chronic heart failure: Metoprolol CR/XL Randomised Intervention Trial in Congestive Heart Failure (MERIT-HF). Lancet 1999; 353:2001–7.
8. Dickstein K, Cohen-Solal A, Filippatos G, et al. ESC guidelines for the diagnosis and treatment of acute and chronic heart failure 2008: the Task Force for the diagnosis and treatment of acute and chronic heart failure 2008 of the European Society of Cardiology. Developed in collaboration with the Heart Failure Association of the ESC (HFA) and endorsed by the European Society of Intensive Care Medicine (ESICM). Eur J Heart Fail 2008;10:933–89.
9. Malmberg K, Herlitz J, Hjalmarson A, et al. Effects of metoprolol on mortality and late infarction in diabetics with suspected acute myocardial infarction. Retrospective data from two large studies. Eur Heart J 1989;10:423–8.
10. Chen J, Radford MJ, Wang Y, et al. Effectiveness of beta-blocker therapy after acute myocardial infarction in elderly patients with chronic obstructive pulmonary disease or asthma. J Am Coll Cardiol 2001;37:1950–6.
11. Radack K, Deck C. Beta-adrenergic blocker therapy does not worsen intermittent claudication in subjects with peripheral arterial disease. A meta-analysis of randomized controlled trials. Arch Intern Med 1991;151:1769–76.
12. Solomon SA, Ramsay LE, Yeo WW, et al. Beta blockade and intermittent claudication: placebo controlled trial of atenolol and nifedipine and their combination. BMJ 1991;303:1100–4.
13. Thadani U, Whitsett TL. Beta-adrenergic blockers and intermittent claudication. Time for reappraisal. Arch Intern Med 1991;151:1705–7.
14. Sinha S, Goldstein M, Penrod J, et al. Brief report: beta-blocker use among veterans with systolic heart failure. J Gen Intern Med 2006;21:1306–9.

15. Michael BF, Allen JF, Pincus HA. DSM-IV-TR handbook of differential diagnosis. Washington, DC: American Psychiatric Publishing; 2007.
16. Alonso J, Lepine JP. Overview of key data from the European Study of the Epidemiology of Mental Disorders (ESEMeD). J Clin Psychiatry 2007;68(Suppl 2):3–9.
17. van Melle JP, de Jonge P, Spijkerman TA, et al. Prognostic association of depression following myocardial infarction with mortality and cardiovascular events: a meta-analysis. Psychosom Med 2004;66: 814–22.
18. Rutledge T, Reis VA, Linke SE, et al. Depression in heart failure a meta-analytic review of prevalence, intervention effects, and associations with clinical outcomes. J Am Coll Cardiol 2006;48:1527–37.
19. Murray CJ, Lopez AD. Global mortality, disability, and the contribution of risk factors: Global Burden of Disease Study. Lancet 1997;349:1436–42.
20. Waal HJ. Propranolol-induced depression. Br Med J 1967;2:50.
21. McNeil GN, Shaw PK, Dock DS. Substitution of atenolol for propranolol in a case of propranolol-related depression. Am J Psychiatry 1982;139:1187–8.
22. Cremona-Barbaro A. Propranolol and depression. Lancet 1983;1:185.
23. Parker WA. Propranolol-induced depression and psychosis. Clin Pharm 1985;4:214–8.
24. Petrie WM, Maffucci RJ, Woosley RL. Propranolol and depression. Am J Psychiatry 1982;139:92–4.
25. Pollack MH, Rosenbaum JF, Cassem NH. Propranolol and depression revisited: three cases and a review. J Nerv Ment Dis 1985;173:118–9.
26. Nolan BT. Acute suicidal depression associated with use of timolol. JAMA 1982;247:1567.
27. Schweitzer I, Maguire K. A case of melancholic depression induced by beta-blocker antiglaucoma agents. Med J Aust 2008;189:406–7.
28. Rao MR, O'Brien J, Dening TR, et al. Systemic hazards of ocular timolol. Br J Hosp Med 1993;50: 553.
29. Kohn R. Beta-blockers an important cause of depression: a medical myth without evidence. Med Health R I 2001;84:92–5.
30. Naranjo CA, Fornazzari L, Sellers EM. Clinical detection and assessment of drug induced neurotoxicity. Prog Neuropsychopharmacol 1981;5:427–34.
31. Steffensmeier JJ, Ernst ME, Kelly M, et al. Do randomized controlled trials always trump case reports? A second look at propranolol and depression. Pharmacotherapy 2006;26:162–7.
32. McAinsh J, Cruickshank JM. Beta-blockers and central nervous system side effects. Pharmacol Ther 1990;46:163–97.
33. Koella WP. CNS-related (side-)effects of beta-blockers with special reference to mechanisms of action. Eur J Clin Pharmacol 1985;28(Suppl):55–63.
34. Pazos A, Probst A, Palacios JM. Beta-adrenoceptor subtypes in the human brain: autoradiographic localization. Brain Res 1985;358:324–8.
35. Direct evidence for an interaction of beta-adrenergic blockers with the 5-HT receptor. Nature 1977;267: 289–90.
36. Costain DW, Green AR. Beta-adrenoceptor antagonists inhibit the behavioural responses of rats to increased brain 5-hydroxytryptamine. Br J Pharmacol 1978;64:193–200.
37. Cruickshank JM. Beta-blocking agents. Lancet 1980;1:1415.
38. Kohn R. Beta-blockers an important cause of depression: a medical myth without evidence. Med Health RI 2001;84(3):92–5.
39. Avorn J, Everitt DE, Weiss S. Increased antidepressant use in patients prescribed beta-blockers. JAMA 1986;255:357–60.
40. Thiessen BQ, Wallace SM, Blackburn JL, et al. Increased prescribing of antidepressants subsequent to beta-blocker therapy. Arch Intern Med 1990;150:2286–90.
41. Johnson JA, Wallace SM. Investigating the relationship between beta-blocker and antidepressant use through linkage of the administrative databases of Saskatchewan Health. Pharmacoepidemiol Drug Saf 1997;6:1–11.
42. Johnell K, Fastbom J. The association between use of cardiovascular drugs and antidepressants: a nationwide register-based study. Eur J Clin Pharmacol 2008;64:1119–24.
43. Bright RA, Everitt DE. Beta-blockers and depression. Evidence against an association. JAMA 1992; 267:1783–7.
44. Hallas J. Evidence of depression provoked by cardiovascular medication: a prescription sequence symmetry analysis. Epidemiology 1996;7:478–84.
45. Coope JR, Warrender TS. Randomised trial of treatment of hypertension in elderly patients in primary care. Br Med J (Clin Res Ed) 1987;294:179.
46. Dahlöf B, Lindholm LH, Hansson L, et al. Morbidity and mortality in the Swedish Trial in Old Patients with Hypertension (STOP-Hypertension). Lancet 1991;338:1281–5.
47. Perez-Stable EJ, Coates TJ, Baron RB, et al. Comparison of a lifestyle modification program with propranolol use in the management of diastolic hypertension. J Gen Intern Med 1995; 10:419–28.
48. Hansteen V, Moinichen E, Lorentsen E, et al. One year's treatment with propranolol after myocardial infarction: preliminary report of Norwegian multicentre trial. Br Med J (Clin Res Ed) 1982;284: 155–60.
49. Julian DG, Jackson FS, Szekely P, et al. A controlled trial of sotalol for 1 year after myocardial infarction. Circulation 1983;67:I61–2.

50. A randomized trial of propranolol in patients with acute myocardial infarction. I. Mortality results. JAMA 1982;247:1707–14.
51. A trial of the beta-blocker bucindolol in patients with advanced chronic heart failure. N Engl J Med 2001; 344:1659–67.
52. Stoudemire A, Brown JT, Harris RT, et al. Propranolol and depression: a reevaluation based on a pilot clinical trial. Psychiatr Med 1984;2:211–8.
53. Griffin SJ, Friedman MJ. Depressive symptoms in propranolol users. J Clin Psychiatry 1986;47: 453–7.
54. Blumenthal JA, Madden DJ, Krantz DS, et al. Short-term behavioral effects of beta-adrenergic medications in men with mild hypertension. Clin Pharmacol Ther 1988;43:429–35.
55. Sorgi P, Ratey J, Knoedler D, et al. Depression during treatment with beta-blockers: results from a double-blind placebo-controlled study. J Neuropsychiatry Clin Neurosci 1992;4:187–9.
56. Adler L. CNS effects of beta blockade: a comparative study. Psychopharmacol Bull 1988;24:232–7.
57. Head A, Kendall MJ, Ferner R, et al. Acute effects of beta blockade and exercise on mood and anxiety. Br J Sports Med 1996;30:238–42.
58. Goldstein G, Materson BJ, Cushman WC, et al. Treatment of hypertension in the elderly: II. Cognitive and behavioral function. Results of a Department of Veterans Affairs Cooperative Study. Hypertension 1990;15:361–9.
59. Crane PB, Oles KS, Kennedy-Malone L. Beta-blocker medication usage in older women after myocardial infarction. J Am Acad Nurse Pract 2006;18:463–70.
60. Wurzelmann J, Frishman WH, Aronson M, et al. Neuropsychological effects of antihypertensive drugs. Cardiol Clin 1987;5:689–701.
61. Prisant LM, Spruill WJ, Fincham JE, et al. Depression associated with antihypertensive drugs. J Fam Pract 1991;33:481–5.
62. Ried LD, Tueth MJ, Handberg E, et al. A Study of Antihypertensive Drugs and Depressive Symptoms (SADD-Sx) in patients treated with a calcium antagonist versus an atenolol hypertension Treatment Strategy in the International Verapamil SRTrandolapril Study (INVEST). Psychosom Med 2005;67: 398–406.
63. Perez-Stable EJ, Halliday R, Gardiner PS, et al. The effects of propranolol on cognitive function and quality of life: a randomized trial among patients with diastolic hypertension. Am J Med 2000;108:359–65.
64. Carney RM, Rich MW, Tevelde A, et al. Major depressive disorder in coronary artery disease. Am J Cardiol 1987;60:1273–5.
65. Bartels D, Glasser M, Wang A, et al. Association between depression and propranolol use in ambulatory patients. Clin Pharm 1988;7:146–50.
66. Schleifer SJ, Slater WR, Macari-Hinson MM, et al. Digitalis and beta-blocking agents: effects on depression following myocardial infarction. Am Heart J 1991;121:1397–402.
67. van Melle JP, Verbeek DE, van den Berg M, et al. Beta-blockers and depression after myocardial infarction: a multicenter prospective study. J Am Coll Cardiol 2006;48:2209–14.
68. Ried LD, McFarland BH, Johnson RE, et al. Beta-blockers and depression: the more the murkier? Ann Pharmacother 1998;32:699–708.
69. Lama PJ. Systemic adverse effects of beta-adrenergic blockers: an evidence-based assessment. Am J Ophthalmol 2002;134:749–60.
70. Ko DT, Hebert PR, Coffey CS, et al. Beta-blocker therapy and symptoms of depression, fatigue, and sexual dysfunction. JAMA 2002;288:351–7.
71. Patten SB, Barbui C. Drug-induced depression: a systematic review to inform clinical practice. Psychother Psychosom 2004;73:207–15.
72. Dimsdale JE, Newton RP, Joist T. Neuropsychological side effects of beta-blockers. Arch Intern Med 1989;149:514–25.
73. Lindholm LH, Carlberg B, Samuelsson O. Should beta blockers remain first choice in the treatment of primary hypertension? A meta-analysis. Lancet 2005;366:1545–53.
74. Rothman KJ. Causes. Am J Epidemiol 1976;104: 587–92.
75. Russell JW, Schuckit NA. Anxiety and depression in patient on nadolol. Lancet 1982;2:1286–7.
76. Kaiserman I, Kaiserman N, Elhayani L, et al. Topical beta-blockers are not associated with an increased risk of treatment for depression. Ophthalmology 2006;113:1077–80.
77. Yudofsky SC. Beta-blockers and depression. The clinician's dilemma. JAMA 1992;1(267):1826–7.
78. Gerstman BB, Jolson HM, Bauer M, et al. The incidence of depression in new users of beta-blockers and selected anti-hypertensives. J Clin Epidemiol 1996;49:809–15.
79. Mabuchi F, Yoshimura K, Kashiwagi K, et al. High prevalence of anxiety and depression in patients with primary open-angle glaucoma. J Glaucoma 2008;17:552–7.

50. A randomized trial of propranolol in patients with acute myocardial infarction. II. Morbidity results. JAMA 1983;250:2814–9.
51. A trial of the beta-blocker bucindolol in patients with advanced chronic heart failure. N Engl J Med 2001;344:1659–67.
52. Stoudemire A, Brown JT, Harris RT, et al. Propranolol and depression: a reevaluation based on a pilot clinical trial. Psychiatr Med 1984;2:211–8.
53. Griffin SJ, Friedman MJ. Depressive symptoms in propranolol users. J Clin Psychiatry 1986;47:453–7.
54. Blumenthal JA, Madden DJ, Krantz DS, et al. Short-term behavioral effects of beta-adrenergic medications in men with mild hypertension. Clin Pharmacol Ther 1988;43:429–35.
55. Sorgi P, Ratey J, Knoedler D, et al. Depression during treatment with beta-blockers: results from a double-blind placebo-controlled study. J Neuropsychiatry Clin Neurosci 1992;4:187–9.
56. Adler L. CNS effects of beta blockade: a comparative study. Psychopharmacol Bull 1988;24:232–7.
57. Head A, Kendall MJ, Ferner R, et al. Acute effects of beta blockade and exercise on mood and anxiety. Br J Sports Med 1996;30:238–42.
58. Goldstein G, Materson BJ, Cushman WC, et al. Treatment of hypertension in the elderly: II. Cognitive and behavioral function. Results of a Department of Veterans Affairs Cooperative Study. Hypertension 1990;15:361–9.
59. Gleason PP, Giles KS, Kennedy-Malone LM. Beta-blocker medication usage in elderly women after myocardial infarction. J Am Acad Nurse Pract 2006;18:463–70.
60. Vuurzeltrinho J, Eastman WH, Atkinson M, et al. Neuropsychological effects of antihypertensive drugs. Cardiol Clin 1995;13:583–701.
61. Prisant LM, Spruill WJ, Fincham JE, et al. Depression associated with antihypertensive drugs. J Fam Pract 1991;33:481–5.
62. Ried LD, Tueth MJ, Handberg E, et al. A Study of Antihypertensive Drugs and Depressive Symptoms (SADD-Sx) in patients treated with a calcium antagonist versus an atenolol hypertension treatment strategy in the International Verapamil SR-Trandolapril Study (INVEST). Psychosom Med 2005;67:398–406.
63. Dimsdale JE, Halloran L, Bergner L, et al. The effect of propranolol on cognitive function and mood of hypertensive patients with borderline hypertension. Am J Med 2002;13:280–3.
64. Carney RM, Rich MW, Tevelde A, et al. Major depressive disorder in coronary artery disease. Am J Cardiol 1987;60:1273–5.
65. Bartels D, Glasser M, Wang A, et al. Association between depression and propranolol use in elderly patients. Clin Pharm 1988;7:146–50.
66. Schleifer SJ, Slater WR, Macari-Hinson MM, et al. Digitalis and beta-blocking agents: effects on depression following myocardial infarction. Am Heart J 1991;121:1397–402.
67. van Melle JP, Verbeek DE, van den Berg MP, et al. Beta-blockers and depression after myocardial infarction: a multicenter prospective study. J Am Coll Cardiol 2006;48:2209–14.
68. Ried LD, McFarland BH, Johnson RE, et al. Beta-blockers and depression: the more the murkier? Ann Pharmacother 1998;32:699–708.
69. Lama PJ. Systemic adverse effects of beta-adrenergic blockers: an evidence-based assessment. Am J Ophthalmol 2002;134:749–60.
70. Ko DT, Hebert PR, Coffey CS, et al. Beta-blocker therapy and symptoms of depression, fatigue, and sexual dysfunction. JAMA 2002;288:351–7.
71. Patten SB, Barbui C. Drug-induced depression: a systematic review to inform clinical practice. Psychother Psychosom 2004;73:207–15.
72. Dimsdale JE, Newton RP, Joist T. Neuropsychological side effects of beta-blockers. Arch Intern Med 1989;149:514–25.
73. Lindholm LH, Carlberg B, Samuelsson O. Should beta blockers remain first choice in the treatment of primary hypertension? A meta-analysis. Lancet 2005;366:1545–53.
74. Rothman KJ. Causes. Am J Epidemiol 1976;104:587–92.
75. Russell JW, Schuckit MA. Anxiety and depression in patient on nadolol. Lancet 1982;2:1286–7.
76. Kaiserman I, Kaiserman N, Elhayany A, et al. Topical beta-blockers are not associated with an increased risk of treatment for depression. Ophthalmology 2006;113:1077–80.
77. Adelson SC. Beta-blockers and depression: the [illegible]
78. [illegible]
79. Mabuchi F, Yoshimura K, Kashiwagi K, et al. High prevalence of anxiety and depression in patients with primary open-angle glaucoma. J Glaucoma 2008;17:552–7.

An Updated Review of Implantable Cardioverter/ Defibrillators, Induced Anxiety, and Quality of Life

J. Michael Bostwick, MD, Christopher L. Sola, DO*

KEYWORDS

• Anxiety • Depression • Psychopathology

Irrespective of its psychologic effects, the implantable cardioverter-defibrillator (ICD) has become the reference standard for treatment of potentially life-threatening ventricular arrhythmias.[1] Since the Food and Drug Administration (FDA) approved ICDs for treatment of ventricular fibrillation in 1985,[2] large-scale trials have demonstrated a survival benefit,[3–9] resulting in increased use of the device in a variety of conditions and broadening FDA indications that include resistance to pharmacologic treatment and ventricular arrhythmias associated with cardiac arrest or hemodynamic compromise.[10] During the same period, technologic advances have included shrinking device size and improved firing specificity.[2]

Despite overall good acceptance of ICDs,[11–13] patients may experience discharges as frightening and painful. Moreover, a significant percentage of patients who have ICDs experience a shock in the first year after implantation, with estimates ranging from 10% to 54% of recipients.[14,15] Worsened quality of life may result, and a substantial proportion of patients develop psychologic disturbances.[16–18]

The authors reviewed ICD-induced psychopathology in 2005,[19] concluding that the literature showed depression and anxiety to be unfortunate products of these devices in a substantial minority of patients, with recency and frequency of firing the best predictors of incipient psychopathology. Since then, coincident with the rapid increase in the use of implanted devices, dozens of studies addressing psychologic sequelae have appeared, warranting an update of that review. Using the search terms "implantable cardioverter-defibrillator," "ICD," "psychopathology," " anxiety," "depression," and "quality of life," the authors queried the MEDLINE database for articles dealing with psychologic sequelae to ICD implantation and use. Bibliographies of those articles yielded additional publications. They identified more than 50 articles of interest, most of which were published after the authors submitted their original review in late 2004.

Since then, researchers have expended considerable effort identifying potential risk factors and—to a lesser extent—mitigating factors for the development of psychopathology in ICD recipients. Commonly occurring categories of inquiry include age, gender, number of shocks experienced, predictability and perceived control of shocks, perception of support, family response, anger, anxiety, optimism, and somatization. In almost no category is there consensus on the degree of risk.

This article originally appeared in *Psychiatric Clinics of North America,* Volume 30, Number 4.

Department of Psychiatry and Psychology, Mayo Clinic College of Medicine, 200 First Street SW, Rochester, MN 55905, USA

* Corresponding author.

E-mail address: sola.christopher@mayo.edu

Heart Failure Clin 7 (2011) 101–108

doi:10.1016/j.hfc.2010.10.003

AGE

In their original review, the authors reported that youth (age <50 years) was a risk factor for increased anxiety, reduced quality of life, and compromised adjustment to the device. They have found six additional studies, four of which refute this conclusion, and two of which concur with it, at least in part.

The first study to disagree found neither anxiety nor depression to be increased in 20 patients aged 9 to 19 years, despite worsened physical functioning.[20] These children and adolescents do not escape unscathed, however, experiencing "a greater need for social acceptance" than the normative sample. Crossmann and colleagues[21] showed that ICD discharges, age, and gender did not predict anxiety levels in 35 ICD recipients age 35 to 65 years. In their study of 91 ICD patients, Bilge and colleagues[22] found "no significant relation between age and depression or anxiety scores." Yarnoz and Curtis[23] arrived at a similar conclusion, noting that "older patients reported a less active lifestyle, less satisfaction with their physical fitness, and more anxiety, while younger patients demonstrated improvements in the same categories."

On the other hand, Hamilton and Carroll[24] examined 70 patients aged 21 to 84 years, finding that anxiety scores in younger subjects are significantly higher than in older ones, although scores for the younger decrease at 6 months before rising again at 1 year. Although calmer than the younger subjects, the older group perceives little improvement in health and functioning, whereas the anxious younger group reports some improvement. These seemingly contradictory findings suggest a reciprocal relationship between quality of life and level of anxiety. Despite functional gains, younger adults with ICDs are thought to have "worse quality of life and more psychological distress than older adults".[25]

GENDER

Female gender has been thought to be an independent risk factor, although the literature is limited by the consistent finding that most study participants are male. Six studies update the understanding of this risk factor; like the studies of the effect of age, they either fail to achieve consensus or frankly contradict one another.

Thomas and colleagues[25] showed women reporting lower scores on the emotional subscale of the SF-36 than men. Two groups of investigators[26,27] found women reporting clinically significant depression and anxiety nearly twice as often as men and link this distress to body image concerns and loss of social roles. Both recommend altering approaches to management of female ICD recipients. Walker and colleagues[26] propose reframing the ICD scar as "a sign of 'survivorship' and a symbol of the ability to cope with adversity." Sowell and colleagues[27] suggest reducing disfigurement by developing alternate techniques such as submammary implantation. They also recommend involving the family in preoperative decisions and encouraging ongoing psychologic support for both patient and family.

On multivariate analysis, depression and anxiety in women do not travel together reliably or increase predictably. Bilge and colleagues[22] found female gender independently to predict elevated anxiety but not depression. Luyster and colleagues[28] found the reverse. In yet another study, women experienced more pain and worse sleep but no more depression or anxiety than men.[29] Making this finding particularly robust is the relative disadvantages of the women in other respects. Compared with the men, they are younger, less functional, and less likely to have a spouse' support.

NUMBER AND FREQUENCY OF SHOCKS

Most investigators in the authors' earlier review found that increasing numbers of ICD shocks corresponded to elevated rates of psychopathology.[19,25] One such study of 167 ICD recipients revealed both increased depression and anxiety in those experiencing shock and also decreased adaptation to living with the device.[15]

Although a representative early paper stated unequivocally that "multiple shocks were a clear precipitant for the psychiatric disorders",[30] more recent reports disagree partly or completely with this assertion. In their 91 subjects, Bilge and colleagues[22] found worsened anxiety but not depression in those who experienced shock, whereas Luyster and colleagues[28] observed the opposite in 100 subjects.

Three studies discern no relationship at all between shock frequency and psychopathology. Among all ICD recipients living in Iceland (44 patients), no differences in anxiety or depression occurred, regardless of shock history, and ICD and pacemaker recipients were indistinguishable in terms of anxiety, depression, and quality of life.[31] Agreeing with the Iceland study, Godemann and colleagues[32] evaluated 93 patients and ascertained no effect on quality of life from ICD discharges. Finally, even though 5 of 14 patients in another study received more than five shocks in a 24-hour period, the occurrence of shocks—appropriate or not—bore no relationship to depression or anxiety scores or quality of life.[33]

When shock, or the possibility of it, does worsen quality of life, it generally does so in the context of premorbid psychologic traits. Multiple authors recommend psychologic referral for those who experience shock.[34] In general, however, patients who actually are shocked are only slightly more likely to suffer from anxiety. It is the patients who have a high level of concern about being shocked, even if they have not been, who manifest heightened anxiety.[35] Indeed, even as cardiologists interrogate devices for objective evidence of a discharge, the belief that one has experienced a shock may be more important than actually having received a shock. Of 75 ICD recipients, the 19 who experienced "phantom shocks" (a sensation of shock in the absence of verified discharge) were noted to be more anxious and depressed than the other 56, even those actually shocked.[36]

For ICD recipients who have anxious temperaments, the unpredictability of the ICD shocks is likely to be associated with negative emotions.[15,31] Such patients may attempt to mitigate potential distress from shocks by trying to control their actions or environment to prevent discharges.[19] Avoidant behaviors and symptoms of hypervigilance in these patients can reach the proportions of posttraumatic stress disorder.[37]

PERCEPTION OF SUPPORT AND FAMILY RESPONSE

In the authors' original review, excessive family anxiety and poor social support led to worse quality of life and emergent psychopathology. In a more recent review, Thomas and colleagues[25] reinforce this finding, stating "low anxiety, high social support and no shocks were predictive of the best quality of life." It is not necessarily the recipient's own anxiety that is the problem. Eight of 12 patients voiced frustration with "overprotective" family members, with one reportedly moving away from home to escape a parent's vigilance.[38] Although social support has been deemed "imperative in managing stress and rehabilitation," it needs to be the right kind of support.[39] Because family members also are affected by the ICD, they can benefit from education and encouragement to provide the calm and steady emotional and physical environment these patients need.[35]

Marriage is considered a proxy for social support, although Walker and colleagues[26] note that the protective effects of marriage against heart disease are more marked in men than in women. Sears and colleagues[34] observe that psychologic variables such as social support "account for as much, if not more, of the variance in quality of life outcomes [than] age and ejection fraction." The lower levels of anxiety and depression reported by the married people in Bilge's cohort report did not reach statistical significance, however.[22]

ANGER AND ANXIETY

The authors previously found that baseline state and traits of anger and anxiety may be higher in ICD recipients before implantation, with anxiety improving after implantation, and they noted that elevated anxiety predicts worse quality of life. ICD recipients commonly report anger and anxiety.[15,40] Thirty-five ICD recipients scored higher on the Beck Anxiety Inventory than did controls, although not as high as patients who had a full-blown anxiety disorder.[21] The authors concluded that anxiety in these patients remains "remarkably stable over a period of 2.5 years," despite their surprising finding that trait anxiety as measured by the Trait Anxiety Inventory decreases during that same period.[21]

Illustrating the power of psychosomatic interactions, Burg and colleagues[41] have studied 240 ICD recipients, finding that individuals with high trait anger and anxiety are significantly more likely to experience ICD-treated ventricular arrhythmias.

One specific anxiety manifestation is avoidance. Of 143 ICD recipients in one study,[40] 55% had begun to avoid activities, objects, or places they feared might cause ICD discharge, significantly diminishing quality of life. Some patients consider the price required to maintain physical health not worth the cost in mental health. Frustrated by being unable to discern whether sexual activity triggered shock, one man asked that his ICD be turned off.[38] Unwilling to give up sex and equally unwilling to risk being shocked, he states, "I just don't want to take the chance." A similar request to deactivate the ICD, although to avoid noxious memories rather than engage in pleasurable stimuli, is described in a man experiencing flashbacks of childhood physical abuse when his device fired.[37]

Anxiety may also manifest as nonspecific somatic worry. Through multivariate analysis, Godemann and colleagues[32] tease out that "somatization" (defined as the summation of ratings of nonspecific physical complaints such as pain, nausea, numbness, weakness, and tingling) is the most potent contributor to poor quality of life. As seems to be case throughout the recent ICD literature, however, the findings of another research team diametrically oppose Godemann's work. In 49 patients in whom anxiety sensitivity (a measure of the intolerance of somatic symptoms of anxiety) was associated with elevations in anxiety, depression, and stress at baseline, Lemon and Edelman[42] conclude that ICDs provide reassurance, with concomitant improvement in adaptation to life with the device.

OPTIMISM AND POSITIVE HEALTH EXPECTATIONS

Just as elevated anxiety can lead to pessimism, a fundamentally optimistic outlook can generate reduced anxiety and positive health expectations. Two recent trials address this possibility. The first, looking at 88 patients who had newly implanted ICDs, demonstrated that patients who had higher baseline positive health expectations, defined as "patient beliefs specifically related to the likelihood of a positive health outcome," reported better general physical health at follow-up than patients who had lower baseline positive health expectations.[43] Additionally, patients who had high optimism ("a trait or disposition, capturing more of a generalized expectancy") reported better mental health and social functioning at follow-up. The authors concluded that these "resilience factors" warrant more attention, because they may direct eventual interventions. Trait optimism since has been suggested to be among the psychologic variables in ICD recipients "most important in predicting mental health quality of life".[34]

TREATMENT OPTIONS

Psychoeducation

In the authors' original review, as now, there is consensus as to the importance of patient education. Recent researchers would all agree with Bourke and colleagues'[30] 1997 assertion that "appropriate interventions should begin with education as to the nature and purpose of the defibrillator." Although several distinct approaches are advocated,[28,44,45] commonalities include providing education about the nature of ICDs, including (1) their survival advantage over antiarrhythmic medications, (2) setting realistic expectations that shocks cannot be eliminated by avoiding such basic activities as exercise and sex, and (3) preparing a plan for dealing with the aftermath when a shock occurs. Nearly all recommend teaching relaxation techniques and problem-solving skills and encouraging rapid return to daily activities. Proposed teaching modalities range from individual therapy[38] and support groups[46] to telephone discussions,[44] computer-based instruction,[47] consumer newsletters such as "The Zapper",[48] and patient-centered articles.[45] Support groups are particularly favored for facilitating social interactions that help members share common experiences, normalize concerns, and exchange emotional support.[28,40]

Psychotherapy

Although it has been advocated that "provision of psychological interventions to all ICD recipients presenting with known risk factors ... may be beneficial",[34] limited literature explores the efficacy of modalities other than cognitive behavioral therapy (CBT). A Cochrane review is underway to weigh CBT's benefits in ICD recepients, although results are not yet available.[49] A focus on reducing catastrophic interpretations has been recommended,[19,30] as has using other techniques like cognitive reframing and changing counterproductive thoughts to reduce anxiety, improve communication skills, and teach relaxation training and stress management skills.[39,47] One case report describes a patient successfully reducing his anxiety during a 4-day intensive CBT-based program on an inpatient psychiatry unit.[37]

In addition to reducing depression and anxiety, CBT also may contribute to improved physical functioning. After randomly assigning half of 70 ICD recipients to CBT and half to conventional care, Chevalier and colleagues[50] found that fewer patients receiving CBT sustained shocks. Whether improved physical functioning results from undergoing CBT or experiencing fewer instances of aversive stimuli is unknown. In either case, the difference was neither statistically significant nor persistent at 1-year follow-up. Anxiety, however, was significantly lower in the CBT group at both 3 and 12 months. A second study compares 10 ICD recipients getting conventional care and 12 ICD recipients receiving a 12-week educational program incorporating exercise, relaxation, and specific training about the cognitive modes of anxiety, phobia, and panic. The treatment group experienced decreased anxiety and depression and improved quality of life.[51] Although only 26% of the patients approached actually enrolled in the group, it was "overwhelmingly popular" among attendees. Neither study attempted to parse the proportion of benefit from CBT alone. One non-CBT study showed that prescribed exercise augmented functional capacity and quality of life in 30 ICD recipients.[52]

Pharmacology

As in the authors' original review, the literature continues to offer minimal guidance on choices of psychotropic medication for this population. Noting the dearth of ICD-specific literature addressing cardiac-safe antidepressants and anxiolytics, one case report outlines a plan for short-term anxiolysis with a benzodiazepine and longer-term treatment with a serotonin reuptake inhibitor because of its relatively benign side-effect profile.[37] Tricyclic antidepressants, which prolong cardiac conduction, should be avoided, and caution should be observed with venlafaxine, which was shown in five of five subjects in one study to lower defibrillation thresholds by an order of magnitude, possibly through blocking cardiac sodium-channel activity.[53]

NEW DIRECTIONS

Since the authors' original review, several areas of inquiry have emerged. Stutts and colleagues[54] note "increasing attention given to psychological factors in cardiac disease subgroups is representative of a broader trend ... in most chronic diseases." These factors include the curious experience of feeling the ICD firing when it has not, called "phantom shock" and associated with depression and anxiety.[36,46] The literature increasingly references ICD-induced posttraumatic stress disorder,[36,37,46] although a formal study has yet to determine its prevalence.

Two studies have evaluated the psychologic impact of product recalls.[55,56] One suggests that not all ICD recipients are equally affected by a product recall, reminding physicians to include recall risk as part of informed consent.[55] The other highlights that pathologic anxiety risk increases in ICD recipients during a recall, with ventricular arrhythmias a potential consequence.[56]

An additional line of inquiry achieving recent prominence is ICD costs, both financial and psychologic. Although implantation costs have decreased substantially, to about $30,000 currently, with average ICD-related annual health care costs ranging from $5000 to $17,000, hidden costs to ICD recipients are increasingly acknowledged.[32] These costs include worsened quality of life,[57] failure to return to work,[32] hesitancy to return to sexual activity,[32,38] and decreased self-efficacy stemming from driving restrictions.[32]

Assessment Tools

Since the authors' original review, two new scales have been introduced in response to a void in the literature regarding assessments specific to the unique experience of living with an ICD. The ICD Patient Concerns Questionnaire is a 20-item questionnaire detailing concerns about living with an ICD and addressing the number and severity of new-onset concerns patients who have ICDs may experience.[58] The Florida Shock Anxiety Scale[14] is a 10-item scale that operationalizes device-specific fears in two dimensions: consequences of device firing and triggers of discharge. The authors recommend using this instrument to identify patients at risk for emotion-triggered shock. This brief but useful instrument can recognize and track anxiety both before and after implantation.

SUMMARY

During the past 2 years the number of studies examining psychopathology and quality of life after ICD implantation has increased dramatically. Variables assessed have included recipient age, gender, and social support network. How recipients respond to having the device, particularly after experiencing firing, has been evaluated in light of new depression and anxiety disorder diagnoses as well as premorbid personality structure. Now the picture of what is known is, if anything, cloudier than it was 2 years ago, with little definitive and much contradictory data emerging in most of these categories. It still seems clear that in a significant minority of ICD recipients the device negatively affects quality of life, probably more so if it fires. Education about life with the device before receiving it remains paramount.

Reports continue to appear of patients developing new-onset diagnosable anxiety disorders such as panic and posttraumatic stress disorder. Until recently the strongest predictors of induced psychopathology were considered to be the frequency and recency of device firing. It now seems that preimplantation psychologic variables such as degree of optimism or pessimism and an anxious personality style may confer an even greater risk than previously thought.

Certainly many variables factor into the induction of psychopathology in these patients. Among these factors are age, gender, and perception of control of shocks, as well as the predictability of shocks and psychologic attributions made by the patient regarding the device. Another source of variability is this population's medical heterogeneity. Some patients receive ICDs after near-death experiences; others get them as anticipatory prophylaxis. Some have longstanding and entrenched heart disease; others were apparently healthy before sudden dangerous arrhythmias. Diagnoses as diverse as myocardial infarction in the context of advanced coronary artery disease and dilated cardiomyopathy after acute viral infection may warrant ICD placement. Moreover the course of cardiac disease after ICD placement may vary from relative stability to continuing disease progression and severe functional compromise. Unless these and other pre- and postimplantation differences are taken into account, it is almost impossible to make meaningful comparisons between studies.

Ideally, future research would consist either of large-scale, randomized, prospective studies using validated structured-interview tools to supplement a literature dominated by self-report measures, unstructured assessments, and anecdotal reports, or of smaller studies designed to focus on particular diagnostic subsets.

As ICDs become the standard of care for potentially life-threatening arrhythmias, the rate of implantations continues to increase. Because negative emotions have been linked to an increased incidence of arrhythmias, and untreated or unrecognized psychiatric illness can interfere with adaptation to an ICD, assessing and managing both pre-existing and induced psychiatric disorders becomes even more critical. Greater research attention should be paid to determining which patients meet criteria for anxiety disorders before and after implantation and what premorbid traits predispose to postimplantation psychopathology. The authors predict that psychiatrists will be involved increasingly in caring for this population, offering insights into treatment options that increase the likelihood of successful ICD acceptance and decrease the psychosocial costs of these devices.

REFERENCES

1. DiMarco JP. Implantable cardioverter-defibrillators. N Engl J Med 2003;349(19):1836–47.
2. Glikson M, Friedman PA. The implantable cardioverter defibrillator. Lancet 2001;357(9262): 1107–17.
3. Moss AJ, Hall WJ, Cannom DS, et al. Improved survival with an implanted defibrillator in patients with coronary disease at high risk for ventricular arrhythmia. Multicenter Automatic Defibrillator Implantation Trial Investigators. N Engl J Med 1996;335(26):1933–40.
4. A comparison of antiarrhythmic-drug therapy with implantable defibrillators in patients resuscitated from near-fatal ventricular arrhythmias. The Antiarrhythmics Versus Implantable Defibrillators (AVID) Investigators. N Engl J Med 1997;337(22): 1576–83.
5. Connolly SJ, Gent M, Roberts RS, et al. Canadian Implantable Defibrillator Study (CIDS): a randomized trial of the implantable cardioverter defibrillator against amiodarone. Circulation 2000;101(11): 1297–302.
6. Kuck KH, Cappato R, Siebels J, et al. Randomized comparison of antiarrhythmic drug therapy with implantable defibrillators in patients resuscitated from cardiac arrest: the Cardiac Arrest Study Hamburg (CASH). Circulation 2000;102(7):748–54.
7. Bokhari F, Newman D, Greene M, et al. Long-term comparison of the implantable cardioverter defibrillator versus amiodarone: eleven-year follow-up of a subset of patients in the Canadian Implantable Defibrillator Study (CIDS). Circulation 2004;110(2): 112–6.
8. Greenberg H, Case RB, Moss AJ, et al. Analysis of mortality events in the Multicenter Automatic Defibrillator Implantation Trial (MADIT-II). J Am Coll Cardiol 2004;43(8):1459–65.
9. Bardy GH, Lee KL, Mark DB, et al. Amiodarone or an implantable cardioverter-defibrillator for congestive heart failure. N Engl J Med 2005;352(3):225–37.
10. U.S. Food and Drug Administration Center for Devices and Radiological Health. Available at: http://www.accessdata.fda.gov/scripts/cdrh/devicesatfda/index.cfm. Accessed June 8, 2007.
11. Vlay SC. The automatic internal cardioverter-defibrillator: comprehensive clinical follow-up, economic and social impact—the Stony Brook experience. Am Heart J 1986;112(1):189–94.
12. Luderitz B, Jung W, Deister A, et al. Patient acceptance of the implantable cardioverter defibrillator in ventricular tachyarrhythmias. Pacing Clin Electrophysiol 1993;16(9):1815–21.
13. Eads AS, Sears SF Jr, Sotile WM, et al. Supportive communication with implantable cardioverter defibrillator patients: seven principles to facilitate psychosocial adjustment. J Cardiopulm Rehabil 2000;20(2):109–14.
14. Kuhl EA, Dixit NK, Walker RL, et al. Measurement of patient fears about implantable cardioverter defibrillator shock: an initial evaluation of the Florida Shock Anxiety Scale. Pacing Clin Electrophysiol 2006; 29(6):614–8.
15. Kamphuis HC, de Leeuw JR, Derksen R, et al. Implantable cardioverter defibrillator recipients: quality of life in recipients with and without ICD shock delivery: a prospective study. Europace 2003;5(4):381–9.
16. Namerow PB, Firth BR, Heywood GM, et al. Quality-of-life six months after CABG surgery in patients randomized to ICD versus no ICD therapy: findings from the CABG Patch Trial. Pacing Clin Electrophysiol 1999;22(9):1305–13.
17. Irvine J, Dorian P, Baker B, et al. Quality of life in the Canadian Implantable Defibrillator Study (CIDS). Am Heart J 2002;144(2):282–9.
18. Sears SE Jr, Conti JB. Understanding implantable cardioverter defibrillator shocks and storms: medical and psychosocial considerations for research and clinical care. Clin Cardiol 2003;26(3):107–11.
19. Sola CL, Bostwick JM. Implantable cardioverter-defibrillators, induced anxiety, and quality of life. Mayo Clin Proc 2005;80(2):232–7.

20. DeMaso DR, Lauretti A, Spieth L, et al. Psychosocial factors and quality of life in children and adolescents with implantable cardioverter-defibrillators. Am J Cardiol 2004;93(5):582–7.
21. Crossmann A, Pauli P, Dengler W, et al. Stability and cause of anxiety in patients with an implantable cardioverter-defibrillator: a longitudinal two-year follow-up. Heart Lung 2007;36(2):87–95.
22. Bilge AK, Ozben B, Demircan S, et al. Depression and anxiety status of patients with implantable cardioverter defibrillator and precipitating factors. Pacing Clin Electrophysiol 2006;29(6):619–26.
23. Yarnoz MJ, Curtis AB. Why cardioverter-defibrillator implantation might not be the best idea for your elderly patient. Am J Geriatr Cardiol 2006;15(6):367–71.
24. Hamilton GA, Carroll DL. The effects of age on quality of life in implantable cardioverter defibrillator recipients. J Clin Nurs 2004;13(2):194–200.
25. Thomas SA, Friedmann E, Kao CW, et al. Quality of life and psychological status of patients with implantable cardioverter defibrillators. Am J Crit Care 2006;15(4):389–98.
26. Walker RL, Campbell KA, Sears SF, et al. Women and the implantable cardioverter defibrillator: a lifespan perspective on key psychosocial issues. Clin Cardiol 2004;27(10):543–6.
27. Sowell LV, Kuhl EA, Sears SF, et al. Device implant technique and consideration of body image: specific procedures for implantable cardioverter defibrillators in female patients. J Womens Health (Larchmt) 2006;15(7):830–5.
28. Luyster FS, Hughes JW, Waechter D, et al. Resource loss predicts depression and anxiety among patients treated with an implantable cardioverter defibrillator. Psychosom Med 2006;68(5):794–800.
29. Smith G, Dunbar SB, Valderrama AL, et al. Gender differences in implantable cardioverter-defibrillator patients at the time of insertion. Prog Cardiovasc Nurs 2006;21(2):76–82.
30. Bourke JP, Turkington D, Thomas G, et al. Florid psychopathology in patients receiving shocks from implanted cardioverter-defibrillators. Heart 1997; 78(6):581–3.
31. Leosdottir M, Sigurdsson E, Reimarsdottir G, et al. Health-related quality of life of patients with implantable cardioverter defibrillators compared with that of pacemaker recipients. Europace 2006;8(3):168–74.
32. Godemann F, Butter C, Lampe F, et al. Determinants of the quality of life (QoL) in patients with an implantable cardioverter/defibrillator (ICD). Qual Life Res 2004;13(2):411–6.
33. Newall EG, Lever NA, Prasad S, et al. Psychological implications of ICD implantation in a New Zealand population. Europace 2007;9(1):20–4.
34. Sears SF, Lewis TS, Kuhl EA, et al. Predictors of quality of life in patients with implantable cardioverter defibrillators. Psychosomatics 2005;46(5):451–7.
35. Pedersen SS, van Domburg RT, Theuns DA, et al. Concerns about the implantable cardioverter defibrillator: a determinant of anxiety and depressive symptoms independent of experienced shocks. Am Heart J 2005;149(4):664–9.
36. Prudente LA, Reigle J, Bourguignon C, et al. Psychological indices and phantom shocks in patients with ICD. J Interv Card Electrophysiol 2006;15(3):185–90.
37. Hoecksel K, Bostwick J. Getting to the heart of his shocking trauma. Current Psychiatry 2007;6: 84–91.
38. Steinke EE, Gill-Hopple K, Valdez D, et al. Sexual concerns and educational needs after an implantable cardioverter defibrillator. Heart Lung 2005; 34(5):299–308.
39. Sears SF Jr, Stutts LA, Aranda JM Jr, et al. Managing congestive heart failure patient factors in the device era. Congest Heart Fail 2006;12(6): 335–40.
40. Lemon J, Edelman S, Kirkness A. Avoidance behaviors in patients with implantable cardioverter defibrillators. Heart Lung 2004;33(3):176–82.
41. Burg MM, Lampert R, Joska T, et al. Psychological traits and emotion-triggering of ICD shock-terminated arrhythmias. Psychosom Med 2004; 66(6):898–902.
42. Lemon J, Edelman S. Psychological adaptation to ICDs and the influence of anxiety sensitivity. Psychol Health Med 2007;12(2):163–71.
43. Sears SF, Serber ER, Lewis TS, et al. Do positive health expectations and optimism relate to quality-of-life outcomes for the patient with an implantable cardioverter defibrillator? J Cardiopulm Rehabil 2004;24(5):324–31.
44. Dougherty CM, Lewis FM, Thompson EA, et al. Short-term efficacy of a telephone intervention by expert nurses after an implantable cardioverter defibrillator. Pacing Clin Electrophysiol 2004;27(12): 1594–602.
45. Sears SF Jr, Shea JB, Conti JB. Cardiology patient page. How to respond to an implantable cardioverter-defibrillator shock. Circulation 2005; 111(23):e380–2.
46. Prudente LA. Psychological disturbances, adjustment, and the development of phantom shocks in patients with an implantable cardioverter defibrillator. J Cardiovasc Nurs 2005;20(4):288–93.
47. Kuhl EA, Sears SF, Conti JB. Using computers to improve the psychosocial care of implantable cardioverter defibrillator recipients. Pacing Clin Electrophysiol 2006;29(12):1426–33.
48. The Zapper online newsletter. Available at: http://www.zaplife.org/. Accessed June 8, 2007.
49. Johnson B, Francis J. Cognitive behavourial therapy for patients with implantable cardioverter-defibrillators [protocol]. The Cochrane Library, Issue

3, 2007. Available at: http://www.thecochranelibrary.com. Accessed May 29, 2007.
50. Chevalier P, Cottraux J, Mollard E, et al. Prevention of implantable defibrillator shocks by cognitive behavioral therapy: a pilot trial. Am Heart J 2006; 151(1):191, e1–191.e6.
51. Frizelle DJ, Lewin RJ, Kaye G, et al. Cognitive-behavioural rehabilitation programme for patients with an implanted cardioverter defibrillator: a pilot study. Br J Health Psychol 2004;9(Pt 3):381–92.
52. Belardinelli R, Capestro F, Misiani A, et al. Moderate exercise training improves functional capacity, quality of life, and endothelium-dependent vasodilation in chronic heart failure patients with implantable cardioverter defibrillators and cardiac resynchronization therapy. Eur J Cardiovasc Prev Rehabil 2006;13(5):818–25.
53. Carnes CA, Pickworth KK, Votolato NA, et al. Elevated defibrillation threshold with venlafaxine therapy. Pharmacotherapy 2004;24(8):1095–8.
54. Stutts LA, Cross NJ, Conti JB, et al. Examination of research trends on patient factors in patients with implantable cardioverter defibrillators. Clin Cardiol 2007;30(2):64–8.
55. Sears SF Jr, Conti JB. Psychological aspects of cardiac devices and recalls in patients with implantable cardioverter defibrillators. Am J Cardiol 2006; 98(4):565–7.
56. van den Broek KC, Denollet J, Nyklicek I, et al. Psychological reaction to potential malfunctioning of implantable defibrillators. Pacing Clin Electrophysiol 2006;29(9):953–6.
57. Noyes K, Corona E, Zwanziger J, et al. Health-related quality of life consequences of implantable cardioverter defibrillators: results from MADIT II. Med Care 2007;45(5):377–85.
58. Frizelle DJ, Lewin B, Kaye G, et al. Development of a measure of the concerns held by people with implanted cardioverter defibrillators: the ICDC. Br J Health Psychol 2006;11(Pt 2):293–301.

Psychiatric Aspects of Heart and Lung Disease in Critical Care

Peter A. Shapiro, MD[a,b,*], David A. Fedoronko, MD[a,b], Lucy A. Epstein, MD[a,b], Elsa G.E. Mirasol, MD[c], Chirag V. Desai, MD[a,b]

KEYWORDS

- Anxiety • Depression • Agitation • Delirium
- Chronic lung disease • Substance withdrawal

Heart and lung diseases are associated with a high prevalence of psychiatric disorders. These psychiatric disorders may occur as premorbid risk factors, as comorbidities, and as complications of the heart and lung conditions. In intensive and critical care settings, appropriate diagnosis and management of psychiatric problems can alter the medical outcome. The most common issues are anxiety, depression, and agitation and delirium. This article addresses differential diagnosis and management, with an emphasis on the intensive care and critical care settings.

DIFFERENTIAL DIAGNOSIS OF ANXIETY AND DEPRESSION IN SERIOUSLY ILL HEART AND LUNG DISEASE PATIENTS

Although unpleasant feeling states of fear, anxiety, and sadness may be normal responses to stressful and unfortunate life events, not all anxious and depressed moods in patients with new or exacerbated chronic illness are normal reactions to a stressful life event. Depending on diagnosis, some patients who seem to be anxious or unhappy may benefit from reassurance and observation alone, whereas others need additional intervention.

In general, psychiatric disorders are differentiated from normal mental functioning by the presence of significant subjective distress or impairment in adaptive functioning caused by the mental state itself.[1] This criterion helps to define the set of "adjustment disorders," in which clinically significant emotional distress occurs following a stressful circumstance, and persists for more than a few days, but does not meet criteria for another psychiatric disorder. Adjustment disorders with depressed mood or anxious mood are common in medically ill patients. They often remit spontaneously or in response to brief supportive interventions, such as clarification of the patient's concerns, education about his or her condition, or provision of social support.

More severe depression problems occur in major depressive disorder and bipolar affective disorder. The cardinal feature of major depressive disorder (**Box 1**) is the presence of a major depressive episode. A major depressive episode is defined by the presence of at least five of the following: persistent depressed mood most of the day; persistent loss of interest in usually enjoyable activities; sleep disturbance; appetite disturbance; difficulty thinking, concentrating, or making decisions; fatigue or loss of energy; inability to experience

This article is supported in part by the Nathaniel Wharton Fund, New York, NY.
This article originally appeared in *Critical Care Clinics*, Volume 24, Number 4.

[a] Department of Psychiatry, Columbia University, 622 West 168 Street, Box 427, New York, NY 10032, USA
[b] Consultation-Liaison Psychiatry Service, New York Presbyterian Hospital-Columbia University Medical Center, 622 West 168 Street, Box 427, New York, NY 10032, USA
[c] Department of Psychiatry, Veterans Administration Medical Center, 79 Middleville Road, Northport, NY 11768, USA
* Corresponding author. Department of Psychiatry, NYPH-CUMC, 622 West 168 Street, Box 427, New York, NY 10032.
E-mail address: pas3@columbia.edu

Heart Failure Clin 7 (2011) 109–125
doi:10.1016/j.hfc.2010.10.002
1551-7136/11/$ – see front matter

Box 1
Diagnostic criteria for major depressive disorder

A. Five (or more) of the following symptoms have been present during the same 2-week period and represent a change from previous functioning; at least one of the symptoms is either (1) depressed mood or (2) loss of interest or pleasure. **Note:** Do not include symptoms that are clearly caused by a general medical condition, or mood-incongruent delusions or hallucinations.
   (1) Depressed mood most of the day, nearly every day, as indicated by either subjective report (eg, feels sad or empty) or observation made by others (eg, appears tearful). **Note:** in children and adolescents, can be irritable mood.
   (2) Markedly diminished interest or pleasure in all, or almost all, activities most of the day, nearly every day (as indicated by either subjective account or observation made by others).
   (3) Significant weight loss when not dieting or weight gain (eg, a change of more than 5% of body weight in a month), or decrease or increase in appetite nearly every day. **Note:** In children, consider failure to make expected weight gains.
   (4) Insomnia or hypersomnia nearly every day.
   (5) Psychomotor agitation or retardation nearly every day (observable by others, not merely subjective feelings of restlessness or being slowed down)
   (6) Fatigue or loss of energy nearly every day
   (7) Feelings of worthlessness or excessive or inappropriate guilt (which may be delusional) nearly every day (not merely self-reproach or guilt about being sick)
   (8) Diminished ability to think or concentrate, or indecisiveness, nearly every day (either by subjective account or as observed by others)
   (9) Recurrent thoughts of death (not just fear of dying), recurrent suicidal ideation without a specific plan, or a suicide attempt or a specific plan for committing suicide

B. The symptoms do not meet criteria for a mixed episode.
C. The symptoms cause clinically significant distress or impairment in social, occupational, or other important areas of functioning.
D. The symptoms are not caused by the direct physiologic effects of a substance (eg, a drug of abuse, a medication) or a general medical condition (eg, hypothyroidism).
E. The symptoms are not better accounted for by bereavement (ie, after the loss of a loved one), the symptoms persist for longer than 2 months or are characterized by marked functional impairment, morbid preoccupation with worthlessness, suicidal ideation, psychotic symptoms, or psychomotor retardation.

Data from American Psychiatric Association. Diagnostic and statistical manual of mental disorders, 4th edition, revised. Washington: American Psychiatric Association; 2000.

pleasure; psychomotor retardation or agitation; and thoughts of death or suicidal ideation. Either depressed mood or persistent loss of interest must be included among the features of the episode. The symptoms must persist for at least 2 weeks. Major depressive disorder is defined by the occurrence of a major depressive episode that cannot be better ascribed to another mental disorder or to another medical condition, and is not substance-induced, and in which the symptoms cause significant subjective distress or impairment in functioning. In bipolar affective disorder, significant depressive symptoms may occur, including major depressive episodes, but the patient also has episodes of abnormal, clinically significant mood elevation or irritability (mania or hypomania). In dysthymic disorder, mood symptoms that are below the threshold of a major depressive episode are persistent chronically over at least 2 years. Mood disorders are designated "secondary" when they are attributed to a medical condition, substance, or substance withdrawal. Other mood disorders may occur that do not meet criteria for any of these specific diagnoses because they are below the severity or duration thresholds or have atypical features.

Panic disorder and generalized anxiety disorder are the most common anxiety disorders associated with cardiac and pulmonary diseases. The sine qua non of panic disorder (**Box 2**) is the occurrence of recurring panic attacks, which are episodes of acute fear or anxiety with abrupt onset and numerous associated physical symptoms, such as shortness of breath, choking sensations, chest discomfort, palpitations, dizziness, lightheadedness, nausea, paresthesias, chills, hot flushes, and sweating, and fears of death, loss of control, or of going crazy; these symptoms are not caused by another medical condition or induced by a substance. They may also be accompanied by a sense of detachment from oneself (ie, depersonalization) or from reality (ie, derealization). In

Box 2
Diagnostic criteria for panic disorder

A. Both (1) and (2):
  (1) Recurrent unexpected panic attacks
  (2) At least one of the attacks has been followed by 1 month (or more) of one (or more) of the following:
    (a) Persistent concern about having additional attacks
    (b) Worry about the implications of the attack or its consequences (eg, losing control, having a heart attack, "going crazy")
    (c) A significant change in behavior related to the attacks

B. Presence or absence of agoraphobia.
C. The panic attacks are not caused by the direct physiologic effects of a substance (eg, a drug of abuse, a medication) or a general medical condition (eg, hyperthyroidism).
D. The panic attacks are not better accounted for by another mental disorder, such as social phobia (eg, occurring on exposure to feared social situations); specific phobia (eg, on exposure to a specific phobic situation); obsessive-compulsive disorder (eg, on exposure to dirt in someone with an obsession about contamination); posttraumatic stress disorder (eg, in response to stimuli associated with a severe stressor); or separation anxiety disorder (eg, in response to being away from home or close relatives).

Data from American Psychiatric Association. Diagnostic and statistical manual of mental disorders, 4th edition, revised. Washington: American Psychiatric Association; 2000.

generalized anxiety disorder, the primary feature is persistent nervousness, worry, or fearfulness, associated with fatigue, irritability, restlessness, difficulty concentrating, muscle tension, or sleep disturbance, which continues over a period of months, cannot be controlled, causes distress or impairs function, and is neither caused by a medical condition nor substance-related (**Box 3**). Secondary forms of these disorders may be caused by medical conditions, as side effects of substances including medications, or as effects of withdrawal from substances.

PSYCHIATRIC DISORDERS ASSOCIATED WITH CHRONIC LUNG DISEASE

Anxiety symptoms commonly accompany many pulmonary disorders.[2] These have been best

Box 3
Diagnostic criteria for generalized anxiety disorder

A. Excessive anxiety and worry (apprehensive expectation), occurring more days than not for at least 6 months, about a number of events or activities (eg, work or school performance).
B. The person finds it difficult to control the worry.
C. The anxiety and worry are associated with three (or more) of the following six symptoms (with at least some symptoms present for more days than not for the past 6 months). **Note:** Only one item is required in children.
  (1) Restlessness or feeling keyed up or on edge
  (2) Being easily fatigued
  (3) Difficulty concentrating or mind going blank
  (4) Irritability
  (5) Muscle tension
  (6) Sleep disturbance (difficulty falling or staying asleep, or restless unsatisfying sleep)

D. The focus of the anxiety and worry is not confined to features of an axis I disorder (eg, the anxiety or worry is not about having a panic attack [as in panic disorder], being embarrassed in public [as in social phobia], being contaminated [as in obsessive-compulsive disorder], being away from home or close relatives [as in separation anxiety disorder], gaining weight [as in anorexia nervosa], having multiple physical complaints [as in somatization disorder], or having a serious illness [as in hypochondriasis], and the anxiety and worry do not occur exclusively during posttraumatic stress disorder.
E. The anxiety, worry, or physical symptoms cause clinically significant distress or impairment in social, occupational, or other important areas of functioning.
F. The disturbance is not caused by the direct physiologic effects of a substance (eg, a drug of abuse, a medication) or a general medical condition (eg, hyperthyroidism) and does not occur exclusively during a mood disorder, a psychotic disorder, or a pervasive developmental disorder.

Data from American Psychiatric Association. Diagnostic and statistical manual of mental disorders. 4th edition, revised. Washington: American Psychiatric Association; 2000.

studied in chronic conditions, such as asthma and chronic obstructive pulmonary disease.[3,4] The anxiety experienced by affected patients may be described as either generalized anxiety or panic. Some patients with respiratory disease have a combination of both types of anxiety. Patients with acute respiratory failure seem even more anxious that those with stable chronic disease. Most of this increase seems to be panic rather than generalized anxiety.[5] Given the description of a panic attack, there may be some overlap between these symptoms and those of acute respiratory failure. Many patients with acute respiratory failure experience shortness of breath, choking, and chest discomfort. There are others, however, who are overwhelmed by these and the other classic symptoms of panic including fear of dying, losing control, going crazy, depersonalization, or derealization.

Various models have been offered to explain this apparent connection between pulmonary symptoms and the experience of panic (**Box 4**).[6] One model involves the psychological theory that some patients are prone to misinterpreting physical sensations within their bodies or "interoceptive cues" that may be associated with dyspnea. These include hyperventilation, chest tightness, tachycardia, and other physical symptoms. They may "catastrophize" the significance of these physical symptoms, leading them to believe that the symptoms are much more dangerous than is actually the case. This misinterpretation escalates their sense of anxiety. This anxiety heightens their focus on and sensitivity to somatic sensations, likely leading them to become even more preoccupied with their physical symptoms. These are again misinterpreted, leading to even more anxiety. This positive feedback cycle continues, leading to a heightened sense of anxiety and even more physical symptoms of panic.[7] Some patients with acute respiratory failure are likely prone to this cycle. For them, the primary issue is fear and the catastrophic misinterpretation of unexpected physical symptoms.

Box 4
Contributing factors in anxiety associated with lung disease

Catastrophizing cognitions

CO_2 sensitivity

Medication side effects

a. Corticosteroids
b. Methylxanthines
c. β_2-adrenergic agonists
d. Substance abuse (eg, cocaine)
e. Substance withdrawal (eg, alcohol)

Other models for the connection between acute respiratory failure and panic focus more directly on pulmonary pathophysiology. Various researchers have demonstrated a connection between sodium lactate infusion and the experience of panic symptoms.[8,9] They theorize that the metabolism of lactate to carbon dioxide is likely the key in producing panic symptoms. Others have demonstrated a connection between inhalation of exogenous carbon dioxide and the experience of panic symptoms.[10,11] The exact connection between the elevation of carbon dioxide and the development of panic symptoms remains unclear, although some patients are likely more vulnerable to experience anxiety in this setting than others.[12] One theory is that in vulnerable individuals the medullary chemoreceptors are abnormally sensitive to even small increases in carbon dioxide level in the bloodstream. This leads to activation of the locus coeruleus, which leads in turn to autonomic activation.[13] This leads to increased plasma norepinephrine, increased diastolic blood pressure, and an exaggerated ventilatory response, which leads to the symptomatic experience of a panic attack.[14] Patients with acute respiratory failure with resultant changes in blood carbon dioxide levels are vulnerable to experiencing panic symptoms according to this model.

There are likely other factors to consider in patients with acute respiratory failure who are experiencing panic symptoms. Many medications that are used to treat pulmonary disease produce anxiety as a side effect. Corticosteroids are used to treat numerous acute and chronic pulmonary conditions. Their use may contribute to a variety of psychiatric symptoms including anxiety. These side effects are dose-dependent. Some patients experience a spectrum of psychiatric symptoms, with irritability and insomnia at low doses. This may progress to anxiety at moderate doses and psychosis at large doses.[15] Other pulmonary medications are also associated with anxiety. These include β_2-adrenergic agonists and methylxanthines. β_2-Adrenergic agonists frequently cause restlessness, apprehension, anxiety, and tremor.[16] Again, there is a dose and time relationship. Inhaled medications tend to have less of an effect than systemic ones. Methylxanthines are associated with anxiety, fear, and panic.[16] Blood levels may be useful in diagnosing theophylline toxicity. Recreational drug use may also contribute to anxiety experienced by patients with acute respiratory failure during medical hospitalizations. Patients who are acutely intoxicated on stimulants, such as cocaine or amphetamines, often seem very anxious.[17] Others who are withdrawing from sedatives including alcohol, benzodiazepines, barbiturates, or opioids may also seem very anxious.[18,19]

Treatment of anxiety in this setting should focus on identification of these possible secondary causes of anxiety. Therapeutic medications, such as steroids, β_2-adrenergic agonists, and methylxanthines, that are contributing to anxiety may be tapered or switched to alternative therapies. Treatment of withdrawal from sedative drugs is also essential, whether these are drugs of abuse or those prescribed for the management of a pre-existing anxiety disorder. There may be some concern about the use of benzodiazepines in the setting of acute respiratory failure. Some benzodiazepines have been shown to decrease patient performance in some pulmonary function tests including forced expiratory volume in 1 second. They also have been shown to increase Pco_2 and decrease responsiveness to carbon dioxide challenge.[20] These may be of significant concern in patients with acute respiratory failure. Some patients with acute respiratory failure seem to benefit from benzodiazepines; however, the literature is mixed regarding efficacy.[21,22] Small doses of short-acting benzodiazepines, such as alprazolam and lorazepam, may be suited to a safe trial in patients with respiratory disease. If the patient is in a closely monitored setting or already requires mechanical ventilation, there may be less need for concern. Antidepressant medications including tricyclics and serotonin reuptake inhibitors seem safe and effective in treating anxiety in patients with respiratory failure.[6] It is generally accepted, however, that these take weeks to achieve a full antianxiety effect; their use in acute respiratory failure is often limited. Buspirone seems safe and may also be effective in relieving anxiety and obsessive symptoms in patients with respiratory failure, but also may take weeks to reach its full effect.[23] Other medications may be used in the acute setting, but these are generally poorly studied regarding safety and efficacy in this patient population. There may be a role for antipsychotics, antihistamines, gabapentin, or pregabalin in select patients.

Nonpharmacologic interventions may also be effective in relieving anxiety. These include controlled breathing exercises, progressive relaxation, guided imagery, hypnosis, biofeedback, and participation in pulmonary rehabilitation.[6] Cognitive behavioral therapy techniques may also be effective. This approach targets anxiety that is caused by the misinterpretation of "interoceptive cues," which leads to the escalating cycle of anxiety and panic. Patients learn to assign new meanings to unexpected and disturbing bodily perceptions. This leads them to feel more confident and in control of their breathing and, consequently, less anxious.[24]

Psychiatric factors may play a role in patients who seem difficult to wean from mechanical ventilation. These include delirium, anxiety, and depression. Delirium is characterized by global cerebral dysfunction caused by a patient's medical condition. This manifests as a temporary disturbance in consciousness and cognitive ability (**Box 5**).[1] This may make the patient unaware of his or her medical condition or unable to understand or coordinate full participation in the weaning process from mechanical ventilation. Delirium may be related to metabolic disarray as a direct physiologic consequence of pulmonary dysfunction (hypoxia, hypercapnia) or a number of other comorbid medical conditions common in critically ill patients. Isolated hypoxia has been shown to have a significant impact on cognitive function, including loss of judgment, inattention, and motor incoordination with even a slight decrease in oxygenation, and progressing to memory impairment with moderate decrease, and loss of

Box 5
Diagnostic criteria for delirium

A. Disturbance of consciousness (ie, reduced clarity of awareness of the environment) with reduced ability to focus, sustain, or shift attention.
B. A change in cognition (eg, memory deficit, disorientation, language disturbance) or the development of a perceptual disturbance that is not better accounted for by a pre-existing, established, or evolving dementia.
C. The disturbance develops over a short period of time (usually hours to days) and tends to fluctuate during the course of the day.
D. There is evidence from the history, physical examination, or laboratory findings that the disturbance is caused by the direct physiologic consequences of a general medical condition; or, symptoms developed during substance intoxication or were etiologically related to medication use; or, developed during or shortly after a withdrawal syndrome. (More than one etiology may be present, and in some instances no specific etiology, or a cause other than those listed above, may be identified.)

Data from American Psychiatric Association. Diagnostic and statistical manual of mental disorders. 4th edition, revised. Washington: American Psychiatric Association; 2000.

consciousness with significant decrease in oxygenation. Hypercapnia rarely presents in isolation, but is usually accompanied by hypoxia and acidosis. Slight increases in Pco_2 cause inattention, forgetfulness, drowsiness, and psychomotor slowing. This may progress to loss of consciousness at significantly increased levels.[25] Other contributors to delirium must also be considered, and may include other metabolic abnormalities, infections, toxic effects of medications or recreational drugs, and withdrawal from medications or recreational drugs.

Anxiety sometimes interferes with the ability to wean from mechanical ventilation. This anxiety may be directly related to pulmonary pathophysiology. It may be related to side effects of prescribed medications or the rapid tapering of intravenous sedatives. Patients may become physiologically dependent on intravenous sedatives that are used to treat agitation or discomfort associated with mechanical ventilation. If these medications are stopped or tapered too rapidly for a planned weaning trial, significant withdrawal symptoms may occur, including significant anxiety.[26]

There are a range of psychologic reactions to mechanical ventilation that may also contribute to a patient's emotional state. One should consider the practical limitations on one's life and experience during mechanical ventilation. Patients may not be able to communicate fully because of tracheal intubation, sedatives, or neuromuscular blockade. It has been reported that the inability to talk is the single greatest contributor to anxiety in mechanically ventilated patients.[27] Associated sleep disruption can intensify feelings of anxiety. Patients may also experience frightening nightmares. Some report never being able truly to rest. This complaint is supported by studies that have found that the average amount of sleep in ICU patients is as low as 1.8 hours per 24-hour period and that, while sleeping, awakenings from sleep typically occur more than six times per hour, resulting in absence of deep, restorative sleep.[28,29] Pain may be another factor that can have substantial psychologic impact, leading to feelings of anxiety or depression. Loss of independence is a common worry because many patients must depend on others for suctioning, moving, or toileting.[30] Sensory alteration may also be a concern, and this may involve deprivation or overstimulation. Staff or visitors may withdraw from the patient, perhaps because the patient cannot communicate or does not seem alert. Others withdraw because of fear of critical illness or end-of-life issues. Many patients experience sensory overload because of the activity, noise, and light present in the ICU throughout day and night.[31]

These factors sometimes limit the patient's fully understanding what mechanical ventilation means to them. For some, it means the conscious and continuous fear of death or disability. For others, it means the loss of independence. They may have the sense that they are entirely dependent on a machine or other people for the most basic bodily functions, and they sense that they have no control. They may not know or trust all of the people involved in their care. Nursing staff may change several times each day. The struggle with independence is a common theme for patients both during mechanical ventilation and at the time of attempted wean.

Patients who only become anxious when weaning is attempted may fear change or have a lack of confidence in the weaning process or themselves. Some fear that they will not be capable of spontaneous breathing after a prolonged period of reliance on the mechanical ventilator. Other emotions commonly experienced are anger, frustration, discouragement, and loneliness.[32] Intervening with these psychologic reactions before attempted weaning may prove effective. Taking time to talk can mitigate patients' anxiety about their limited communication. Allowing the patient to write or use an alphabet or picture board may be helpful. Allowing patients to make choices when possible and keeping them informed of planned procedures and test results may give them more of a sense of control or independence. Continuity of nursing and other care with frequent visits may reduce their sense of isolation or fear of strangers. Frequent orientation and visits with friends and family may address sensory alteration.[31] Many patients have feelings of sadness, but one should also consider the diagnosis of depression in the patient who is difficult to wean. Prospective studies of patient's mood states before attempted weaning have demonstrated increased symptoms of depression compared with controls, cardiac surgery patients, and cancer patients.[33] The connection between mood symptoms and difficulty weaning from mechanical ventilation, however, remains unclear.

In evaluating patients who are difficult to wean from mechanical ventilation, one should evaluate for the presence of delirium, anxiety, and depression. The distinction between these diagnoses can sometimes be challenging and more than one may coexist in the same patient. Delirium may resemble anxiety, especially when the patient is agitated, or depression, especially when the patient is hypoactive. Cognitive testing should be part of the evaluation process. New-onset or fluctuating cognitive deficits or a fluctuating level of arousal or responsiveness are indicative of delirium. Interview should be attempted when sedation has been minimized or discontinued. Feelings of sadness, worthlessness, hopelessness, anhedonia, and wish for death may all support a diagnosis of depression. Reversal of any identified causes of delirium is critical so that the presence of anxiety or depression can be clarified. Once delirium is resolved, patients are much better able actively to participate in the weaning process.

Antipsychotic medication may be effective in managing delirium, especially when the patient is agitated or has psychotic symptoms.[34] Anxiety may be treated with benzodiazepines, such as lorazepam, with due attention to the impact on respiratory status, as previously discussed. If some aspect of anxiety is caused by the rapid taper of intravenous sedatives, these may be replaced with longer-acting oral agents of the same class that can subsequently be tapered at a more gradual pace. Antipsychotic medication may also be effective in the management of anxiety and may present less concern for impact on respiratory status. These too can be added as intravenous sedatives are tapered. The antipsychotic medication can then be tapered over subsequent days as tolerated. Antidepressant medication may play a role in the treatment of patients with severe depression,[35] but their benefits may be limited because of the prolonged length of time necessary for them to reach full effect. Because of this, stimulants may be preferred for the treatment of depression in the acute setting. There have been case reports of patients who seemed depressed, had difficulty weaning from mechanical ventilation, and were successfully treated with methylphenidate in doses of 5 to 30 mg/day.[36,37] Nonpharmacologic treatments may also be effective in relieving anxiety and depression in patients on mechanical ventilation, thereby assisting with weaning. These include hypnosis, guided imagery, biofeedback, and music therapy.[38]

PSYCHIATRIC DISORDERS ASSOCIATED WITH HEART DISEASE

Certain psychologic factors and psychiatric disorders are associated with increased risk for the development of heart disease. A high level of anxiety symptoms, especially phobic anxiety, has been linked particularly to elevated risk of sudden cardiac death, but not nonfatal coronary disease, in large-scale prospective epidemiologic studies.[39,40] High levels of anger and hostility have been linked to increased atherosclerosis, earlier age of onset of clinical coronary disease symptoms, and higher risk of major adverse cardiac events in patients with diagnosed coronary artery disease, but the strength of the association has been questioned in the face of some negative studies.[41–46] A robust association of previous depressive symptoms and major depressive disorder with incident coronary artery disease (nonfatal myocardial infarction [MI], acute coronary syndromes, cardiac death) has been demonstrated in numerous epidemiologic studies in nonclinical samples; the increase in risk associated with depression has been estimated as approximately 70%.[47–49] "Negative affect states" related to depression, including "vital exhaustion" and "type D personality" (negative affectivity combined with social inhibition) also demonstrate increased risk for coronary artery disease.[50–52] An in-depth review of psychologic factors as risk factors for heart disease is beyond the scope of this article but is available elsewhere.[53,54]

The most common psychiatric problems in patients hospitalized for an acute coronary event are anxiety and depression. Patients may not bring these symptoms to the attention of their physicians on their own initiative, and several studies have shown that emotional disturbances are underrecognized in usual cardiac care.[55,56] Early recognition offers opportunity to reduce psychiatric morbidity and may have benefits for cardiac outcomes. Although such symptoms as fatigue, low energy, and sleep and appetite disturbance may discriminate poorly between acute coronary patients with and without clinically meaningful psychiatric problems, other symptoms, such as feeling persistently sad, loss of self-esteem, and feeling unable to experience interest or pleasure about ordinarily pleasurable matters (ie, anhedonia), are effective discriminators of depression.[57] It is probably worthwhile for clinicians caring for patients in acute cardiac care settings to inquire specifically about such symptoms, because they suggest that intervention might be indicated.

Two studies have demonstrated that anxiety in the period immediately after an acute coronary event is associated with adverse cardiac outcomes. Moser and Dracup[58] measured anxiety symptoms with a self-report questionnaire in the first 48 hours of hospitalization in 86 post-MI patients. The rate of in-hospital complications including reinfarction, new-onset ischemia, ventricular fibrillation, sustained ventricular tachycardia, and in-hospital death was 19.6% in patients with anxiety symptoms above the median, compared with 6% for patients with lower levels of anxiety ($P<.01$). Adjusting for other prognostic risk factors, these investigators estimated that anxiety was associated with a 4.9-fold increased relative risk of cardiac complications in the post-MI period. Likewise, Frasure-Smith and colleagues[59] found that a high self-reported anxiety symptom level in 222 post-MI patients was associated with a greater than twofold increased risk of recurrent acute coronary syndromes, even after adjusting for other prognostic factors. Recently, Frasure-Smith and Lesperance[60] extended this observation in a 2-year follow-up study of patients with stable coronary artery disease 2 months after MI. Of 804 subjects, over 5% met criteria for a diagnosis of generalized anxiety disorder, and over 40% had self-reported anxiety symptoms in the clinically significant range. Major adverse cardiac events in the follow-up period were significantly associated with both generalized anxiety disorder (odds ratio, 2.09; 95% confidence interval [CI], 1.08–4.05) and elevated anxiety symptoms (odds ratio, 1.67; 95% CI, 1.18–2.37).

There have been no large-scale trials directed primarily at treatment of anxiety disorders or high levels of anxiety symptoms specifically in cardiac patients, although some smaller-scale studies suggest that counseling or relaxation training interventions may be beneficial in reducing anxiety outcomes.[61–63] Benzodiazepines (eg, lorazepam), serotonin reuptake inhibitors, and buspirone are generally well-tolerated for pharmacotherapy of anxiety disorders and have little to no cardiovascular effect, other than a tendency to lower heart rate by one to two beats per minute. Drug-drug interactions between serotonin reuptake inhibitors that inhibit the cytochrome P-450 2D6 system and β-adrenergic blockers may exacerbate the negative chronotropic effects of β-blockers.[64]

Depression seen in patients after acute coronary events may be a transient adjustment response, but may also be a manifestation of previous history of depressive disorder, continuation of a first episode of depression with onset before the coronary event, or onset of major depression after the coronary event. Major depressive episodes are common, with point-prevalence of about 15%, compared with a lifetime prevalence of 6% to 10% in the general population in the United States.[49,65,66] Moreover, only a minority of major depressive episodes seen in the early aftermath of an acute coronary syndrome quickly remit without intervention.[55–57]

Depression after an acute coronary syndrome is associated with a markedly increased risk of recurrent cardiac events and cardiac death, even after adjusting for other prognostic factors.[49,65,67] Frasure-Smith and colleagues[56] demonstrated a greater than threefold increased risk of death over 6-month follow-up associated with major depression immediately after MI. An elevated level of depression symptoms after acute coronary syndromes predicts major adverse events and cardiac mortality up to 5 years after the acute event, in a dose-dependent manner.[68–70] Depression has a similarly negative prognostic impact for patients admitted to hospital for congestive heart failure, whether or not of ischemic etiology.[71,72] Mechanisms mediating these effects of depression and impairing survival include abnormalities in platelet function; autonomic derangements; increased inflammatory activation; and impaired adherence to lifestyle modification (smoking cessation, adherence to medication, exercise, diet modification) (**Box 6**).[73–76] Effective treatment of depression after acute coronary syndromes is an important goal.

In this regard, four large trials in recent years have examined treatment of depression in coronary patients. Of these, the SADHART trial, a randomized, placebo-controlled, double-blind trial of sertraline treatment for major depression following admission for acute coronary syndromes, enrolled patients who were still in the hospital, and active medication treatment began within 30 days of the index event.[77,78] In the remaining studies, active treatment began several weeks to several months after a previous coronary event. The SADHART trial showed that sertraline treatment for depression immediately after an acute coronary event (dose range, 50–200 mg/day) had no adverse effect on heart rate, blood pressure, cardiac conduction measures, and left ventricular function, and was not associated with an increase in adverse events, compared with placebo treatment. Sertraline was modestly effective in treatment of depression, particularly for

Box 6
Possible mechanisms linking depression and coronary disease[a]

A. Physiologic

1. Platelet activation
2. Sympathetic nervous system activation
3. Increased circulating inflammatory factors

B. Behavioral

1. Smoking
2. Reduced adherence to medication regimen
3. Reduced adherence to recommendations for exercise and diet

[a] See text for references.

patients with recurrent or more severe depression, or onset of depression before the index cardiac event. These findings suggest that antidepressant treatment with sertraline need not be withheld from patients even early in the post–acute coronary syndrome period. There was no difference in efficacy or safety profile for patients with left ventricular ejection fraction above versus below 30%, suggesting safety in congestive heart failure and in acute coronary syndromes.

The ENRICHD trial, a large randomized trial of a cognitive behavioral psychotherapy intervention in acute post-MI patients with either major depression or a history of major depression and current minor depression, demonstrated that, compared with usual care, a relatively low-intensity intervention (generally, 6–10 psychotherapy sessions over 6 months) was associated with a statistically significant although clinically modest effect on depression symptoms. The intervention had no effect, however, on the study's principal outcome measure, survival free of recurrent MI or cardiac death over 3.5-year (mean) follow-up.[79] Complicating the analysis of the ENRICHD study, some patients with severe depression received sertraline or other antidepressants. Patients who received sertraline had a 42% lower rate of death than patients who did not receive antidepressant therapy, but because psychopharmacologic treatment was not randomized, the meaning of this finding is uncertain.

In the CREATE trial, 284 patients with stable coronary artery disease and major depression were doubly randomized to receive either interpersonal psychotherapy or clinical management visits without psychotherapy, and to receive the serotonin reuptake inhibitor citalopram or placebo. Citalopram treatment was superior to placebo treatment, whereas interpersonal psychotherapy showed no greater efficacy than clinical management visits in reducing depression symptoms.[80] Citalopram was not associated with a higher rate of adverse events than placebo.

Finally, a European study of post-MI depression intervention (MIND-IT) found significant differences in most depression outcome measures for therapy with the antidepressant mirtazepine compared with placebo.[81] Mirtazepine's safety profile was favorable. Another interesting aspect of this study was the finding that persistence of depression, in comparison with good treatment response, was associated with worse cardiac outcomes at 18-month follow-up: treatment nonresponders had a recurrent event rate (cardiac-related hospitalization or cardiac death) of 25.6%, versus 7.4% for responders. By intention-to-treat analysis, however, a cardiac benefit was not significantly associated with antidepressant treatment.[82] A similar result was noted in the ENRICHD trial.[83]

These results leave the field in an unsettled state: treatment of depression after an acute coronary event seems to be at least modestly effective with respect to depression outcome, and recovery from depression seems to be associated with favorable cardiac outcome, yet it remains to be demonstrated that treatment of depression has a favorable effect on cardiac outcome. Still, for the patient in an acute treatment setting, the available data suggest that treatment of depression with either cognitive behavior therapy, citalopram, or sertraline can be undertaken with a reasonable expectation of safety and with the goal of improvement in mood.

POST–CORONARY ARTERY BYPASS GRAFT DEPRESSION

Depressive disorders and elevated depression symptoms are common after coronary artery bypass graft (CABG) surgery, with prevalence of about 15% for depressive disorder at 1 to 2 weeks after surgery, and a substantially higher rate of elevated depressive symptoms.[84,85] These depressive syndromes are associated with increased morbidity and mortality. Major depression at 1 week after CABG surgery was associated with doubled risk of recurrent cardiac events in a 12-month follow-up study of 302 consecutive patients. Depression was as strong a predictor of adverse outcome as low ejection fraction, diabetes, and prior MI.[84] Development of new depression symptoms after surgery, failure to achieve remission of depression symptoms over 6 months after surgery, and severe symptoms were all associated with more mortality in a 5-year follow-up study of over 800 patients.[85]

There have been no controlled trials of depression treatment, however, specifically in post-CABG patients. An observational study[86] found that patients undergoing CABG while on SSRI antidepressant therapy actually had worse prognosis than patients not taking antidepressants, but because treatment assignment was not randomized it cannot be determined whether this effect was caused by more severe depression or medical conditions in the treated patients, an adverse effect of the treatment, or another confounding factor.

POST–CARDIAC SURGERY DELIRIUM AND NEUROPSYCHOLOGIC IMPAIRMENT

Delirium is an acute condition characterized by a waxing and waning disturbance in level of consciousness, reduced awareness of the environment, inability to sustain and focus attention, and impaired cognition, sometimes associated with disorientation, hallucinations, or delusions. Patients may be agitated or hypoactive. By definition, delirium is a direct physiologic consequence of an underlying medical problem, intoxication, or withdrawal (see **Box 5**).[1] Delirium occurs in 10% to 50% of cardiac surgery patients, and may be unrecognized, especially in those patients who are not overtly agitated (so-called "hypoactive" delirium).[87,88] Delirium after cardiac surgery is associated with risk of self-harm (eg, because of self-extubation, inappropriate removal of lines, and falls) and with substantially longer length of stay in the ICU and heightened mortality.[88–93] Its prevention and treatment is important for improved outcomes.

Kornfeld and coworkers,[94] pioneers in the description of delirium after cardiac surgery, recognized two syndromes, one characterized by confusion immediately on regaining consciousness, and one developing after a so-called "lucid interval." Kornfeld identified the combination of long cardiopulmonary bypass time along with postoperative sleep loss, the combination of sensory overload and sensory monotony, and the absence of clear-cut day and night periods as contributing factors for delirium arising in the ICU after a lucid interval, and recognized that human contact, reassurance, quiet, an opportunity to sleep, and transfer out of the ICU were helpful in many cases. In both forms of delirium, however, Kornfeld recognized the "organic" etiology of the disturbance of consciousness. The unfortunate term "ICU psychosis" is a misnomer that may have the unintended effect of misleading care providers to attribute delirium solely to the ICU environment, while neglecting the role of toxic, metabolic, infectious, and cerebrovascular etiologic factors.

In contemporary practice, risk factors for delirium in cardiac surgery patients include older age; prior cerebrovascular disease or cognitive impairment; alcohol abuse or dependence; azotemia; hyponatremia; infection; and prolonged sedation with narcotics, benzodiazepines, or propofol. Depression, peripheral vascular disease, and atrial fibrillation are also identified as risk factors in some studies.[88,95–98] In a study of 1267 CABG surgery patients, patients with low cardiac output in the perioperative period had a significantly greater risk for postoperative delirium.[92] Another large (N = 8139) Scandinavian study of CABG and valve surgery patients, focusing specifically on the development of psychotic symptoms (hallucinations, delusions), identified a similar list of independent risk factors including older age; preoperative renal failure, dyspnea, heart failure, and left ventricular hypertrophy; perioperative hypothermia; and postoperative hypoxemia, low hematocrit, renal failure, hypernatremia, infection, and stroke. "Off-pump" surgery was not associated with a lower incidence of delirium.[93]

In addition to correction of underlying causes of delirium, treatment of postcardiac surgery delirium often requires use of antipsychotic medication to reduce psychotic symptoms and agitation.[64] Although rigorous clinical trials are lacking, widespread clinical practice embraces the off-label use of a variety of antipsychotic agents including haloperidol, olanzapine (which can be given as an orally disintegrating tablet), and quetiapine, despite the acknowledged metabolic, infectious, and cardiovascular risks of this class of medications. All of these agents have potential to provoke torsade de pointes, although the incidence of this complication is quite low. Parameters to be monitored before and during antipsychotic treatment of delirium should include blood pressure, QTc interval, and potassium and magnesium levels. The prophylactic effect of another antipsychotic medication, risperidone, was tested in a randomized, double-blinded, placebo-controlled study. A total of 126 patients undergoing cardiac surgery with cardiopulmonary bypass were randomized to receive either risperidone, 1 mg, or placebo on regaining consciousness after surgery. The incidence of delirium was 11.1% in risperidone-treated patients versus 31.7% in placebo-treated patients ($P = .009$; relative risk = 0.35; 95% CI, 0.16–0.77).[99] Aripiprazole, a drug with less propensity for QT prolongation and metabolic side effects, may be a reasonable alternative agent for antipsychotic treatment of delirium,[100] but controlled studies have not been reported.

Recent studies indicate that substitution of dexmedetomidine, a centrally acting, selective α_2-adrenergic agonist, for other sedative agents also may substantially reduce the incidence or duration of delirium after cardiac surgery.[101–104] In the early report of Maldonado and coworkers,[101] the incidence of delirium after cardiac valve surgery was reduced from 50% to under 5%, and the recent MENDS trial demonstrated a reduction in the incidence of delirium from over 30% to about 10%.[104] In an open trial in 20 cases, introduction of dexmedetomidine facilitated weaning and extubation in 65% of patients who had failed previous weaning trials because of agitation.[103] Problems noted with dexmedetomidine include inadequate sedation, excessive pain, bradycardia, hypotension, and a case of cardiac arrest.[105,106] There are conflicting reports about its use to reduce opioid requirements for pain.[107,108]

Chronic neuropsychological impairment may occur after cardiac surgery; prevalence reports vary. In what may be the largest follow-up study, impairment in multiple domains of neuropsychological function was noted in almost half of patients at discharge following surgery, but the prevalence of impairment fell sharply over the next 6 months. The prevalence of impairment was somewhat higher when the same patients were re-examined 5 years after surgery; cognitive impairment at the point of discharge after surgery was a predictor of impairment at 5-year follow-up.[109] The list of risk factors for chronic neuropsychologic impairment after cardiac surgery includes many of the same factors as that for delirium: advanced age, prior neuropsychologic impairment, prior head injury, prior cerebrovascular events including transient ischemic attacks, and history of alcohol abuse or dependence.[110,111] The hoped-for cognitive benefit of "off-pump" surgery has not been established.[112–114]

PSYCHIATRIC COMPLICATIONS AFTER LEFT VENTRICULAR ASSIST DEVICE

In addition to the problems common to cardiac surgery patients in general, patients who undergo implantation of ventricular assist devices experience discomfort and anxiety related to the device. Depending on the specific type of device, noise, the pressure of the device on the stomach, tethering to a machine, and the visible extracorporeal circulation of blood are disturbing features. Once out of the ICU setting, the need to change batteries, master the control panel, and respond to alarms can be cognitively difficult challenges for ventricular assist device patients, many of whom have pre-existing or new neuropsychologic deficits secondary to prior cerebrovascular disease or hypoperfusion, hypoxic episodes, embolic events, or metabolic disarray.[111,115] The ongoing risks of infection, bleeding, and thromboembolic complications (especially stroke) contribute to anxiety associated with ventricular assist device treatment.

SUBSTANCE WITHDRAWAL

Alcohol and benzodiazepine withdrawal is a common problem in the ICU, and often unrecognized, although life-threatening if untreated.[19,116] Alcohol-related medical conditions affect the hospital course of up to 12% to 30% patients in all medical settings.[117] Consequences of alcohol use account for nearly 25% of hospitalizations for traumatic injury, and many of these patients require intensive care.[118] In one study, alcohol use was directly responsible for approximately 20% of all ICU admissions.[119]

Withdrawal syndromes can arise from a number of clinical circumstances. Physicians may already be aware of the patient's alcohol use and anticipate withdrawal. Occult alcohol abuse is not uncommon, and it may be diagnosed only when the patient starts to manifest classic symptoms. Patients may also manifest withdrawal symptoms from known or occult sedative-hypnotic dependence, as from lorazepam or alprazolam. Patients may also withdraw from sedative or anesthetic agents specific to the critical care setting, such as propofol.[120] Last, barbiturate withdrawal may also occur with similar manifestations.

Alcohol, benzodiazepines, and barbiturates all interact with the γ-aminobutyric acid $(GABA)_A$ receptor, a neurotransmitter receptor with a chloride ion channel and several binding sites.[121,122] Benzodiazepines bind to the benzodiazepine site on the $GABA_A$ receptor, which increases the frequency of the chloride channel opening in the presence of GABA.[121] Barbiturates increase the duration of time this channel is open; at high doses, sustained channel opening can occur even in the absence of GABA, which contributes to the substantial lethality risk of barbiturate overdose.[121,123,124] Ethanol also acts as an agonist at the GABA receptor. This common pathway can result in similar behavioral effects, cross-tolerance, and additive properties when used concurrently.[125]

Management of alcohol-benzodiazepine withdrawal includes a rapid replenishing of medications that target the GABA receptor. Typically, this involves the administration of benzodiazepine medications at a dose high enough to control the agitation and autonomic response of withdrawal, limited by the need to prevent oversedation and respiratory depression. Many institutions have developed protocols and guidelines for the management of withdrawal syndromes in the ICU, which typically include a stratified system of management with oral or intravenous benzodiazepines.[126] Phenobarbital is also occasionally used in this setting, especially in complicated cases where benzodiazepines have proved ineffective.[127] Adjustments may need to be made for patients with significant liver dysfunction.

Several specific aspects of withdrawal may affect the course of patients with pre-existing cardiopulmonary disease. The autonomic effects of withdrawal, including prolonged hypertension or tachycardia, can precipitate cardiac ischemia, pump failure, and abnormalities in heart rhythm caused by increased myocardial oxygen demand.[128] This is balanced by the tendency of benzodiazepines to cause hypotension, which can also increase cardiac demand by reflex tachycardia. Management of withdrawal can be especially difficult if the patient also requires the use of antihypertensive or cardioprotective agents (eg, β-blockers), because the autonomic manifestations of withdrawal may be masked. Also, there is some evidence to suggest that medications used to treat hypertension, such as nitrates, β-blockers, and calcium channel blockers, have different effects in patients undergoing alcohol withdrawal.[129] During early stages of withdrawal, negative inotropic effects of β-blockers may be reduced, but negative chronotropic effects increased, whereas vasodilator effects of nitrates may be reduced. Antipsychotic medications are necessary at times to address severe agitation associated with withdrawal, despite the risk of adverse cardiac rhythm effects, such as QT prolongation and torsade de pointes.[128] Patients with underlying lung disease have an increased risk of respiratory compromise (because of underlying restrictive or obstructive processes) and may be more difficult to extubate. For these patients, one of the main complications of alcohol withdrawal lies with the benzodiazepine-mediated reduction in ventilatory drive associated with hypoxia, especially at higher doses.[128,130]

CHILDREN WITH SEVERE HEART AND LUNG DISEASE

Children with heart and lung diseases including bronchopulmonary dysplasia, asthma, cystic fibrosis, α_1-antitrypsin deficiency, congenital heart diseases, familial cardiomyopathy, and acute myocarditis may require critical and intensive care. Intensive and critical care of the pediatric patient requires understanding not only of disease pathophysiology and medical and surgical intervention, but also of the developmental level of the patient. Child psychiatrists are trained to assess the children with regard to their physical, motor, language, cognitive, sexual, and emotional development. In medically ill children, this assessment takes on a greater level of complexity, because there can be a disruption in the normal developmental progression and a regression to more developmentally primitive and at times less adaptive cognitive functioning and coping mechanisms.[131,132] In addition, work with the medically ill child necessitates work with the parents and other significant figures in the child's life. Young children fear separation from their parents, whereas older children and teenagers balance the need for their parents with desires for acceptance into their peer group, a sense of autonomy, and a feeling of mastery of age-appropriate tasks and social roles. At times these desires can overwhelm the ability of the growing child to accept and constructively participate in his or her medical care. Respect for the importance of these normal feelings in the psychological lives of young patients is essential, even in intensive and critical care settings.

Although a comprehensive review is not possible here, the importance of exaggerated anxiety over body image and issues of identity in pediatric heart and lung transplant patients are highlighted. In evaluation of seriously ill children with heart and lung disease for possible transplantation, one is concerned with the patient's degree of understanding of the procedure, based on age, developmental level, and cognitive status; parents, too, must be assessed to ascertain their comprehension of the procedure, and the risks, benefits, and alternatives available, to enable them to make an informed decision. Those providing care must also be mindful of the psychological, social, and emotional resources that the parents are able to contribute in helping the child cope with the transplant process.

Given a particular child's developmental level, his or her conceptualization of illness, body image, and medical procedures can vary tremendously. For example, discussing heart transplantation with a 7 year old is considerably different than with a 15 year old. Each requires a tailored approach, however, in assessing his or her level of understanding and appreciating developmentally appropriate concerns that may arise. In cases of cardiac transplantation, it is not only young children who can experience magical thinking. Pediatric patients may develop all varieties of fantasy regarding the new heart and what impact it may have on their own thoughts and feelings. Children may fear, in a conscious, literal, and concrete sense, the replacement of their pretransplant identity with the identifying characteristics of the organ donor (eg, language spoken, religious beliefs, emotional attachment to significant others, sex). In older children, anxiety over body image, threats to self-esteem because of the facts of being ill, taking medication, scars and changes in appearance and habitus, and limited ability to participate in school and physical activity, combined with a nearly overwhelming need to fit in with peers, is developmentally typical.[133] Awareness of this constellation of feelings should be helpful in working with young patients and their reactions toward their illness, and may also serve to guide the clinician in anticipating and resolving issues with noncompliance that inevitably arise. One survey estimated that 25% to 40% of pediatric transplant survivors have been found to have some psychiatric issues.[134] Additionally, there are different outcomes based on whether the patient had received the transplant as a result of congenital cardiac disease rather than an acquired cardiac condition.[135]

END-OF-LIFE CARE

Physicians who care for chronically and critically ill patients with cardiopulmonary disease routinely confront the challenge of providing both effective and compassionate end-of-life care. This can be further complicated by the presence of psychiatric comorbidities, such as major depression and anxiety. Psychiatrists can assist in the effective management of these patients. This topic is addressed elsewhere in this issue.

REFERENCES

1. American Psychiatric Association. Diagnostic and statistical manual of mental disorders. 4th edition. [Text Revision]. Washington, D.C.: American Psychiatric Association; 2000.
2. Goodwin RD, Pine DS. Respiratory disease and panic attacks among adults in the United States. Chest 2002;122:645–50.
3. Karajgi B, Rifkin A, Doddi S, et al. The prevalence of anxiety disorders in patients with chronic obstructive pulmonary disease. Am J Psychiatry 1990;147:200–1.
4. Janson C, Björnsson E, Hetta J, et al. Anxiety and depression in relation to respiratory symptoms and asthma. Am J Respir Crit Care Med 1994; 149:930–4.
5. Yellowlees PM, Alpers JH, Bowden JJ, et al. Psychiatric morbidity in patients with chronic airflow obstruction. Med J Aust 1987;146:305–7.
6. Smoller JW, Pollack MH, Otto MW, et al. Panic anxiety, dyspnea, and respiratory disease. Am J Respir Crit Care Med 1996;154:6–17.
7. Clark DM. A cognitive approach to panic. Behav Res Ther 1986;24:461–70.
8. Pitts FN, McClure JN. Lactate metabolism in anxiety neurosis. N Engl J Med 1967;277:1329–36.
9. Cowley DS, Arana GW. The diagnostic utility of lactate sensitivity in panic disorder. Arch Gen Psychiatry 1990;47:277–84.
10. Van Den Hout MA, Griez E. Panic symptoms after inhalation of CO_2. Br J Psychiatry 1984;144:503–7.
11. Papp LA, Klein DF, Martinez J, et al. Diagnostic and substance specificity of carbon dioxide induced panic. Am J Psychiatry 1993;150:250–7.
12. Papp LA, Klein DF, Gorman JM. Carbon dioxide hypersensitivity, hyperventilation and panic disorder. Am J Psychiatry 1993;150:1149–57.
13. Elam M, Yao T, Thorén P, et al. Hypercapnia and hypoxia: chemoreceptor-mediated control of locus coeruleus neurons and splanchnic, sympathetic nerves. Brain Res 1981;222:373–81.
14. Gorman JM, Fyer MR, Goetz R, et al. Ventilatory physiology of patients with panic disorder. Arch Gen Psychiatry 1988;45:31–9.
15. Thompson WL, Thompson TL. Use of medications in patients with chronic pulmonary disease. Adv Psychosom Med 1985;14:136–48.
16. Brunton LL, editor. Goodman & Gilman's the pharmacologic basis of therapeutics. New York: McGraw Hill; 2006. p. 253, 729.
17. Cox BJ, Norton GR, Swinson RP, et al. Substance abuse and panic related anxiety: a critical review. Behav Res Ther 1990;28:385–93.
18. Cosci F, Schruers KR, Abrams K, et al. Alcohol use disorders and panic disorder: a review of the evidence of a direct relationship. J Clin Psychiatry 2007;68:874–80.
19. O'Brien CP. Benzodiazepine use, abuse, and dependence. J Clin Psychiatry 2005;66(Suppl 2): 28–33.
20. Geddes DM, Rudolf M, Saunders KB. Effect of nitrazepam and flurazepam on the ventilatory response to carbon dioxide. Thorax 1976;31: 548–51.
21. Mitchell-Heggs P, Murphy K, Minty K, et al. Diazepam in the treatment of the pink puffer syndrome. Q J Med 1980;49:9–20.
22. Man GC, Hsu K, Sproule B. Effect of alprazolam on exercise and dyspnea in patients with chronic obstructive pulmonary disease. Chest 1986;90: 832–6.
23. Argyropoulou P, Patakas D, Koukou A, et al. Buspirone effect on breathlessness and exercise performance in patients with chronic obstructive pulmonary disease. Respiration 1993;60:216–20.
24. Brenes G. Anxiety and chronic obstructive pulmonary disease: prevalence, impact, and treatment. Psychosom Med 2003;65:963–70.
25. Ropper AH, Brown RH, editors. Adams and Victor's principles of neurology. New York: McGraw-Hill; 2005. p. 964.
26. Murray MJ, DeRuyter ML, Harrison BA. Opioids and benzodiazepines. Crit Care Clin 1995;11: 849–73.
27. Bergbom-Engberg I, Haljamae H. Assessment of patients' experience of discomfort during respirator therapy. Crit Care Med 1989;17:1068–72.
28. Aurell J, Elmqvist D. Sleep in the surgical intensive care unit: continuous polygraphic recording of sleep in nine patients receiving postoperative care. Brit Med J (Clin Res Ed) 1985;290:1029–32.

29. Friese RS, Diaz-Arrastia R, McBride D, et al. Quantity and quality of sleep in the surgical intensive care unit: are our patients sleeping? J Trauma 2007;63:1210–4.
30. Johnson MM, Sexton DL. Distress during mechanical ventilation: patient's perceptions. Crit Care Nurse 1990;10:48–57.
31. Gale J, O'Shanick GJ. Psychiatric aspects of respirator treatment and pulmonary intensive care. Adv Psychosom Med 1985;14:93–108.
32. Castillo A, Egan H. How it feels to be a ventilator patient. Respiratory Care 1974;19:289–93.
33. Connelly B, Gunzerath L, Knebel A. A pilot study exploring mood state and dyspnea in mechanically ventilated patients. Heart Lung 2000;29:173–9.
34. Rea RS, Battistone S, Fong JJ, et al. Atypical antipsychotics versus haloperidol for treatment of delirium in acutely ill patients. Pharmacotherapy 2007;27:588–94.
35. Mendel J, Kahn F. Psychological aspects of weaning from mechanical ventilation. Psychosomatics 1980;21:465–71.
36. Johnson CJ, Auger WR, Fedullo PF, et al. Methylphenidate in the hard to wean patient. J Psychosom Res 1994;39:63–8.
37. Rothenhäusler HB, Ehrentraut S, von Degenfeld G, et al. Treatment of depression with methylphenidate in patients difficult to wean from mechanical ventilation in the intensive care unit. J Clin Psychiatry 2000;61:750–5.
38. Fontaine DK. Nonpharmacologic management of patient distress during mechanical ventilation. Crit Care Clin 1994;10:695–708.
39. Kawachi I, Colditz GA, Ascherio A, et al. Prospective study of phobic anxiety and risk of coronary heart disease in men. Circulation 1994; 89:1992–7.
40. Kawachi I, Sparrow D, Vokonas PS, et al. Symptoms of anxiety and risk of coronary heart disease: the Normative Aging Study. Circulation 1994;90: 2225–9.
41. Barefoot JC, Dahlstrom WG, Williams RB. Hostility, CHD incidence, and total mortality: a 25-year follow-up study of 255 physicians. Psychosom Med 1983;45:59–63.
42. Shekelle RB, Gale M, Ostfeld AM, et al. Hostility, risk of coronary heart disease, and mortality. Psychosom Med 1983;45:109–14.
43. Kawachi I, Sparrow D, Spiro A III, et al. A prospective study of anger and coronary heart disease: the Normative Aging Study. Circulation 1996;94:2090–5.
44. Williams JE, Paton CC, Siegler IC, et al. Anger proneness predicts coronary heart disease risk: prospective Analysis from the Atherosclerosis Risk In Communities (ARIC) study. Circulation 2000;101:2034–9.
45. Matthews KA, Gump BB, Harris KF, et al. Hostile behaviors predict cardiovascular mortality among men enrolled in the multiple risk factor intervention trial. Circulation 2004;109:66–70.
46. Schulman JK, Muskin PR, Shapiro PA. Psychiatry and cardiovascular disease. Focus 2005;3: 208–24.
47. Anda R, Williamson D, Jones D, et al. Depressed affect, hopelessness, and the risk of ischemic heart disease in a cohort of U.S. adults. Epidemiology 1993;4:285–94.
48. Shapiro PA, Lidagoster L, Glassman AH. Depression and heart disease. Psychiatr Ann 1997;27: 347–52.
49. Glassman AH, Shapiro PA. Depression and the course of coronary artery disease. Am J Psychiatry 1998;155:4–11.
50. Appels A, Otten F. Exhaustion as precursor of cardiac death. Br J Clin Psychol 1992;31:351–6.
51. Denollet J, Sys SU, Brutsaert DL. Personality and mortality after myocardial infarction. Psychosom Med 1995;57:582–91.
52. Denollet J, Brutsaert D. Personality, disease severity, and the risk of long-term cardiac events with a decreased ejection fraction after myocardial infarction. Circulation 1998;97:167–73.
53. Rozanski A, Blumenthal JA, Kaplan J. Impact of psychological factors on the pathogenesis of cardiovascular disease and implications for therapy. Circulation 1999;99:2192–217.
54. Rozanski A, Blumenthal JA, Davidson KW, et al. The epidemiology, pathophysiology, and management of psychosocial risk factors in cardiac practice: the emerging field of behavioral cardiology. J Am Coll Cardiol 2005;45:637–51.
55. Hance M, Carney RM, Freedland KE, et al. Depression in patients with coronary heart disease. Gen Hosp Psychiatry 1996;18:61–5.
56. Frasure-Smith N, Lesperance F, Talajic M. Depression following myocardial infarction: impact on 6-month survival. JAMA 1993;270:1819–25.
57. Lesperance F, Frasure-Smith N, Talajic M. Major depression before and after myocardial infarction: its nature and consequences. Psychosom Med 1996;58:99–110.
58. Moser DK, Dracup K. Is anxiety early after myocardial infarction associated with subsequent ischemic and arrhythmic events? Psychosom Med 1996;58:395–401.
59. Frasure-Smith N, Lesperance F, Talajic M. The impact of negative emotions on prognosis following myocardial infarction: is it more than depression? Heath Psychol 1995;14:388–98.
60. Frasure-Smith N, Lesperance F. Depression and anxiety as predictors of 2-year cardiac events in patients with stable coronary artery disease. Arch Gen Psychiatry 2008;65:62–71.

61. Bambauer KZ, Aupont O, Stone PH, et al. The effect of a telephone counseling intervention on self-rated health of cardiac patients. Psychosom Med 2005;67:539–45.
62. Kanji N, White AR, Ernst E. Autogenic training reduces anxiety after coronary angioplasty: a randomized clinical trial. Am Heart J 2004;147: E10.
63. Lie I, Arnesen H, Sandvik L, et al. Effects of a home-based intervention program on anxiety and depression 6 months after coronary artery bypass grafting: a randomized controlled trial. J Psychosom Res 2007;62:411–8.
64. Shapiro PA. Heart disease. In: Levenson JL, editor. APPI Textbook of Psychosomatic Medicine. Washington, DC: APPI; 2004. p. 423–44.
65. Shapiro PA. Psychiatric aspects of cardiovascular disease. Psychiatr Clin North Am 1996;19:613–29.
66. Kessler RC, Berglund P, Demler O, et al. The epidemiology of major depressive disorder: results from the National Comorbidity Survey Replication (NCS-R). JAMA 2003;289:3095–105.
67. Wulsin LR, Vaillant GE, Wells VE. A systematic review of the mortality of depression. Psychosom Med 1999;61:6–17.
68. Frasure-Smith N, Lesperance F, Talajic M. Depression and 18-month prognosis following myocardial infarction. Circulation 1995;91:999–1005.
69. Lesperance F, Frasure-Smith N, Juneau M, et al. Depression and 1-year prognosis in unstable angina. Arch Intern Med 2000;160:1354–60.
70. Lesperance F, Frasure-Smith N, Talajic M, et al. Five-year risk of cardiac mortality in relation to initial severity and one-year changes in depression symptoms after myocardial infarction. Circulation 2002;105:1049–53.
71. Jiang W, Alexander J, Christopher E, et al. Relationship of depression to increased risk of mortality and rehospitalization in patients with congestive heart failure. Arch Intern Med 2001;161:1849–56.
72. Faris R, Purcell H, Henein MY, et al. Clinical depression is common and significantly associated with reduced survival in patients with non-ischaemic heart failure. Eur J Heart Fail 2002;4: 541–51.
73. Musselman DL, Evans DL, Nemeroff CB. The relationship of depression to cardiovascular disease. Arch Gen Psychiatry 1998;55:580–92.
74. Carney RM, Freedland KE, Miller GE, et al. Depression as a risk factor for cardiac mortality and morbidity: a review of potential mechanisms. J Psychosom Res 2002;53:897–902.
75. Ziegelstein RC, Fauerbach JA, Stevens SS, et al. Patients with depression are less likely to follow recommendations to reduce cardiac risk during recovery from a myocardial infarction. Arch Intern Med 2000;160:1818–23.
76. Kronish IM, Rieckmann N, Halm EA, et al. Persistent depression affects adherence to secondary prevention behaviors after acute coronary syndromes. J Gen Intern Med 2006;21:1178–83.
77. Glassman AH, O'Connor CM, Califf RM, et al. Sertraline treatment of major depression in patients with acute MI or unstable angina. JAMA 2002; 288:701–9.
78. Glassman AH, Bigger JT Jr, Gaffney M, et al. Onset of major depression associated with acute coronary syndromes: relationship of onset, major depressive disorder history, and episode severity to sertraline benefit. Arch Gen Psychiatry 2006; 63:283–8.
79. Writing Committee for the ENRICHD Investigators. Effects of treating depression and low perceived social support on clinical events after myocardial infarction: the Enhancing Recovery In Coronary Heart Disease Patients (ENRICHD) randomized trial. JAMA 2003;289:3106–16.
80. Lesperance F, Frasure-Smith N, Koszycki D, et al. Effects of citalopram and interpersonal psychotherapy on depression in patients with coronary artery disease: the Canadian Cardiac Randomized Evaluation of Antidepressant and Psychotherapy Efficacy (create) trial. JAMA 2007;297: 367–79.
81. Honig A, Kuyper AM, Schene AH, et al. Treatment of post-myocardial infarction depressive disorder: a randomized, placebo-controlled trial with mirtazapine. Psychosom Med 2007;69:606–13.
82. de Jonge P, Honig A, van Melle JP, et al. Nonresponse to treatment for depression following myocardial infarction: association with subsequent cardiac events. Am J Psychiatry 2007;164:1371–8.
83. Carney RM, Blumenthal JA, Freedland KE, et al. Depression and late mortality after myocardial infarction in the Enhancing Recovery In Coronary Heart Disease (ENRICHD) study. Psychosom Med 2004;66:466–74.
84. Connerney I, Shapiro PA, McLaughlin JS, et al. Relation between depression after coronary artery bypass surgery and 12-month outcome: a prospective study. Lancet 2001;358:1766–71.
85. Blumenthal JA, Lett HS, Babyak MA, et al. Depression as a risk factor for mortality after coronary artery bypass surgery. Lancet 2003;362:604–9.
86. Xiong GL, Jiang W, Clare R, et al. Prognosis of patients taking selective serotonin reuptake inhibitors before coronary artery bypass grafting. Am J Cardiol 2006;98:42–7.
87. Mittal D, Majithia D, Kennedy R, et al. Differences in characteristics and outcome of delirium as based on referral patterns. Psychosomatics 2006;47: 367–75.
88. Mirasol EG, Shapiro PA, Fang Y. Delirium in the cardiothoracic ICU: prevalence, predictors, and

effect on length of stay. Amelia Island (FL): Academy of Psychosomatic Medicine; 2007.

89. Ely EW, Shintani A, Truman B, et al. Delirium as a predictor of mortality in mechanically ventilated patients in the intensive care unit. JAMA 2004; 291:1753–62.
90. Leslie DL, Marcantonio ER, Zhang Y, et al. One-year health care costs associated with delirium in the elderly population. Arch Intern Med 2008;168: 27–32.
91. van der Mast RC, Roest FH. Delirium after cardiac surgery: a critical review. J Psychosom Res 1996; 41:13–30.
92. Norkiene I, Ringaitiene D, Misiuriene I, et al. Incidence and precipitating factors of delirium after coronary artery bypass grafting. Scand Cardiovasc J 2007;41:180–5.
93. Giltay EJ, Huijskes RV, Kho KH, et al. Psychotic symptoms in patients undergoing coronary artery bypass grafting and heart valve operation. Eur J Cardiothorac Surg 2006;30:140–7.
94. Kornfeld DS, Zimberg S, Malm JR. Psychiatric complications of open heart surgery. N Engl J Med 1965;273:287–92.
95. Inouye SK, Charpenter PA. Precipitating factors for delirium in hospitalized elderly persons: predictive model and interrelationship with baseline vulnerability. JAMA 1996;275:852–7.
96. Gunther ML, Morandi A, Ely EW. Pathophysiology of delirium in the intensive care unit. Crit Care Clin 2008;24:45–65.
97. Young J, Inouye SK. Delirium in older people. BMJ 2007;334:842–6.
98. Kazmierski J, Kowman M, Banach M, et al. Preoperative predictors of delirium after cardiac surgery: a preliminary study. Gen Hosp Psychiatry 2006;28: 536–8.
99. Prakanrattana U, Prapaitrakool S. Efficacy of risperidone for prevention of postoperative delirium in cardiac surgery. Anaesth Intensive Care 2007;35: 714–9.
100. Straker DA, Shapiro PA, Muskin PM. Aripiprazole in the treatment of delirium. Psychosomatics 2006;47: 385–91.
101. Maldonado J, Wysong A, van der Starre PJA, et al. Dexmedetomidine and the reduction of postoperative delirium after cardiac surgery. Psychosomatics, in press.
102. Gerlach AT, Dasta JF. Dexmedetomidine: an updated review. Ann Pharmacother 2007;41:245–52.
103. Arpino KA, Kalafatas K, Thompson BT. Feasibility of dexmedetomidine in facilitating extubation in the intensive care unit. J Clin Pharm Ther 2008; 33:25–30.
104. Pandharipande PP, Pun BT, Herr DL, et al. Effect of sedation with dexmedetomidine vs lorazepam on acute brain dysfunction in mechanically ventilated patients: the MENDS randomized controlled trial. JAMA 2007;298:2644–53.
105. MacLaren R, Forrest L, Kiser TH. Adjunctive dexmedetomidine therapy in the intensive care unit: a retrospective assessment of impact on sedative and analgesic requirements, levels of sedation and analgesia, and ventilatory and hemodynamic parameters. Pharmacotherapy 2007;27:351–9.
106. Shah AN, Koneru J, Nicoara A, et al. Dexmedetomidine related cardiac arrest in a patient with permanent pacemaker: a cautionary tale. Pacing Clin Electrophysiol 2007;30:1158–60.
107. Corbett SM, Rebuck JA, Greene CM, et al. Dexmedetomidine does not improve patient satisfaction when compared to propofol during mechanical ventilation. Crit Care Med 2005;33:940–5.
108. Herr DL, Sum-Ping ST, England M. ICU sedation after coronary artery bypass surgery: dexmedetomidine-based versus propofol-based sedation regimens. J Cardiothorac Vasc Anesth 2003;17:576–84.
109. Newman MF, Kirchner JL, Phillips-Bute B, et al. Longitudinal assessment of neurocognitive function after coronary-artery bypass surgery. N Engl J Med 2001;344:395–402.
110. Roach GW, Kanchuger M, Mangano CM, et al. Adverse cerebral outcomes after coronary bypass surgery. N Engl J Med 1996;335:1857–63.
111. Shapiro PA, Levin HR, Oz MC. Left ventricular assist devices: psychosocial burden and implications for heart transplant programs. Gen Hosp Psychiatry 1996;18:30S–5S.
112. Diegeler A, Hirsch R, Schneider F, et al. Neuromonitoring and neurocognitive outcome in off-pump versus conventional coronary bypass operation. Ann Thorac Surg 2000;69:1162–6.
113. Van Dijk D, Jansen EW, Hijman R, et al. Cognitive outcome after off-pump and on-pump coronary artery bypass graft surgery: a randomized trial. JAMA 2002;287:1405–12.
114. Sellke FW, DiMaio JM, Caplan LR, et al. Comparing on-pump and off-pump coronary artery bypass grafting: numerous studies but few conclusions: a scientific statement from the American Heart Association Council on cardiovascular surgery and anesthesia in collaboration with the interdisciplinary working group on quality of care and outcomes research. Circulation 2005;111: 2858–64.
115. Lazar RM, Shapiro PA, Jaski BE, et al. Neurological events during long-term mechanical circulatory support for heart failure: the REMATCH experience. Circulation 2004;109:2423–7.
116. O'Brien JM, Lu B, Ali NA, et al. Alcohol dependence is independently associated with sepsis, septic shock, and hospital mortality among adult

intensive care unit patients. Crit Care Med 2007;35: 345–50.

117. Moore RD, Bone L, Geller G, et al. Prevalence, detection, and treatment of alcoholism in hospitalized patients. JAMA 1989;261:403–7.
118. Blondell RD, Looney SW, Hottman LM, et al. Characteristics of intoxicated trauma patients. J Addict Dis 2002;21:1–12.
119. Marik P, Mohedin B. Alcohol-related admissions to an inner city hospital intensive care unit. Alcohol Alcohol 1996;31:393–6.
120. Cammarano WB, Pittet JF, Weitz S, et al. Acute withdrawal syndrome related to the administration of analgesic and sedative medications in adult intensive care patients. Crit Care Med 1998;26: 676–84.
121. Bateson AN. Basic pharmacologic mechanisms involved in benzodiazepine tolerance and withdrawal. Curr Pharm Des 2002;8:5–21.
122. Katzung BG, Trevor A. Sedative-hypnotic drugs: examination and board review pharmacology. New York: McGraw-Hill; 1998. p. 171–8.
123. Morgan WW. Abuse liability of barbiturates and other sedative-hypnotics. Adv Alcohol Subst Abuse 1990;9:67–82.
124. Zawertailo LA, Busto UE, Kaplan HL, et al. Comparative abuse liability and pharmacological effects of meprobamate, triazolam, and butabarbital. J Clin Psychopharmacol 2003;23:269–89.
125. Krystal JH, Staley J, Mason G, et al. Gamma-aminobutyric acid type A receptors and alcoholism: intoxication, dependence, vulnerability, and treatment. Arch Gen Psychiatry 2006;63:957–68.
126. DeCarolis DD, Rice KL, Ho L, et al. Symptom-driven lorazepam protocol for treatment of severe alcohol withdrawal delirium in the intensive care unit. Pharmacotherapy 2007;27:510–8.
127. Gold JA, Rimal B, Nolan A, et al. A strategy of escalating doses of benzodiazepines and phenobarbital administration reduces the need for mechanical ventilation in delirium tremens. Crit Care Med 2007;35:724–30.
128. Crippen D. Life-threatening brain failure and agitation in the intensive care unit. Crit Care 2000;4: 81–90.
129. Kahkonen S. Responses to cardiovascular drugs during alcohol withdrawal. Alcohol Alcohol 2006; 41:11–3.
130. Lineaweaver WC, Anderson K, Hing DN. Massive doses of midazolam infusion for delirium tremens without respiratory depression. Crit Care Med 1988;16:294–5.
131. Pao M, Ballard ED, Raza H, et al. Pediatric psychosomatic medicine: an annotated bibliography. Psychosomatics 2007;48:195–204.
132. Pao M, Ballard ED, Rosenstein DL. Growing up in the hospital. JAMA 2007;297:2752–5.
133. Shapiro PA. Life after heart transplantation. Prog Cardiovasc Dis 1990;32:405–18.
134. Weill CM, Rodgers S, Rubovits S. School re-entry of the pediatric heart transplant recipient. Pediatr Transplant 2006;10:928–33.
135. Collier JA, Nathanson JW, Anderson CA. Personality functioning in adolescent heart transplant recipients. Clin Child Psychol Psychiatry 1999;4: 367–77.

Cognitive Therapy for Depression in Patients with Heart Failure: A Critical Review

Rebecca L. Dekker, PhD, ARNP, ACNS-BC

KEYWORDS

- Heart failure • Congestive • Depression
- Cardiovascular diseases • Cognitive therapy • Stroke
- Diabetes

Depression is a significant problem in patients with heart failure (HF). One in 5 people with HF has clinical depression,[1] and up to 48% have clinically significant depressive symptoms.[2] According to the Diagnostic and Statistical Manual of Mental Disorders, Fourth Edition (DSM-IV-TR), a major depressive episode, sometimes referred to as clinical depression, consists of 5 or more symptoms that are present for most of the day, almost daily, for at least 2 weeks. One of these symptoms must be depressed mood or loss of interest or pleasure in usual activities, and the symptoms must cause significant distress in social, occupational, or other areas of functioning (**Box 1**).[3] However, patients can experience clinically significant depressive symptoms without the presence of major depressive disorder.[4] Depressive symptoms may include depressed mood, irritability, guilt, hopelessness, low self-esteem, fatigue, sleep disturbances, appetite change, and inability to concentrate.[5]

The adverse effects of clinical depression and depressive symptoms on mortality and hospitalizations in patients with HF have been well documented.[1,2,6–8] Results from a meta-analysis demonstrated that patients with HF who have depressive symptoms are more than twice as likely to die or experience a cardiac event compared with patients without depressive symptoms.[1] Moreover, the presence of depressive symptoms has a negative impact on every dimension of health-related quality of life in patients with HF, including physical functioning, social functioning, and mental health.[2]

The problems associated with depression and depressive symptoms in patients with HF are well described. It is time for researchers to test interventions. There is a lack of research on nonpharmacologic interventions for depressive symptoms in patients with HF.[9] Cognitive therapy (CT) has been used successfully to treat depression in multiple populations.[10,11] Therefore, it may also be useful for treating depression in patients with cardiovascular illnesses, including HF. The purpose of this critical review was to examine the empirical support for the use of CT in treating depression and depressive symptoms in patients with cardiovascular-related illnesses.

Beck, a psychiatrist, developed the Cognitive Model of depression in 1967 to explain the psychological processes that occur in depression. The underlying assumption behind the Cognitive Model was that human minds are biased and cannot interpret stimuli objectively. This bias leads to cognitive errors, or dysfunctional thinking.[10] The Cognitive Model holds that dysfunctional thinking influences the emotions, behaviors, and psychosomatic symptoms associated with depression. Thus, interventions aimed at changing dysfunctional thinking should improve the emotional, behavioral, and somatic symptoms of depression.[11]

Disclosure: The author has nothing to disclose.
A version of this article originally appeared in *Nursing Clinics of North America*, Volume 43, Number 1.
University of Kentucky College of Nursing, 760 Rose Street, Lexington, KY 40536-0232, USA
E-mail address: rdekker@uky.edu

Heart Failure Clin 7 (2011) 127–141
doi:10.1016/j.hfc.2010.10.001

Box 1
DSM-IV-TR criteria for a major depressive episode

At least 5 of the following symptoms have been present most of the day, nearly every day, during the same 2-week period and represent a change from previous functioning; at least one of the symptoms is depressed mood or loss of interest or pleasure:

1. Depressed mood
2. Loss of interest or pleasure
3. Weight loss or changes in appetite
4. Insomnia or hypersomnia
5. Psychomotor agitation or retardation
6. Fatigue
7. Feelings of worthlessness or guilt
8. Decreased ability to concentrate
9. Thoughts of death, suicidal ideation, or suicide attempt.

- The symptoms must cause significant impairment in functioning (ie, work, social)
- The symptoms must not be directly due to a medical condition (ie, hypothyroidism) or a medication
- The episode is not better accounted for by a different diagnosis, such as bereavement, bipolar disorder, or schizoaffective disorder

Data from Diagnostic and statistical manual of mental disorders (DSM-IV-TR), 4th edition. Washington, DC: American Psychiatric Association; 2000.

CT, also called cognitive behavioral therapy, is the psychotherapeutic intervention based on the Cognitive Model of depression. The primary goal of CT is to alter emotions and behavior by redirecting negative cognitive processes. CT is typically a short-term therapy that consists of 4 to 14 sessions, depending on the individual's progress. The role of the therapist is to develop a collaborative, therapeutic relationship with clients and to teach them to become their own therapists. The therapist teaches the client to identify, analyze, and question dysfunctional thinking. For example, the therapist may help the client to identify negative thoughts, such as "I'm a burden to others". Together, the therapist and the client explore the evidence behind this negative thought. After evaluating the rationale for the thought, the therapist then guides the client to challenge the thought and, eventually, to a change in thinking. By creating changes in thinking, the client may modify negative emotions and behaviors.[11]

CT offers several potential advantages for the treatment of depression and depressive symptoms in patients with HF. First, CT is a nonpharmacologic intervention. Nonpharmacologic interventions may have several advantages over pharmacologic treatments, such as a lack of drug-drug interactions, immediate short-term relief of symptoms, and greater involvement of patients in their own self-care. Second, CT is an intervention that many health care professionals, including nurses, can be trained to administer. CT is compatible with common nursing interventions of teaching patients to accurately appraise stressors, determining the best coping method, and increasing perceived control. Despite the potential benefits of CT, its effectiveness in patients with cardiovascular illness, including HF, remains unknown. The following review provides a critical analysis of the existing research on the effectiveness of CT for treating depression or depressive symptoms in patients with cardiovascular illnesses.

METHODS

The databases searched for relevant literature were PubMed, PsychInfo, Cumulative Index to Nursing and Allied Health Literature (CINAHL), and MEDLINE. Keywords included depress* and cognitive therapy (or cognitive behavioral therapy) and cardiovascular (or heart failure, chronic illness, coronary artery disease, cardiac, stroke, or diabetes). The search was limited to English-language papers published between 1980 and December 2009.

Studies were included in the review if they met the following criteria: randomized controlled trial (RCT); cognitive therapy intervention; depression or depressive symptoms measured as an outcome; and sample consisting of patients with cardiovascular disease, nonhemorrhagic stroke, or diabetes. Diabetes mellitus commonly coexists with HF[12] and is an important risk factor for the development of HF,[13] Thus, samples that contained patients with diabetes were also included. The search resulted in 335 articles of which the titles or abstracts were screened for inclusion criteria. Reference lists of relevant articles were screened for additional studies. Fourteen papers met the inclusion criteria and were extracted for review.

RESULTS

Cardiovascular Disease

Eight studies were identified for evaluation of the impact of CT on depression in patients with cardiovascular illness (**Table 1**).

In the largest RCT on CT in cardiovascular disease to date, the ENRICHD (Enhancing Recovery in Coronary Heart Disease) investigators[14] compared the impact of CT with usual care on depressive symptoms and event-free survival in 2481 patients with a recent myocardial infarction (MI). Patients were eligible to participate if they were defined as depressed on a diagnostic interview or if they had low perceived social support. Patients in the intervention group attended 6 to 19 individual or group CT sessions (median of 11 sessions) over 6 months with the use of selective serotonin-reuptake inhibitor when indicated. The intervention group experienced a statistically significant decrease in depressive symptoms compared with the control group at 6 months. However, this difference was no longer present at 30 or 42 months of follow-up. There was no difference in event-free survival between the intervention and control groups.

The lack of impact on event-free survival may have been due to several factors. The ENRICHD investigators assumed that CT should begin as soon as possible (within 28 days) after an MI. Thus, the study may have included patients in the control group who had transient rather than clinical depression and recovered without intervention. The investigators also assumed that the usual-care group would not receive treatment for depression, but this was not the case. Antidepressant use was comparable in the control group (21%) and intervention group (28%).[14–16] It is not known why a decrease in depressive symptoms in the intervention group in this study did not translate into improved outcomes. It may be that this decrease was insufficient to affect clinical outcomes. This conclusion is supported by the observation that although depressive symptoms in the intervention group decreased by 49%, depressive symptoms in the control group also decreased by 33%.[14]

More recently, Freedland and colleagues[17] compared the effects of CT, supportive stress management, and usual care for the treatment of depression in 123 patients after coronary artery bypass graft (CABG) surgery. Patients were included if they scored 10 or higher on the Beck Depression Inventory (BDI) and met the DSM-IV criteria for depression based on a diagnostic interview. The investigators tested 2 separate interventions: 12 weeks of CT and 12 weeks of supportive stress management (progressive relaxation, controlled breathing, and imagery); both interventions were delivered in individual sessions by a trained clinical social worker or psychologist. Follow-up information on depression was collected at 3, 6, and 9 months using the BDI and the Hamilton Rating Scale for Depression.

The investigators found that patients in both intervention groups were more likely to experience remission from depression at all time points compared with patients in the usual-care group. At 9 months, 73% of the CT group and 57% of the stress management group experienced remission from depression, compared with 23% of patients in the usual-care group ($P = .003$). This study was underpowered to detect differences between the CT and stress management arms of the study. Therefore, it is difficult to draw conclusions as to whether CT or stress management was superior for the treatment of depression in patients who are post-CABG. However, patients who received CT experienced greater improvement in secondary outcomes, such as lower anxiety, hopelessness, and perceived stress; these results suggest that CT may offer more benefits to patients compared with stress management.

Twenty years ago, Burgess and colleagues[18] reported that an intervention combining CT, social support, and job-return counseling failed to reduce depressive symptoms in patients who had recently experienced an acute MI. In this RCT, 180 patients were randomized to the intervention group or usual care. There were no differences in depression scores between the groups at baseline, 3 months, or 13 months of follow-up. The authors did not offer any explanations for the null effects on depression. Women were underrepresented in the study; thus, it is not known whether the intervention would have been effective for women.

CT may be effective in reducing depressive symptoms in survivors of sudden cardiac death. Cowan and colleagues[19] tested the impact of CT, biofeedback therapy, and health education on depressive symptoms and mortality in 133 survivors of sudden cardiac death.[20] Only 11% of the sample had depressive symptoms at baseline and all were men. Approximately half the sample had chronic heart failure (New York Heart Association [NYHA] functional class II–IV). The treatment group experienced a significant decrease in depressive symptoms compared with the control group. Although the study was not originally powered to detect differences in mortality, it reported that the treatment group experienced an 86% reduction in the risk of cardiac death compared with the control group. Therefore, the results suggest that CT and biofeedback may be beneficial for survivors of sudden cardiac death, whether or not they are experiencing depressive symptoms.

Limited evidence suggests that CT may be more effective than exercise at reducing depressive

Table 1
Study characteristics and findings

First Author (Year)	Design, Follow-up Time	Sample	Measurement of Depression	Treatment	Control	Results
Cardiovascular Disease						
ENRICHD[14] (2003)	RCT 2 arms 30 months	N = 2481 28 days post-MI Eligible if classified as depressed or low perceived social support Women 44% Minorities 34%	DISH, BDI, HRSD	Eleven tailored CT sessions over 6 months, group therapy as needed, referral to psychiatry for antidepressants as needed	Usual care; physicians were notified if patients were depressed or had low perceived social support	The CT group had a lower BDI score compared with controls (9.1 vs 12.2, $P<.001$), and a lower HRSD score (7.6 vs 9.4, $P<.001$) at 6 mo. This difference was not present at 30 or 42 mo
Freedland et al[17] (2009)	RCT 3 arms 9 months	N = 123 CABG surgery within the past year Eligible if scored ≥10 on the BDI and met DSM-IV criteria for major or minor depression based on the DISH Women 50% Minorities 19%	HRSD score derived from the DISH; BDI	1. CT: 12 weekly, individual, 50–60 min sessions with a therapist 2. Supportive stress management: 12 weekly, individual, 50–60 min session. Training included progressive relaxation, imagery, and controlled breathing	Usual care	Patients in the CT and stress management group were more likely to experience remission from depression at 3, 6, and 9 mo compared with patients in the usual care group

Burgess et al[18] (1987)	RCT 2 arms 13 months	N = 180 Postacute MI Women 14% Minorities not reported	ZDS	A mean of 6.32 CT visits per patient, social support, facilitation of job return	Usual care	There were no differences between groups on depression scores at baseline or follow-up
Cowan et al[19,20] (2001)	RCT 2 arms 3 months	N = 133 Sudden cardiac death survivors Women 27% Minorities 10%	SCR-90: depression subscale	Eleven sessions of combined CT, biofeedback, and health education, administered biweekly for 6 wk	Health education class (90 min)	Depressive symptoms decreased in the treatment group when compared with the control group
Black et al[21] (1998)	RCT 2 arms 6 months	N = 60 Recently hospitalized for angina, MI, angioplasty, or CABG Eligible if scored as distressed Women 12% Minorities not reported	SCR-90: depression subscale	One to 7 weekly sessions with a psychologist including relaxation training, stress management, reduction of risk factors, efforts to improve adherence, and CT intervention; antidepressants if necessary	Cardiac rehabilitation with monitored exercise 1–3 times per wk, for 8 wk, daily home exercise; education on stress management, support group meeting with spouses, individual nutritional counseling	The CT group had significant reductions in depressive symptoms compared with the control group (−5.2 vs −0.2, *P*<.034)
Frizelle et al[22] (2004)	RCT 2 arms 3 months	N = 22 Patients with ICD's Women not reported Minorities not reported	HADS	Group-based therapy, 6 sessions, 1 h each: home-based exercise, education, relaxation, behavioral goal setting, education on identifying and challenging negative thoughts	Wait list	The treatment group experienced decreases in depressive symptoms compared with the control group (−4.25 vs −0.2, *P* = .001)

(*continued on next page*)

Table 1
(continued)

First Author (Year)	Design, Follow-up Time	Sample	Measurement of Depression	Treatment	Control	Results
Kohn et al[23] (2000)	RCT 2 arms 9 months	N = 49 Post-ICD implantation Women 35% African American 8%	BDI version II; Four biologic measures of depression: sexual functioning, appetite, weight change, and sleep patterns	Nine sessions ranging from 15- to 90-min, sessions included psycho-education on anxieties about ICD, avoidance behavior, fear of shocks, stress management, work and social activities, distorted cognitions	Usual care	The CT group had lower levels of depressive symptoms at follow-up compared with the control group (6.9 vs 15, $P = .037$), but depressive symptoms were not measured at baseline
Lewin et al[24] (2007)	Clustered RCT 2 arms 6 months	N = 192 Patients undergoing ICD implantation Eight implantation centers in the United Kingdom were randomized to intervention or control Women 20% Minorities 3%	HADS: depression subscale	Intervention consisted of 2 booklets for patients, 1 booklet for family, goal-setting diary, and relaxation tape. The first booklet targeted fears before ICD implantation. The second booklet consisted of a self-help CT program. The intervention was delivered by health care staff that underwent a half day of training.	Usual care and contact by a study facilitator to discuss postoperative progress	The intervention group experienced a greater reduction in the proportion of patients with depression at 6 mo compared with the control group (−13.2% vs −2.1%, *P* value not reported)

Kostis et al[25] (1994)	RCT 3 arms 3 months	N = 20 Patients with congestive heart failure Women 30% Minorities not reported	BDI	12 wk of exercise training at a cardiac rehabilitation facility for 1 h, 3 times per wk; weekly meetings with a dietician; group-based CT intervention: twice weekly for 60–90 min (relaxation, positive imagery, appraisal of negative cognitions)	1. Lanoxin titrated to achieve levels between 0.8 2.0 ng/mL 2. Placebo	There was a 52% decrease in BDI scores in the intervention group compared with a 15% and 25% increase in the control groups at follow-up ($P = .04$)
Stroke						
Lincoln and Flannaghan[26] (2003)	RCT 3 arms 6 months	N = 123 1–6 mo poststroke Eligible if scored as depressed Women 49% Minorities not reported	BDI WDI	Ten 1-h sessions over 3 mo; tailored CT intervention: education, task assignment, activity scheduling, identification and modification of inaccurate thoughts	1. No intervention 2. Attention placebo: Ten 1 h visits over 3 mo	No significant differences between groups in depression scores
Diabetes						
Lustman et al[27] (1998)	RCT 2 arms 6 months	N = 51 Type II diabetes and major depression Women 60% Minorities 19%	DIS BDI	One h/wk of individual CT for 10 wk; strategies included: behavioral strategies, problem solving, and cognitive techniques to change cognitive errors	Attention placebo: 1 h, biweekly, individual sessions with a diabetes educator	The CT group had a higher rate of remission from depression compared with the control group (58.3% vs 25.9%, $P = .03$)

(*continued on next page*)

Table 1
(continued)

First Author (Year)	Design, Follow-up Time	Sample	Measurement of Depression	Treatment	Control	Results
Snoek et al[28] (2008)	RCT 2 arms 12 months	N = 86 Adults with poorly controlled type I diabetes Women 58% Minorities: not reported	CES-D	Six weekly group sessions of CT delivered by a diabetes nurse educator and a psychologist; sessions focused on cognitive restructuring, behavior change, and stress management	Blood glucose awareness training focused on symptom management and diabetes education, delivered by a diabetes nurse educator and a psychologist	There were no differences between groups with regard to change in depressive symptoms over time
Henry et al[29] (1997)	RCT 2 arms 7 wk	N = 19 Type II Diabetes Women 53% Minorities not reported	BDI	Six sessions of 1.5 h: progressive muscle relaxation, cognitive coping training (such as identifying and modifying negative thoughts), problem-solving skills, homework assignments	Wait list	Depressive symptoms decreased across time in both groups; there was no difference between groups

Ismail et al[30] (2008)	RCT 3 arms 12 months	N = 344 Adults with poorly controlled type I diabetes Women 60% Minorities 20%	PHQ-9	1. CT plus motivational enhancement: 4 individual sessions of motivational enhancement therapy (elaborated next) and 8 sessions of CT delivered over 6 mo by trained diabetes nurses 2. Motivational enhancement: 4 individual sessions delivered over 2 months by a diabetes nurse; sessions focused on assessment of readiness to change, diabetes behavior modification, and problem solving	Usual care	Neither group experienced an improvement in depressive symptoms compared with usual care

Abbreviations: BDI, beck depression inventory version I; CABG, coronary artery bypass graft; CES-D, Center for Epidemiologic Studies Depression (Scale); DIS, diagnostic interview schedule; DISH, depression interview and structured Hamilton; ENRICHD, Enhancing Recovery in Coronary Heart Disease; HADS, hospital anxiety & depression scale; HRSD, Hamilton rating scale for depression; ICD, implantable cardioverter defibrillator; MI, myocardial infarction; PHQ-9, Patient Health Questionnaire; RCT, randomized controlled trial; SCR-90, symptom checklist 90 revised; WDI, Wakefield depression inventory; ZDS, Zung depression scale.

symptoms in patients with coronary artery disease. Black and colleagues[21] randomized 60 patients who had recently been hospitalized for a coronary event and were psychologically distressed to one of 2 groups: (1) a special intervention that consisted of stress management, relaxation training, and CT administered by a psychiatrist and (2) a cardiac rehabilitation group that included exercise and risk reduction counseling. At 6 months, the CT group experienced a significant reduction in depressive symptoms compared with the cardiac rehabilitation group. There was no difference between groups with regard to rehospitalizations. There were several limitations to the study, such as low representation of women (12%), exclusion of the elderly (>80 years old), and lack of a true control group. Adherence to the intervention was low. Less than 50% of participants attended more than one intervention session. Crossover between groups was also a problem, because 6 participants in the usual-care group were treated with antidepressants or psychological counseling. Combined, these limitations severely weakened the internal and external validity of the study.

Results from 3 studies suggest that CT may be helpful for reducing depressive symptoms in patients with implanted cardioverter defibrillators (ICDs). Frizelle and colleagues[22] compared the impact of a cardiac rehabilitation and CT on depressive symptoms in patients with ICDs to a wait-list control group. Despite the small sample size (N = 22), the intervention group experienced a significant reduction in depressive symptoms compared with the control group at 3 months. The intervention included exercise, which makes it impossible to ascertain whether the CT alone had an impact on depressive symptoms.

In another study, Kohn and colleagues[23] evaluated the effects of CT on depressive symptoms in 49 patients with ICDs. This study was limited by the lack of a comprehensive measure of depressive symptoms at baseline. Only 3 biologic indicators of depression were measured at baseline: sexual functioning difficulties, changes in appetite, and sleep disturbance. At 9 months follow-up, the CT group reported fewer sexual functioning difficulties than the control group; however, sexual difficulties increased in both groups over time. The BDI version II (BDI-II) was administered only at follow-up. Although the CT group had a lower BDI-II score than the control group at follow-up, the lack of depression score data at baseline limits the conclusions that can be drawn from findings.

Lewin and colleagues[24] tested the effects of a brief, self-help CT booklet on the treatment of depressive symptoms in patients who were undergoing ICD implantation. In this RCT, 8 ICD implantation centers were randomized to intervention or control. The intervention consisted of several booklets that were given to the patient and family by health care providers who had received a half day of training in administering the intervention. One of the booklets consisted of a self-help cognitive behavioral rehabilitation program, but the intervention in this booklet was not described in further detail. Patients in the intervention arm also received 3 phone contacts after ICD implantation to discuss their progress and set goals. The authors defined depression as a Hospital Anxiety and Depression Scale score of 8 or greater, and patients were followed up for 6 months.

In a logistic regression, the investigators found that patients in the intervention group were less likely to experience depression at 6 months compared with patients from control centers, after adjusting for baseline depression score (odds ratio −0.46, Confidence interval −1.93 to 1.00). Furthermore, the intervention group had a greater reduction in the proportion of patients with depression at 6 months compared with the control group (−13.2% vs −2.1%, *P* value not specified). However, this study was limited by the lack of a thorough description of the CT intervention, which limits researchers' ability to replicate the results and translate the study findings to the clinical setting.

Finally, results from a small study suggest that an intense regimen of CT combined with exercise may reduce depressive symptoms in patients with HF.[25] In this study, 20 patients with HF (NYHA class II/III) were randomized to 3 groups: group-based CT plus exercise, digoxin titrated to achieve serum drug levels between 0.8 and 2.0 ng/mL, or placebo. Despite the small sample size, the intervention group experienced a 52% reduction in depressive symptoms, whereas the other groups experienced a 15% and 25% increase in depressive symptoms, respectively. Because exercise with CT were combined, it is not known whether CT alone would have been effective in decreasing depressive symptoms. Also, the follow-up period was short, only 12 weeks, and therefore no conclusions can be drawn regarding the long-term effects of the intervention.

Stroke

There is less evidence regarding the effectiveness of CT on depression in patients with stroke. Lincoln and Flannaghan[26] conducted an RCT in which 123 patients who had recently experienced a stroke and depressive symptoms (scored >10 on the BDI) were assigned to one of 3 groups: CT, an attention placebo group, or a control group. Surprisingly, depressive symptoms improved over time in all the groups. There were no significant differences between the groups at baseline, 3 months, and 6 months of follow-up.

The authors suggested that the intervention, which consisted of 10 one-hour sessions, may not have been intense enough to improve depressive symptoms more than would occur naturally. However, other investigators have tested CT in chronic illness and found positive results using a similar number of CT sessions.[14,27] It is possible that the improvement in depressive symptoms in all 3 groups over time may have reflected the natural improvement of depression that occurs over time after an acute stroke.[26]

Diabetes

The effectiveness of CT for the management of depression in patients with diabetes has been tested in 4 RCTs. Lustman and colleagues[27] conducted an RCT in which 51 patients with type 2 diabetes and clinical depression were assigned to either 10 weeks of CT and diabetes education or an education-only group. As a result of the intervention, the treatment group had a higher rate of remission from depression compared with the control group (58.3% vs 25.9%).

In contrast, investigators from 3 studies have found that CT was not effective for treating depressive symptoms in adults with diabetes. Snoek and colleagues[28] compared the effects of 2 interventions on depressive symptoms in adults with type 2 diabetes. The 2 interventions that were compared were a 6-week group CT intervention and a blood glucose awareness training. The results showed no differences between groups at 6 and 12 months' follow-up. There was no true usual-care group; by comparing 2 active interventions, the investigators may have been less likely to detect a difference in the improvement of depressive symptoms between groups.

Similarly, Henry and colleagues[29] also found that CT did not improve depressive symptoms in patients with type 2 diabetes. The investigators in this small RCT used a wait-list control to evaluate the effects of CT plus progressive muscle relaxation on depressive symptoms in 19 patients with type 2 diabetes and elevated levels of glycosylated hemoglobin. Although there was an overall decrease in depressive symptoms from pre- to post-treatment in both the intervention and wait-list groups, there was no difference between groups. Because of the small sample size, the study probably was underpowered to detect changes in depressive symptoms between groups.

In a much larger study of 344 adults with type 1 diabetes, Ismail and colleagues[30] also found that CT did not improve depressive symptoms. In this RCT, the investigators compared CT plus motivational enhancement therapy and motivational enhancement therapy alone to usual care in the treatment of depressive symptoms. Despite the lengthy intervention (up to 12 sessions over 6 months), a large sample size, and a rigorous design, neither of the intervention groups experienced a greater reduction in depressive symptoms over time than the usual-care group.

DISCUSSION

Fourteen RCTs were identified in which investigators tested the impact of CT on depression or depressive symptoms in patients with cardiovascular-related illnesses. Positive effects of CT on depression or depressive symptoms were reported in 8 of the 14 studies. This section reports possible reasons for the mixed results, as well as limitations that prevent wide generalization of study findings.

The major factors that contributed to the mixed results were that (1) more than one intervention was tested in most studies, (2) a true, no-intervention control group was lacking in most studies, (3) most had small sample sizes, and (4) follow-up periods were short. The consequences of each of these factors are as follows.

The presence of more than one treatment intervention in several studies restricted the ability to determine the effect of CT on outcomes. In 2 studies that found positive outcomes, CT and antidepressant therapy were combined,[14,21] making it impossible to determine the effect of CT alone on depressive symptoms. Similarly, in 2 other studies finding positive outcomes, the intervention consisted of CT plus exercise.[22,25] Although combined interventions may be a valuable addition to the treatment options for depressive symptoms in patients with cardiovascular disease, assessing the value of CT alone is difficult when it is tested in combination with other interventions. For example, a growing body of evidence has demonstrated that exercise is an effective treatment for persons with major depressive disorders or with depressive symptoms.[31,32] Thus, exercise in combination with CT may have yielded a larger effect than CT alone or may obscure the effect of CT.

Six of the 14 studies lacked a true no-intervention group. These studies included various comparison groups. For example, one group of investigators compared patients who received a CT intervention to patients who received a cardiac rehabilitation exercise intervention.[21] Although these investigators found positive results with the CT intervention, the comparison of CT to exercise may have yielded a smaller effect than would have been seen if the investigators compared CT to a third true control group.

Seven of the 14 studies had small sample sizes (total N ranging from 19 to 86), and 8 studies had a follow-up period of 6 months or less. Despite the ENRICHD trial's large sample size and long follow-up period (30 months), the investigators found only modest clinically significant reductions in depressive symptoms. Moreover, this benefit was no longer present by 30 months of follow-up, because all groups improved over time.[14] In contrast, researchers of smaller studies found that CT reduced depressive symptoms at a relatively short follow-up time. It is possible that the improvements in depressive symptoms found in these studies did not persist. Short follow-up times limit the ability of researchers to determine whether CT is a potential long-term treatment for depression.

Researchers' ability to generalize the findings of several of the reviewed studies is compromised by several factors: (1) vaguely described interventions, (2) underrepresentation of women, (3) use of a wide variety of instruments to measure depressive symptoms, and (4) failure to adhere to the Consolidated Standards of Reporting Trials (CONSORT) guidelines for the reporting of clinical trials.

First, researchers often included vague descriptions of the intervention in articles; this limits the ability of future researchers to replicate results from these studies and translate the findings to clinical practice. It is also possible that the investigators tested different forms of CT, which could contribute to the mixed findings.

Second, only 9 of the 14 studies had samples that consisted of at least 30% women. Investigators in 4 of the 9 studies found that CT reduced depressive symptoms. Previous researchers demonstrated that women may react differently to psychological interventions than men. In a post-hoc analysis, the ENRICHD investigators reported that white men who received the CT intervention had a reduced risk of experiencing cardiac mortality or recurrent MI. In contrast, there was no similar beneficial effect for women and minorities.[33] Frasure-Smith and colleagues[34] reported that women who received an intense psychosocial nursing intervention after an MI experienced an increase in all-cause mortality when compared with the control group (10.3% vs 5.4%). This adverse effect was not found in the male participants. The results of these 2 studies suggest that it is important to evaluate the impact of psychological interventions on both men and women. Overall, the studies in this review provide insufficient evidence to determine the impact of CT on depressive symptoms in women with cardiovascular disease.

Third, researchers used various methods to measure clinical depression and depressive symptoms. Many of these measures, such as the BDI, have established reliability and validity. In contrast, Kohn and colleagues[23] used an instrument that measured 3 biologic indicators of depression. The reliability and validity of this instrument was not provided. Overall, there was a lack of consistency in the measurement of depression in the reviewed studies. This limitation may restrict researchers from conducting future meta-analyses to examine the overall effect of CT for the treatment of depression in patients with cardiovascular disease. For this reason, in 2006, a working group of the National Heart, Lung, and Blood Institute made recommendations as to which instruments researchers should use to measure depressive symptoms in clinical trials that include patients with cardiovascular disease.[35]

Finally, of the 12 studies that were published after 1996, only 5 followed all the CONSORT guidelines.[14,26] The CONSORT guidelines were originally published in 1996 and have since been revised.[36,37] These guidelines provide a standardized framework for the reporting of clinical trials. The CONSORT guidelines allow the reader to understand the design, conduct, analysis, and interpretation of an RCT and to judge whether a trial has internal or external validity.[37] A lack of adherence to the CONSORT guidelines in several of the studies reduces the transparency of the reported clinical trials and could contribute to a bias in overestimating the effects of interventions.

Implications for Future Research

The problems associated with depression and depressive symptoms in patients with HF have been adequately described. Interventions such as CT for the treatment of depression in patients with HF are now needed to move us forward. As only one small trial has studied the effects of CT on the treatment of depression in patients with HF, this article reviewed the empirical evidence for CT in the treatment of depression in patients with cardiovascular-related illnesses. Overall, the current evidence to support CT as a treatment for depression or depressive symptoms in patients with cardiovascular-related illnesses is inconclusive because of the limitations of existing studies.

Based on this review, future clinical trials should include the following recommendations. Researchers should test the effect of a CT intervention alone as well as in combination with other treatments. The CT intervention should be replicable in a clinical setting. Careful consideration should be paid to the inclusion of an appropriate comparison group. Given that depression in patients with HF is associated with a high risk for morbidity and mortality, it may be unethical to withhold treatment for depression from patients who are severely depressed. Furthermore, CT alone may not be appropriate for severely depressed individuals. It is suggested that researchers should refer all patients with severe depression to their primary care providers for treatment.

Studies should be designed with sufficient sample sizes to be adequately powered to detect changes in depressive symptoms and related outcomes. Researchers should also make special efforts to include a representative sample of women. Also, trials should include an adequate follow-up time of at least one year to provide information on the long-term effects of CT on depression and other health outcomes, such as morbidity and mortality. It is also important that researchers use consistent methods for measuring depressive symptoms, such as those provided in the National Heart, Lung, and Blood Institute's recommendations.[35] Finally, to improve transparency in the reporting of RCTs, researchers should follow the CONSORT guidelines.[37]

Several gaps in understanding of CT as a treatment for depression in cardiovascular conditions, including HF, remain. It is not known if there is a dose-response relationship between CT and depression in patients with cardiovascular disease. For example, how many CT sessions are necessary to improve depression outcomes and whether the effective dose varies among different cardiovascular populations are unknown. The best time to intervene with patients with depressive symptoms and cardiovascular disease is also unknown. The results of the ENRICHD trial showed that patients who had recently experienced a cardiac event and received a CT intervention only experienced a minimal improvement in depressive symptoms. This led researchers to question whether CT should be offered to patients who have recently experienced a cardiac event or if treatment should be delayed.[15] Likewise, it is not known whether CT should be offered to patients with HF who have been recently hospitalized or whether their depression may remit on its own. Next, it is not known whether CT interventions should be offered only to patients with cardiovascular disease or HF who are clinically depressed or to all patients, regardless of depression status. Finally, it is unknown whether CT can affect outcomes related to depression, such as mortality, morbidity, or health-related quality of life, in patients with cardiovascular disease or HF.

Implications for Practice

CT has been used successfully to treat depression in medically healthy populations. Because there is a scarcity of evidence for patients with HF, this review was broadened to include all patients with cardiovascular-related illnesses. Based on the findings of this review, the current evidence is insufficient to recommend CT as a treatment for depressive symptoms in patients with cardiovascular illness. Although most studies reviewed demonstrated that CT may be effective, the limitations in study design prevent wide generalization of the results. More evidence is needed before it can be recommended that clinicians routinely refer patients with cardiovascular disease to CT for the treatment of depression or depressive symptoms. CT may not be appropriate for all patients with HF or cardiovascular disease, particularly for patients with cognitive impairment or those who may have difficulty adhering to the CT treatment protocol. These patients may benefit from alternative treatments for depression.

SUMMARY

Depression is a significant clinical problem in patients with HF. The time has come for researchers to focus their efforts on designing and testing nonpharmacologic interventions for depression in patients with HF. CT holds promise as an intervention that may decrease depressive symptoms in patients with cardiovascular illness, including HF. Clinicians should continue to monitor the literature for new evidence regarding the effectiveness of CT for treating depression in patients with HF and other cardiovascular disease.

ACKNOWLEDGMENTS

The author would like to acknowledge Susan K. Frazier, PhD, RN, Terry A. Lennie, PhD, RN, and Debra K. Moser, DNSc, RN, from the University of Kentucky College of Nursing for their mentorship during the writing of this article. The intellectual contributions of Dr Frazier, Dr Lennie, and Dr Moser were sponsored by the University of Kentucky College of Nursing Center for Biobehavioral Research on Self-Management, NIH NINR, P20 NR010679. The content is solely the responsibility of the author and does not necessarily represent the official views of the National Institute of Nursing Research or the National Institutes of Health.

This article was written in partial fulfillment of the requirements for the PhD degree in Nursing at the University of Kentucky College of Nursing.

REFERENCES

1. Rutledge T, Reis VA, Linke SE, et al. Depression in heart failure: a meta-analytic review of prevalence, intervention effects, and associations with clinical outcomes. J Am Coll Cardiol 2006;48(8):1527–37.
2. Gottlieb SS, Khatta M, Friedmann E, et al. The influence of age, gender, and race on the prevalence of depression in heart failure patients. J Am Coll Cardiol 2004;43(9):1542–9.
3. American Psychiatric Association. Diagnostic and statistical manual of mental disorders (DSM-IV-TR). 4th edition. Washington, DC: American Psychiatric Association; 2000.
4. Judd LL, Akiskal HS, Zeller PJ, et al. Psychosocial disability during the long-term course of unipolar major depressive disorder. Arch Gen Psychiatry 2000;57(4):375–80.
5. Stuart GW. Emotional responses and mood disorders. In: Stuart GW, Laraia MT, editors. Principles and practice of psychiatric nursing. 7th edition. St Louis (MO): Mosby; 2001. p. 345–80.
6. Jiang W, Kuchibhatla M, Clary GL, et al. Relationship between depressive symptoms and long-term mortality in patients with heart failure. Am Heart J 2007;154(1):102–8.
7. Faris R, Purcell H, Henein MY, et al. Clinical depression is common and significantly associated with reduced survival in patients with non-ischaemic heart failure. Eur J Heart Fail 2002;4(4):541–51.
8. Jiang W, Alexander J, Christopher E, et al. Relationship of depression to increased risk of mortality and rehospitalization in patients with congestive heart failure. Arch Intern Med 2001;161(15):1849–56.
9. Lane DA, Chong AY, Lip GY. Psychological interventions for depression in heart failure. Cochrane Database Syst Rev 2005;1:CD003329.
10. Beck AT. The current state of cognitive therapy: a 40-year retrospective. Arch Gen Psychiatry 2005;62(9):953–9.
11. Beck JS. Cognitive therapy: basics and beyond. New York: Guilford Press; 1995.
12. Masoudi FA, Inzucchi SE. Diabetes mellitus and heart failure: epidemiology, mechanisms, and pharmacotherapy. Am J Cardiol 2007;99(4A):113B–32B.
13. Levy D, Larson MG, Vasan RS, et al. The progression from hypertension to congestive heart failure. JAMA 1996;275(20):1557–62.
14. Berkman LF, Blumenthal J, Burg M, et al. Effects of treating depression and low perceived social support on clinical events after myocardial infarction: The Enhancing Recovery in Coronary Heart Disease Patients (ENRICHD) Randomized Trial. JAMA 2003;289(23):3106–16.
15. Joynt KE, O'Connor CM. Lessons from SADHART, ENRICHD, and other trials. Psychosom Med 2005;67:S63–6.
16. Frasure-Smith N, Lesperance F. Depression–a cardiac risk factor in search of a treatment. JAMA 2003;289(23):3171–3.
17. Freedland KE, Skala JA, Carney RM, et al. Treatment of depression after coronary artery bypass surgery: a randomized controlled trial. Arch Gen Psychiatry 2009;66(4):387–96.
18. Burgess AW, Lerner DJ, D'Agostino RB, et al. A randomized control trial of cardiac rehabilitation. Soc Sci Med 1987;24(4):359–70.
19. Cowan MJ, Pike KC, Budzynski HK. Psychosocial nursing therapy following sudden cardiac arrest: impact on two-year survival. Nurs Res 2001;50(2):68–76.
20. Cowan MJ. Innovative approaches: a psychosocial therapy for sudden cardiac arrest survivors. In: Dunbar SB, Ellenbogen KA, Epstein AE, editors. Sudden cardiac death: past, present, and future. Armonk (NY): Futura Publishing Company, Inc; 1997. p. 371–86.
21. Black JL, Allison TG, Williams DE, et al. Effect of intervention for psychological distress on rehospitalization rates in cardiac rehabilitation patients. Psychosomatics 1998;39(2):134–43.
22. Frizelle DJ, Lewin RJ, Kaye G, et al. Cognitive-behavioural rehabilitation programme for patients with an implanted cardioverter defibrillator: a pilot study. Br J Health Psychol 2004;9(3):381–92.
23. Kohn CS, Petrucci RJ, Baessler C, et al. The effect of psychological intervention on patients' long-term adjustment to the ICD: a prospective study. Pacing Clin Electrophysiol 2000;23(4 Pt 1):450–6.
24. Lewin RJ, Coulton S, Frizelle DJ, et al. A brief cognitive behavioural preimplantation and rehabilitation programme for patients receiving an implantable cardioverter-defibrillator improves physical health and reduces psychological morbidity and unplanned readmissions. Heart 2009;95(1):63–9.
25. Kostis JB, Rosen RC, Cosgrove NM, et al. Nonpharmacologic therapy improves functional and emotional status in congestive heart failure. Chest 1994;106(4):996–1001.
26. Lincoln NB, Flannaghan T. Cognitive behavioral psychotherapy for depression following stroke: a randomized controlled trial. Stroke 2003;34(1):111–5.
27. Lustman PJ, Griffith LS, Freedland KE, et al. Cognitive behavior therapy for depression in type 2 diabetes mellitus. A randomized, controlled trial. Ann Intern Med 1998;129(8):613–21.
28. Snoek FJ, van der Ven NC, Twisk JW, et al. Cognitive behavioural therapy (CBT) compared with blood

glucose awareness training (BGAT) in poorly controlled Type 1 diabetic patients: long-term effects on HbA moderated by depression. A randomized controlled trial. Diabet Med 2008; 25(11):1337–42.
29. Henry JL, Wilson PH, Bruce DG, et al. Cognitive-behavioural stress management for patients with non-insulin dependent diabetes mellitus. Psychol Health Med 1997;2(2):109–18.
30. Ismail K, Thomas SM, Maissi E, et al. Motivational enhancement therapy with and without cognitive behavior therapy to treat type 1 diabetes: a randomized trial. Ann Intern Med 2008;149(10):708–19.
31. Blumenthal JA, Babyak MA, Moore KA, et al. Effects of exercise training on older patients with major depression. Arch Intern Med 1999;159(19):2349–56.
32. Dunn AL, Trivedi MH, Kampert JB, et al. Exercise treatment for depression: efficacy and dose response. Am J Prev Med 2005;28(1):1–8.
33. Schneiderman N, Saab PG, Catellier DJ, et al. Psychosocial treatment within sex by ethnicity subgroups in the Enhancing Recovery in Coronary Heart Disease clinical trial. Psychosom Med 2004; 66(4):475–83.
34. Frasure-Smith N, Lesperance F, Prince RH, et al. Randomised trial of home-based psychosocial nursing intervention for patients recovering from myocardial infarction. Lancet 1997;350(9076): 473–9.
35. Davidson KW, Kupfer DJ, Bigger JT, et al. Assessment and treatment of depression in patients with cardiovascular disease: National Heart, Lung, and Blood Institute working group report. Ann Behav Med 2006;32(2):121–6.
36. Begg C, Cho M, Eastwood S, et al. Improving the quality of reporting of randomized controlled trials. The CONSORT statement. JAMA 1996;276(8): 637–9.
37. Moher D, Schulz KF, Altman D. The CONSORT statement: revised recommendations for improving the quality of reports of parallel-group randomized trials. JAMA 2001;285(15):1987–91.

Index

Note: Page numbers of article titles are in **boldface** type.

Heart Failure Clin 7 (2011) 143–145
doi:10.1016/S1551-7136(10)00125-X

Printed and bound by CPI Group (UK) Ltd, Croydon, CR0 4YY

Printed and bound by CPI Group (UK) Ltd, Croydon, CR0 4YY

03/10/2024

01040354-0016